DRINKING AND CASUALTIES
Accidents, poisonings and violence in an international perspective

Drink-driving accidents and alcohol-induced attacks are a recurrent theme in the media, and the focus of major current debate. *Drinking and Casualties* provides an international survey of those who suffer in alcohol-related incidents, a much neglected area of study.

The contributors address the issues from a wide variety of disciplines, including the fields of biochemistry and epidemiology. They examine the effects of heavy drinking on the victims, friends and relatives of those who have a 'drink problem'. Taking an international perspective, they also analyse theories and practices of treatment from around the world.

The essays' contrasting viewpoints of the role of research and of methods of prevention enable *Drinking and Casualties* to make a major contribution to the current debate and indicate the direction of future policy.

Drinking and Casualties will be a particularly important reference volume for doctors practising in the fields of emergency and acute care, and for alcohol researchers and public health professionals.

The editor

Norman Giesbrecht, a research scientist at the Addiction Research Foundation, Toronto, Canada, is the senior editor of this international team. He has carried out social science research into alcohol-related issues for a number of years, and has also participated in several international research groups.

Drinking
and casualties

Accidents, poisonings and violence in an international perspective

Edited by Norman Giesbrecht, René González,
Marcus Grant, Esa Österberg, Robin Room,
Irving Rootman and Leland Towle

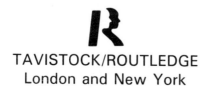

TAVISTOCK/ROUTLEDGE
London and New York

First published 1989 by Routledge
11 New Fetter Lane, London EC4P 4EE

Simultaneously published in the USA and Canada
by Routledge
a division of Routledge, Chapman and Hall, Inc.
29 West 35th Street, New York, NY 10001

Printed and bound in Great Britain by
Mackays of Chatham PLC, Chatham, Kent

British Library Cataloguing in Publication Data
Drinking and casualties: accidents,
poisonings and violence in an international
perspective.
1. Accidents. Role of consumption of
alcoholic drinks
I. Giesbrecht, Norman, *1942–*
363.1

Library of Congress Cataloging in Publication Data
Drinking and casualties: accidents, poisonings, and violence in an
international perspective / edited by Norman Giesbrecht . . . [et al.].
p. cm.
Bibliography: p.
1. Alcoholism – Cross-cultural studies. 2. Alcoholism and crime –
Cross-cultural studies. 3. Drinking and traffic accidents – Cross-
cultural studies. 4. Alcohol – Physiological effect – Cross-cultural
studies. I. Giesbrecht, Norman.
HV5035.D75   1989
364.2'4–dc19   88-29802
CIP

Canadian Cataloguing in Publication Data
Main entry under title:
Drinking and Casualties: Accidents, Poisonings and Violence in an
International Perspective
1.   2.
3.
I. Giesbrecht, Norman II. González, René III. Grant, Marcus, IV.
Österberg, Esa V. Room, Robin VI. Rootman, Irving VII. Towle,
Leland VIII. Routledge (London). HV

ISBN 0-415-00128-5

Table of Contents

Contents

Contents

List of Figures

Figures

List of Tables

Tables

Tables

xiii

Tables

Tables

Acknowledgements

This book would not have been possible without the contributions of the authors who presented material at the International Symposium on Alcohol-Related Casualties, prepared papers after the meeting, or approved requests to have their work, initially published elsewhere, to be reprinted here. This symposium was sponsored by the Addiction Research Foundation of Ontario, Health and Welfare Canada, the US National Institute on Alcohol Abuse and Alcoholism and the World Health Organization.

Special thanks are in order to Ann Marie Aldighieri for her skills in copy-editing and contributions to layout of the manuscript. Jacqui Barker provided invaluable assistance in finalizing bibliographic details, proof-reading and preparing indexes. Debbie Chapman provided information on references. Brian Van Dommele prepared the subject index and checked reference details. John Iskra, Michael-Craig Petersen and Linda Braid of RE:Action Marketing Services Ltd. worked closely with the senior editor in setting up the text, tables and figures for reproduction. Louise Clairemonte, Tim Hardwick, Rosemary Nixon and Elizabeth Tribe of Routledge contributed to the final refinements of the manuscript. The special contributions of all these persons are gratefully acknowledged.

John B. Macdonald supported the plans for publication and was instrumental in arranging a contribution from the Addiction Research Foundation which facilitated the preparation of the manuscript.

Finally, an interest in this endeavour from several key organizations enabled background work which provided a basis for this volume: the Addiction Research Foundation of Ontario, the Alcohol Research Group (Berkeley), the Finnish Foundation for Alcohol Studies, Health and Welfare Canada, the US National Institute on Alcohol Abuse and Alcoholism and the World Health Organization.

Preface

Towards a Clearer Definition of Alcohol's Role in Casualties*

John B. Macdonald

The consumption of alcohol brings pleasure to millions; and to millions it brings misery, illness or death. Its role in society is perceived by different observers as a blessing or a demon.

An amusing example of the difficulties was offered in an address to the legislature by a Mississippi State Senator in 1958:

> You have asked me how I feel about whisky. All right, here is just how I stand on this question:
>
> If, when you say whisky, you mean the devil's brew, the poison scourge, the bloody monster that defiles innocence, yea, literally takes the bread from the mouths of little children; if you mean the evil drink that topples the Christian man and woman from the pinnacles of righteous, gracious living into the bottomless pit of degradation and despair, shame and helplessness and hopelessness, then certainly I am against it with all of my power.
>
> But, if when you say whisky, you mean the oil of conversation, the philosophic wine, the stuff that is consumed when good fellows get together, that puts a song in their hearts and laughter on their lips and the warm glow of contentment in their eyes; if you mean Christmas cheer; if you mean the stimulating drink that puts the spring in the old gentleman's step on a frosty morning; if you mean the drink

* This paper first appeared in *Alcohol-Related Casualties*, edited by Norman Giesbrecht and Honey Fisher, Addiction Research Foundation, Toronto (1987), pp. 13-25. Permission to reprint the paper was granted by the author and publisher.

that enables a man to magnify his joy, and his happiness, and to forget, if only for a little while, life's great tragedies and heartbreaks and sorrows, if you mean that drink the sale of which pours into our treasuries untold millions of dollars, which are used to provide tender care for our little crippled children, our blind, our deaf, our dumb, our pitiful aged and infirm, to build highways, hospitals and schools, then certainly I am in favor of it.

This is my stand. I will not retreat from it; I will not compromise. (Quoted in Goodwin 1976: 4)

One purpose of this volume is to begin a systematic approach to understanding the role that alcohol plays in casualties resulting from accidents, violence, crime and suicidal behaviour. That represents no small task. In spite of the vast literature showing alcohol's involvement in countless morbidities, the relationship of alcohol to disease or casualty has been shown to be quantitatively predictable only in the case of cirrhosis, and then only for large populations and based only on *per capita* consumption. Otherwise the literature, whether dealing with disease, automobile accidents, other accidents or violence, tends to demonstrate that in only a variable proportion of cases alcohol is involved.

The proportion often is high; for example, figures such as 32 per cent of suicides, 42 per cent of homicides and 68 per cent of drownings in New York City had positive blood-alcohol levels (Haberman and Baden 1978). Empirical evidence has been used to support the case that, in the United States,

half of all traffic fatalities are alcohol-related...alcohol use is associated with up to 69 per cent of drownings...alcohol has been found to be involved in up to 70 per cent of all deaths and 63 per cent of all injuries from falls. (US Department of Health, Education and Welfare 1978)

Such figures are startling and the regularity with which they are reported has had no small influence on the passing of laws, the establishment of policies and the promulgation of regulations and interventions. Compulsory breath analysis, random roadside checks, harsh drinking-driving penalties, court-ordered treatment for alcoholism or enrolment in alcohol-education programmes and the growth of employee assistance programmes in business and industry represent common-place examples.

All such policies are well-intended and their introduction by legislators and others is understandable, especially given the escalating public anger in many countries at slaughter on the highways by drinking drivers.

Obviously, one very good reason for improving the quality of statistics on alcohol involvement in casualties is to provide more dependable and more penetrating data for the use of legislators and policy makers. This task is formidable because, as pointed out by a number of critics, there has been in much of the literature a facile leap from the findings of correlations between alcohol consumption and morbid events to conclusions about cause and effect. Judy Roizen put it this way:

> ...critics of these estimates have argued that many studies of alcohol involvement in these 'serious events' do not have appropriate control groups, are poorly designed, are atheoretical, assume a causal role for alcohol when it is found to be present, do not use well-defined measures of either the independent or the dependent variables, and do not attend to the context or situation in which the event occurs. The same studies are cited by those who want to 'enhance' alcohol's role in serious events and by the studies' critics who want to minimize its role. The fact that the same studies can be used either to enhance or to minimize and question alcohol involvement is primarily because most of the research in these areas does not, and in some cases cannot, conform to the standards of epidemiological tradition in which it is rooted. (Roizen 1982)

In my judgement, that statement and its implications are at the very heart of the discussions which led to this book. I reject entirely the notion that we are here to enhance or to discredit the role of alcohol in the causation of serious events. We are here to consider how we can deal with statistical and epidemiological problems in such a way as to illuminate our understanding of the nature of the relationship between alcohol and casualties.

Before turning to some concluding thoughts on this central issue, I want to digress briefly to recognise another very practical reason why it is important to obtain reliable information on alcohol consumption both immediately prior to admission and historically. That reason relates to the importance of good information for diagnosis and medical management. To make the point, let me simply list a number of circumstances in which knowledge of blood alcohol or the history of drinking is highly relevant or crucial.

1. Subdural haemorrhage can be misdiagnosed as alcohol intoxication with fatal consequences.

2. Alcohol increases the action of anaesthetics and its presence increases the risks from anaesthesia.

3. The anaesthetic effect of high blood alcohol can mask the presence of painful and serious injury.

4. The differential diagnosis of stroke, coronary infarct and *grand mal* can be complicated by alcohol intoxication.

5. Liver pathology due to alcohol can create a hazard to the administration of normal doses of acetaminophen.

6. Blood sugar can be depressed when caloric intake has relied on alcohol.

7. Chronic intoxication can result in neuropathy with consequent increased risk of falling.

8. Alcoholism may lead to osteoporosis and increased risk of fractures because of malnutrition, liver impairment and loss of proteins and calcium (Summerhill and Kelly 1963).

9. Liver pathology may complicate the course of recovery of victims of accidental injury, increasing the risk of death.

These examples point out the importance of obtaining and recording blood-alcohol levels in casualty units and of also obtaining and recording good histories of alcohol use and abuse. The point of this digression is to illustrate that beyond questions of the relationship of alcohol to serious injury and the implied legal and policy considerations, there are important medical reasons for routine determinations of blood alcohol and recording of alcohol histories.

I return to my interpretation that the central issue of casualty statistics is to understand the nature of the relationship between alcohol consumption and traumatic events. These relationships are unlikely to be either direct causal relationships or simple relationships applicable to a heterogeneous collection of situations resulting in trauma. It is not easy to imagine a common mechanism for such disparate events as auto accidents, fires, suicides, falls and violence. The problem, however, is the unproven assumption that the high proportion of traumatic events in which the victim (in the case of accidents) or the perpetrator (in the case of violence) has been drinking justifies the conclusion that the alcohol (when present) is probably the cause. The attribution of cause requires much more than mere evidence of juxtaposition.

Drawing from one category of traumatic events, namely violence, Pernanen (1980) has pointed to some of the problems of interpretation. While it is clearly true that alcohol is present in a high proportion of violent crime, other evidence is difficult to reconcile with the notion that alcohol is a cause or even necessarily a contributor to such phenomena. First, there is great variation in behaviour exhibited after alcohol consumption by different cultures. The Camba people of eastern Bolivia drink at festive occasions for days on end. Stupor or coma is common yet there is no increase in aggressive behaviour or violence. Second, a very low proportion of all drinking is accompanied by physical aggression. Third, experimental studies of the effect of alcohol on aggressive be-

4

haviour suggest that factors other than the alcohol consumption are implicated in the alcohol-aggression relationship (Graham 1980). Indeed, overwhelming evidence from many fields has demonstrated that causation is rarely if ever simple. The agent of a particular infectious disease represents only one element in a complex change in which other links such as sanitation, crowding, poverty, vectors, nutrition, immunologic status and even the weather may play crucial roles. Similarly, the role of alcohol in road accidents may be modified by road conditions, lighting, the use of seat belts, speed limits, policing, cultural norms and other factors.

Biological scientists will recall the recorded debates over bacterial causation of disease from the nineteenth century. The debates culminated in a set of postulates formulated by Robert Koch (1891) defining the conditions which must be met to justify concluding that a particular organism was the cause of a particular disease. The postulates stated were:

1. It must be possible to isolate the organism from all victims of the disease.

2. The organism must be grown in pure culture.

3. The pure culture, when injected into a suitable experimental animal, must produce comparable disease in the animal.

4. It must be possible to isolate the organism in pure culture from the infected animal.

Koch's postulates contributed scientific rigor to claims that the cause of various diseases had been identified. It must be noted, however, that it has not always been possible to fulfill the postulates, and other means including immunologic data and epidemiologic studies have had to substitute for one or another step. *Treponema pallidum* is known to be the cause of syphilis though it has never been grown in the laboratory. The acid-fast bacillus found in leprous tissues has not reproduced disease in any experimental animal. Finding the cause of Legionnaire's Disease was heavily dependent on sophisticated epidemiology. In short, Koch's postulates, though highly important, are not a perfect answer. I draw this bit of microbiological history to your attention because I want to suggest that an analogue of Koch's postulates is needed in looking at the role of alcohol in casualties. Obviously, Koch's notions are not directly transferable, but the idea of defining the conditions which must be met to justify claims of an etiological role for alcohol may have merit.

For a starter, I suggest the following:

1. The incidence of the event should be higher among drinkers than non-drinkers in otherwise matched samples.

5

2. The incidence of the event should correlate positively with the blood-alcohol level.

3. The incidence of the event over time should correlate with the availability of alcohol.

4. In populations where the availability of alcohol is temporarily restricted (e.g. strikes, police action), the event should be concurrently reduced in frequency.

5. The behaviour responsible for the event should be consistent with the known pharmacological effects of alcohol.

I make no claim for these proposals except to say that the larger the number of these conditions that can be met, the more justifiable would be the claim that alcohol played an etiological role. Perhaps you will disagree with my suggestions; perhaps you can define better postulates. I look forward to the debate and the prospect of consensus on this important topic.

References

Goodwin, D. (1976) *Is alcoholism hereditary?* Oxford University Press, London

Graham, K. (1980) Theories of intoxicated aggression. *Canadian Journal of Behavioural Science, 12*, 141-58

Haberman, P.W. and M.M. Baden (1978) *Alcohol, other drugs and violent Death.* Oxford University Press, New York

Koch, R. (1891) Uber bakteriologische Forschung. *Verhandlung International Med. Kong.*, 1890, I. Hirschwald, Berlin

Pernanen, K. (1980) Alcohol uses and violence: mapping the problem. Paper presented at the Addiction Research Foundation Conference on Alcohol Use and Family Violence, Toronto, Canada

Roizen, J. (1982) Estimating alcohol involvement in serious events. *Alcohol and Health Monograph 1*, NIAAA US Department of Health and Human Services, DHHS Publication No. (ADM) 82-190, Rockville, MD

Summerhill, W.H.J., and P.J. Kelly (1963) Osteoporosis and fractures in anicteric cirrhosis. *Proc. Mayo Clinic, 38*, 162-79

US Department of Health, Education and Welfare (1978) *Third special report to the U.S. Congress on alcohol and health*, E.P. Noble (ed), DEHW Publication No. (ADM) 78-569, Washington, DC, p. 63

Introduction

Themes and Issues in the Study of Drinking and Casualties

Norman Giesbrecht, René González, Marcus Grant, Esa Österberg, Robin Room, Irving Rootman and Leland Towle

Background

In the late 1970s and early 1980s there were several developments which contributed to the planning activities which eventually led to this volume. In the course of a seven country analysis of post-war developments in control, consumption and drinking-related consequences, participants in the International Study of Alcohol Control Experiences noted gaps and shortcomings in information on alcohol-related complications, particularly with regard to social complications and acute or violent incidents (Mäkelä et al. 1981, Single et al. 1981, Giesbrecht et al. 1983).

Reviews of the literature on casualties and trauma and alcohol, conducted in the late 1970s (Aarens et al. 1977) and early 1980s (Roizen 1982), indicated that with the possible exception of rough prevalence estimates and some linkages to socio-demographic and personal characteristics, research to date provided a fuzzy picture of the dimensions of drinking-related casualties. The research also pointed to the apparent disjunction between, on the one hand, the rough prevalence estimates which suggested that casualties were a major factor in overall morbidity and mortality and that a substantial proportion in some way or other were related to drinking, and, on the other hand, the fact that with the exception of drinking and driving, casualties and alcohol had not been a major theme in alcohol research literature or a focus of prevention initiatives.

Also, in the 1980s major international or regional studies were underway in which alcohol-related casualties were a central or major theme. The Joint Nordic Study of Alcohol Problems, involving participants from Denmark, Finland, Iceland, Norway and Sweden, examined postwar trends in alcohol-related chronic and acute complications in the Nordic countries. Two papers by project participants are provided in this volume (Österberg, *see* Chapter 11; Skog, *see* Chapter 18). Research initiatives already underway at the Alcohol Research Group (Stephens Cherpitel, *see* Chapter 16), the Addiction Research Foundation (Kapur, *see* Chapter 8; Adrian, *see* Chapter 12; Ferrence, *see* Chapter 19) and the Mexican Institute of Psychiatry (Rosovsky, *see* Chapter 14) provided a further basis for framing the plans for this project.

A paper by Robin Room (1982) provided a basis for discussions at a two-day informal meeting on alcohol-related statistics, sponsored by WHO, in Geneva in October 1982. Subsequent discussions in Ottawa, Toronto, Athens, Helsinki and Washington lead to a meeting entitled: International Symposium on Alcohol-Related Casualties, held in Toronto in August 1985. The *Proceedings* of this symposium are presented in another volume (Giesbrecht and Fisher 1987). The majority of the chapters that follow are based on papers initially presented at this meeting.

Themes

The themes can be identified by several questions: What is the scope of alcohol-related casualties, and, specifically, of the contents of this volume? In light of available epidemiological data and the predominant foci in the alcohol literature, are casualties receiving sufficient attention? How are casualties currently documented and what improvements might be made in the systems of registration and documentation? What conclusions can be drawn from studies conducted on casualties about the proportion involving alcohol, the characteristics of those involved in casualties, the casualty event, and the contribution of drinking to type, severity and handling of casualties? What new studies or lines of analysis are suggested by the investigations to date? What methods of monitoring or registration should be encouraged in order to obtain clearer and sounder answers to epidemiological and etiological questions? What policy and prevention initiatives should be encouraged in order to reduce the overall level and severity of casualties?

Scope

This volume is about accidents, violence and poisonings. Specifically it is about the acute, sudden or traumatic events associated with alcohol consumption. However, this indicates only part of the picture. The papers in this collection are also about conceptual models for addressing research questions, about statistical techniques that can be used to isolate and explore relationships, about the impact of culture and political agenda in camouflaging or enhancing the documentation of drinking-related casualties, and about relationships between policy and research. Through the window of casualties, we learn about national or local systems which deliver health care, control public disruptions or prevent trauma. The authors describe cross-cultural variations in drinking, drunken comportment and casualty incidents. Differences in research foci and opportunities are illustrated and debated.

The contributors represent expertise in a number of disciplines, including biochemistry, demography, epidemiology, health planning, medicine, psychology, public health, sociology and statistics. However, on balance, specific papers are not written from the perspective of a particular discipline, but indicate a keen interest by the authors to cross-disciplinary boundaries in their techniques and interpretations. For example, when an analysis focuses on relationship of results based on body fluids, socio-cultural considerations in drinking and trauma are drawn into the interpretation (Papoz *et al.*, *see* Chapter 15). Or when the focus is on temporal variations in aggregate rates of violence, the dose-specific actions of alcohol are acknowledged (Skog, *see* Chapter 18).

The authors also draw on experiences from a number of countries and regions. In addition to the five national systems described in this book (*see* Section III), reviews focus on the USA and Western Europe (Roizen, *see* Chapter 1), Latin America (Medina-Mora and González, *see* Chapter 2), Africa (Haworth, *see* Chapter 3) and Oceania (Casswell, *see* Chapter 4). Overall, the contributors draw on their research experiences in almost a dozen different countries, including Australia, Canada, Finland, France, Mexico, New Zealand, Norway, Poland, Switzerland, the United States and Zambia.

The chapters have been organised into six sections, starting with overviews and reviews (*see* Section I) and ending with two commentaries on research and policy issues (*see* Section VI). The opening section addresses the question of what research tell us about drinking-related casualties, and the concluding section debates how differences in research and policy issues might be addressed.

The four intervening sections deal with topics that are not unique to casualties or studies focusing on the role of drink. Conceptual models and issues are outlined in Section II. Suggestions for improving methods of data collection are provided in Section III. In Section IV the contributors provide an overview of both the type and scope of recording systems and the key substantive findings from these data in Australia, Finland, Canada, Poland and Mexico. Finally, papers with more specific foci and involving exemplary analyses are presented in the last section: this includes papers based on emergency room populations, insurance records of hospitalised alcoholics, long-term trends in violent deaths, gender differences in suicide, and recent casualty research in developing countries.

The book concludes with a report by Fisher (*see* Appendix A) on reporting systems and issues related to how alcohol is handled, and a model for an alcohol-related casualty surveillance system based on explorations with US data systems (Aitken and Zobeck, *see* Appendix B).

Emphasis on Casualties

A central theme is the place of casualties in the alcohol literature, and, conversely, the place of alcohol in the casualty literature. It is generally acknowledged that alcohol has had a relatively marginal place in much of the casualty literature, although, as noted by Roizen (*see* Chapter 1), this has been changing in the years since the mid-1970s.

We might refer to the relative absence of effective and simple documentation or registration methods, but this begs the question. Possibly the wide range of events encompassed by the term casualties, and the competing or divergent foci of agencies categorising these events, have been impediments for more effective monitoring of alcohol. But this is not satisfactory, since it does not explain the relative absence of routine documentation or investigation with regard to specific types of casualties. Finally, the issues of culpability to the injured and related inconvenience to the professional (e.g. doctor) have likely been impediments in either initiating effective routine data recording on drinking and casualties, or obtaining valid data even when systems are in place.

The position of casualties as a topic of study in the alcohol literature probably provides some further hints.

In most developed countries in the postwar era the predominant interest in the alcohol literature on complications has involved two complimentary foci: the alcoholic or problem drinker and the chronic complications related to heavy drinking. An entity perspective of consequences, and an emphasis on the longer-term impact of ethanol on the drinker are derived from these foci. Studies with a more situational or environmental focus, including those examining the drinking event or occasion, while recognised, have been less common. Key findings from the literature on chronic complications depended on data of reasonable quality, usually mortality statistics, some assurance that the majority of the events could be linked to consumption, and the opportunity to proceed at both clinical and aggregated levels of investigation concurrently.

These conditions are more difficult to achieve in the study of casualty, where, not only the alcohol consumed at the time, but other situationally-specific dynamics and event-linked mores play a much more critical role than is the case with chronic consequences (Müller, *see* Chapter 6; Pernanen, *see* Chapter 7). It appears, in principle, to be particularly difficult in the casualty area to move research beyond the preliminary agenda of estimating the proportion of specific events which involve alcohol.

Observations

Several generic conclusions emerge from the chapters that follow about the role of alcohol in casualties.

1. The proportion of casualty events that involve alcohol—the subject was under the influence, had been drinking around the time of the casualty, or was at higher risk because of drinking history—has not been well established. For a variety of reasons involving primarily detection and recording methods, it is nevertheless assumed that the proportions provided by official statistics are considered to be underestimations.

2. Proportions or rates of alcohol-related casualties are crude, preliminary indicators of a relationship. They do not demonstrate that drinking was a contributing cause, and, even with sophisticated analyses (e.g. Skog, *see* Chapter 18), only tentative conclusions about the contribution of drinking to casualties is possible. Even if, for example, it is possible to illustrate that certain types of casualties (such as assaults) have a higher proportion associated with drinking than other incidents (such as industrial accidents), it does not follow that a causal relationship is likely to be stronger — for example, if the person had not been drinking the assault was less likely to have taken place. It is possible that intoxication can be an important precipitating factor even if the overall proportion of incidents is low.

3. Furthermore, there are significant cross-national, regional and situational variations in the role of alcohol in casualties. Even the basic estimates of prevalence indicate that where official statistics are available, the proportions are, for example, considerably lower in developing countries than in developed (*see* Sections I and IV, also Chapter 20). However, this is probably not an accurate reflection of the conditions or experiences of the victims or perpetrators, but strongly influenced by cross-national differences in the priorities or resources of health care and law enforcement institutions.

4. There is considerable variability across types of casualties in the proportion where alcohol is acknowledged, even when the literature is based primarily on one country (*see* Chapter 1). Assaults involving young males have a very high proportion, and industrial incidents have a considerably smaller proportion.

5. Even within one jurisdiction it is possible to note substantial differences in the estimated proportion depending on the methods used. In general those based on official statistics tend to be much lower than those based on self-reports, observations by researchers, or collection of breath or body fluid samples.

6. Within a jurisdiction or country there are differences in the emphasis on alcohol-related casualties. For example, Morawski and Moskalewicz (*see* Chapter 13) indicate that in Poland blaming drink for social ills, a form of problem inflation, may in fact have been out of step with actual trends in consumption and projected rates of problems.

7. The characteristics of those persons turning up with drinking-related casualties varies by casualty and recording methods. Some reports point to certain sectors of a population having a higher risk of alcohol-related casualties: young adult males for drinking-related accidents and violence; older people for falls; chronic heavy drinkers for motor vehicle accidents; middle-aged males and females for suicides. However, a next step of documenting the relative risk based on the frequency of the activity (e.g. fighting) in conjunction with consumption of alcohol may demonstrate quite different findings. For example, per drinking event involving confrontation, the rate of casualties might be quite low for young males. In general, these papers direct our attention to the need for further research contrasting casualty and non-casualty events which involved similar activities.

8. Although there is a temptation to conclude that the more serious the injury or event, the more likely that alcohol is implicated, this is confounded by serious substantive and methodological considerations. Older victims are more likely to suffer serious injury but the relative importance of alcohol may not be a serious consideration. The level and type of documentation, particularly of the alcohol factor, is not consistent across events or even linearly or randomly related to seriousness. For some serious trauma, such as motor vehicle fatalities, BAC is routinely taken in some jurisdictions; in other instances, comatose patients may be under-represented when self-report or objective data on drinking or BAC are obtained.

The catchment of reporting systems is more likely to be comprehensive with regard to mortality than morbidity—in Ontario, for example (Adrian, *see* Chapter 12), extrapolations based on assumptions are required to estimate trauma in emergency departments and the proportions involving alcohol.

Introduction

Current Methods of Documentation and Recommendations for Improvement

A few general points are provided to set the stage for recommendations on improving information on alcohol-related casualties. The reader is referred to specific papers, especially in Sections III, IV and V, for details about documenting casualties in specific jurisdictions, and to Section I for reviews of the literature.

Using Available Data

There are three main resources for routine information on alcohol-related casualties: mortality statistics, morbidity statistics, and police data. In addition, in some jurisdictions there are special data systems focusing on categories of accidents (water-related, industrial, fires), substances (poisonings), or institutional files (health insurance). The key drawbacks of these data systems are clearly illustrated in these chapters: only a very small proportion of mortality statistics in which alcohol may have been involved is actually noted; morbidity data are confounded by the scope of the recording network—for example, out-patient data may be sketchy compared to in-patient data; the under-recording of the alcohol component; and police data are subject to similar generic criticisms—limited scope and problems of validity.

Nevertheless, these are the only resources in contexts where special studies or monitoring procedures are not feasible; therefore, innovative approaches must be taken to seek to by-pass the hurdles they entail. One approach is to limit investigations to those categories where the alcohol component is routinely documented, such as poisoning statistics, or certain motor vehicle incident statistics.

Second, the relative rates of casualties per aggregate volume of alcohol sales can be used to provide an estimate of cross-cultural differences in the covariation of casualties and drinking (Pernanen, *see* Chapter 7). Also, aggregated data on casualties can be used in conjunction with filtering techniques and rates of alcohol sales to demonstrate relationships at general levels and estimate the proportion of casualties attributable to changes in consumption (Skog, *see* Chapter 18).

Third, data from different systems but with a similar substantive focus, such as homicide or suicide, can be used to consider either cross-sectional or temporal variations in comparison with drinking-related variables. This approach requires large jurisdictions in order to have a sufficient number of cases to carry out the study.

Fourth, natural events, such as dramatic or sudden changes in access to alcohol, drinking styles or drinking rates can provide a basis for exploring concomitant developments with regard to aggregated casualty rates (Morawski and Moskalewicz, *see* Chapter 13).

Fifth, comparison and control groups can be created from common institutional files and temporal changes in the documented casualty experiences of the two groups can be plotted—illustrated in Holder's paper on alcoholic and non-alcoholic participants in medical insurance plans (*see* Chapter 17).

Using Original Data

However, if new or revised methods of monitoring, or special primary data collection studies are feasible, even on a pilot basis, a number of other options are available:

1. Self-report data can be combined with official examinations to enhance the estimates obtained from the latter (Rosovsky, *see* Chapter 14).

2. Self-report data can be combined with objective measures using either blood or breath samples (Papoz *et al.*, *see* Chapter 15; Stephens Cherpitel, *see* Chapter 16).

3. Observational techniques by medical staff trained to use a four-point ethyl score can provide an indication of the level of intoxication in patients presenting with casualties (Poikolainen, *see* Chapter 9)

4. Simple and reliable devices for measuring alcohol presence and level of BAC, such as a dipstick, can be used either alone or in combination with other techniques, observational data, or self-reports (Kapur, *see* Chapter 8)

5. Modifications in the ICD E-code could be introduced to allow for cross-referencing of alcohol involvement in all casualties and not only a few categories such as poisoning (Poikolainen, *see* Chapter 9)

Research Issues

A central contribution of these papers is the explicit, or implicit, reference to research issues. The complexity of the topics, the limitations of available data and the strictures of conventional approaches appear to be key stimuli for assessing the models and perspectives used, the foci and design of research endeavours, and the agenda of research.

Models and Perspectives

The unit of analysis ranges from the individual to the sub-culture to the society. A wide range of models or perspectives is evident. In some cases the orientation is to the temporal variation between an intervention, such as treatment for alcoholism, and casualties (Holder, *see* Chapter 17), in others it is social and political developments at the broadest levels which bear on the casualties and alcohol consumption (*see*, for example, Chapters 3, 4 and 20).

A central message, presented in various guises, is that different models are required for different types of casualties (*see* Chapter 7), but, further, that for any of the casualty investigations, models need to take into account the culture, context or system (*see* Chapter 5). Medina-Mora and González (*see* Chapter 2) and Casswell (*see* Chapter 4) point to the variations in cultural mores, specifically those in conjunction with drunken comportment as bearing on casualties. Müller (*see* Chapter 6) notes that norms about risk-taking are part of the puzzle of understanding casualty incidents. Holder (*see* Chapter 5) advocates investigations that include systems of alcohol distribution and control in order to enhance our understanding of casualties.

Systematic examination of the broader contextual and cultural experiences as they bear on casualties is clearly an agenda for studies in the future. To date this has been acknowledged, but the methods for undertaking this need to be explicated.

It appears that many of the studies conducted to date, and referred to by authors of this volume, do not provide sufficient data about the drinking experiences around the time of the casualty and the drinking history of the victim or perpetrator. Further, very little information, if any, is routinely collected about the casualty event so that the relationships can be put into a dynamic context (Roizen, *see* Chapter 1). These agendas — pertaining to the individual and event — need to be addressed in investigations of drinking and casualties. However, progress in these areas is not an adequate substitute for efforts to better appreciate the culturally-linked experiences of work, travel, leisure, recreation and conflict which provide the broader contexts for casualty incidents.

Foci and Design

Several generic recommendations emerge with regard to the appropriate research design and foci. Researchers might take more innovative or sophisticated approaches in manipulating the data available to them from aggregate statistics. In jurisdictions where the number of events is large enough, casualty rates and *per capita* alcohol consumption rates can be analysed. Furthermore, general population surveys which contain information on casualties can provide a referent and also a backdrop against which those casualties which come to official attention can be studied. In general, at the country level a more thorough documentation of the epidemiology of casualties in general, using data from a number of sources, may be a fruitful basis for more focused research, involving original data or estimates using analytical techniques, on the role of alcohol.

Studies based on special populations, such as persons seen in emergency services, are likely to benefit from the application of exclusion and inclusion criteria, for example, excluding children in some studies and including the most severely injured (*see* Chapter 1). Although designs which include a control or comparison group are, in principle, desirable, they may not resolve the issues of volition and lifestyle that are central to interpreting the dynamics of traumatic events.

Along much the same line, investigations based on quasi-experimental designs may provide insights that are closer to the naturalistic experiences of the participants than are available from experimental designs. Natural experiments, based on sudden or major changes in the perceived contributing factors to casualties, are important opportunities that have, at times, been missed or under-utilised.

It is also noteworthy that in a collection which is substantially oriented to tabulations based on secondary data, we also find a number of allusions to the ethnographic methods and to closer scrutiny of the casualty processes, not only the incidents. Special studies of groups or sub-populations which are known to have high rates of casualties involving drinking would be a contribution in this direction. Similarly, special cultural events or ceremonies which typically involve traumatic incidents would also be relevant foci for this type of investigation.

Agenda of Research

What broader agendas of research on drinking and casualties are advocated in this volume? Several themes emerge, illustrating both the current state of knowledge of this field, the linkages to other literature and the diverse backgrounds of the contributors. A basic agenda is to discover the relative proportion of casualty events which in some way or other involve alcohol, and the distinct characteristics of those who are victims or perpetrators.

A related agenda is to improve methods of documentation and measurement, both as a basis for monitoring in order to facilitate treatment, prevention and policy initiatives, but also to enable research with a sounder data base.

Investigations of the contributing causal role of alcohol are a key purpose (Macdonald, *see* the Preface), although there are no illusions that this is a simple task, that the findings are likely to be similar from one type of casualty to the next, or that an underlying objective is to rule out other variables in order to enhance the explanatory status of drinking.

Finally, there is a clear orientation to applied research throughout the volume. While policy initiatives are typically beyond the direct influence of the researcher, the work reported is based on the expectation that further research on drinking and casualties has a bearing on policy decisions.

Policy Issues

The concluding chapters present two perspectives on research and policy. Draper (*see* Chapter 21) proposes that unless researchers become more sensitive to the nature of policy-making and the needs of policy-makers they will continue to generate information which is not central to interventions under consideration. Moskalewicz and Wald (*see* Chapter 22) propose that researchers and policy-makers often do and can continue to have interests in common, but that to expect convergence on all aspects will confound the research enterprise and thus devalue the potential contribution of research findings to policy. It is likely that these perspectives, and their finer points, will continue to be debated in many contexts.

If we consider policy in terms of current local or regional experiences with regard to drinking and casualties, some generalisations may be offered.

Policies on research should be relevant to the needs and experiences, as well as the resources of the host regions or countries. In developing countries, for example, studies that will contribute to putting alcohol and casualties on the agenda of health authorities are probably more useful than replications of studies done in developing countries (Roizen, *see* Chapter 20).

There is sufficient information on the prevalence of drinking and casualties to warrant piloting techniques for routine documentation of alcohol presence in emergency room settings. Such changes do not require proof of etiology, but will nevertheless have immediate benefits in terms of facilitating patient care, or preventing mis-diagnoses, or encouraging follow-up arrangements.

The current levels of vigilance in developed countries with regard to drinking and driving have not emerged overnight, and are not without drawbacks in their orientations and interventions. These developments may be used as models for initiatives with regard to other areas of casualties in which alcohol is implicated. However, both prevention and research endeavours can benefit from these experiences as policies with regard to recreational activities, public transportation and work-site incidents are implemented.

As drinking becomes more closely linked to various events, such as violence or personal damage, this may in fact impede the implementation of effective policies, for at least two reasons: it may narrow the opportunities for and support of research with a broader scope, in which, for example, alcohol is analysed as one variable among many others; findings of drunkenness, for example, may be a basis for circumventing culpability.

Whether the underlying interest of the researcher is to demonstrate that alcohol does indeed play a more significant role in many types of incidents than was previously thought, or to note that it is in fact primarily a spurious variable to which too much importance has been attached, or whether the perspective is somewhere in between, if new areas of inquiry involve an openness to either possibility and methodologies that accommodate such openness, then neither the research or policy opportunities will be seriously compromised.

© 1989 Norman Giesbrecht

References

Aarens, M., T. Cameron, R. Roizen, D. Schneberk, and D. Wingard (eds) (1977) *Alcohol, casualties and crime.* Final Report No. 18, Social Research Group, University of California, Berkeley

Giesbrecht, N., M. Cahannes, J. Moskalewicz, E. Österberg, and R. Room (eds) (1983) *Consequences of drinking: Trends in alcohol problem statistics in seven countries.* Addiction Research Foundation, Toronto

Giesbrecht, N., and H. Fisher (eds) (1987) *Alcohol-related casualties.* Addiction Research Foundation, Toronto

Mäkelä, K., R. Room, E. Single, P. Sulkunen, B. Walsh *et al* (1981) *Alcohol, society, and the state 1: A comparative study of alcohol control.* Addiction Research Foundation, Toronto

Roizen, J. (1982) Estimating alcohol involvement in serious events. In *Alcohol and health monograph*, Lexington Books, Lexington, Mass., pp. 179-219

Room, R. (1982) Improving indicators of alcohol-related problems. Working paper prepared for Informal Consultation on Alcohol Statistics, World Health Organization, Geneva, October 28-29, 1982

Single, E., P. Morgan, and J. de Lint (eds) (1981) *Alcohol, society, and the state 2: The social history of control policy in seven countries.* Addiction Research Foundation, Toronto

Section I:

REVIEWS

1

Alcohol and Trauma

Judy Roizen

Alcohol presence in casualties of all types has been the subject of scientific investigation for nearly a century. In 1976, the then Social Research Group at Berkeley undertook a large-scale review of the literature of alcohol involvement in casualties and crime for the US National Institute of Alcohol Abuse and Alcoholism (Aarens *et al.* 1977). The purpose of undertaking a comprehensive review was not only to identify the literature but, more important, to begin to develop a conceptual framework within which to understand alcohol's role in the events which lead to injury and death.

At that time, the umbrella term 'serious events' was adopted to group together events which actually or potentially result in death, injury or substantial property damage or loss. A number of concepts emerged as being useful in integrating diverse and often large literatures. These included:

1. the 'aspect of alcohol' used in a study (e.g. blood-alcohol concentration or BAC[1], alcoholism, drunken comportment);

2. the 'power of alcohol' — the particular power ascribed to alcohol in a study or an argument (e.g. alcohol as a relaxant, a stimulant, a disinhibitor);

3. 'window' — the vantage point from which a particular social institution views a casualty (e.g. emergency room cases, insurance cases, court cases);

---

1.   Refer to notes following the text of this chapter.

4. the 'event/person' — the degree to which the event or the person is the unit of analysis; and,

5. whether the event was thought to be 'intended' or 'unintended'.

In contrast to the broader Aarens *et al.* study of 1977, this paper will focus on injury rather than death, emergency room studies rather than coroner/mortality studies and drinking in the event rather than alcoholism or problem drinking and its consequences. The question to be addressed is how good a'window' is the emergency room in understanding alcohol's role in injury, and accidental and intentional death?

I intend to look at the role of alcohol in causing traumatic events using the 'window' of the emergency room; to analyze the aspects of drinking and the powers ascribed to alcohol to investigate the causes of these events. The term 'traumatic event' will be used to denote a time-bounded series of actions, and 'trauma' to denote the injury which results from these events. Although the emphasis is on physical trauma in this instance, psychological trauma can be included. While it is of utmost personal and social importance, whether or not the trauma results in death is, in this case, less important. In proportionally few traumatic events — some homicides and most suicides — is death intentional. By and large, therefore, we are looking at 'accidents' in an emergency room. Further, crime *per se* and the role of alcohol in criminal events is not under investigation here although assaults leading to physical trauma are considered.

Perceptions of intention, historically, have played an important part in categorising casualties. The borderline dividing intentional from unintentional acts is far from clear:

> Any 'accident' which is seen as involving human intentions becomes redefined as a crime: thus a fire becomes arson, a black eye becomes assault, a traffic casualty becomes vehicular homicide. Some casualties do not fit on either side: suicide, which no longer is a crime in the US, is by definition not an accident; and inter-family violence, even when intentional and resulting in injury, has not necessarily been a crime either legally or in terms of conventional responses to it. (Aarens *et al.* 1977: p. 2)

The categorisation of an act as intentional or not will often vary from country to country and from analyst to analyst. In Polish, for example, no single word has a meaning and scope equivalent to that of the English word 'casualty' (Morawski and Moskalewicz 1989, *see* Chapter 13).

The International Classification of Disease (ICD)-E codes, used to categorise data on injuries, are subdivided according to apparent intent: unintentional injuries, such as falls and drownings, and intentional injuries, such as suicide and homicide. However, even these categories are often ambiguous. The categorization of a homicide as intentional is based on the intention of the offender, rather than the intentions of all persons in the event, especially the victim. A number of emergency room studies note the difficulty of determining intention in, for example, differentiating falls from assault, and often depend only on the victim's determination of responsibility for the injury. From the perspective of those working in emergency rooms intent is often of little importance.

Prior to this century, the alcohol involvement in accidents was of little social or even medical concern, as Levine (1983) and others have argued. The colonial period in North America saw frequent notices of death from drunkenness. Although the dangers of drinking were acknowledged, little attention, even through the temperance period, was concentrated on preventing accidents by urging the control of drinking. Accidents were not seen as the major social, economic and medical problem they have become in this century.

The first decade of the new century saw the beginnings of a safety movement in the United States. The National Safety Council (1984) was formed in 1913 and about that time attention was turned to the scientific investigation of accidents. Phelps in 1911 used mortality data from insurance records in order to estimate alcohol's role in relation to specific causes of death. The first emergency room study of alcohol and accidents was published in 1915 and it differs little from many of today's studies. The deaths of accident victims treated at Boston's Haymarket Relief Station were analysed for alcohol involvement. An estimated 40 per cent over a three-year period were judged to be 'under the influence of alcohol when they entered' (Brickley 1915). Based on 40,000 patient visits per year, the Boston investigators observed several aspects of alcohol's involvement in accidents: alcohol caused the accident; alcohol retarded the process of repair; alcohol obscured the diagnosis; alcohol increased the danger of infection at the time of the accident; alcohol prevented adequate treatment. Alcohol increased the danger of 'inter-current' complications; alcohol gave a poorer result; or alcohol increased the mortality in accidents; and they noted: ... 'Many alcoholics are quarrelsome and restless. Many persist in undoing the work the surgeon does for them'.

There is little in the contemporary studies reviewed in the present paper that was not already known near the turn of the century. These observations would today form the basis of any reasonable proposal for the study of alcohol and trauma.

Studies of alcohol's involvement in accidental death occurred in any number only from the late 1940s in the United States (Aarens *et al.* 1977). The past decade has seen a developing interest in alcohol's involvement in injury and death and often from unsuspected quarters. Relevant articles are carried in more journals, including journals not usually concerned with alcohol problems, for example, *The International Journal of*

Oral Surgery, Surgery Gynaecology and Obstetrics, Annals of Emergency Medicine, and *The International Journal of Law and Psychiatry*.

In large part, the increasing interest in alcohol and trauma is motivated by concern for the medical management of trauma victims who have been drinking immediately prior to a traumatic event or are known to be chronic drinkers. A review of alcohol effects in medical management mirrors the review by Brickley over half a century earlier. Soderstrom *et al.* (1979) discuss a number of alcohol-related management problems. Alcohol can affect the diagnosis of injuries to the head and neck, thorax, abdomen and extremities. In relation to cardiac disturbances, the authors cite alcoholic cardiomyopathy and arrhythmias caused by alcohol-induced hypothermia. Alcohol intoxication further negatively affects the response to haemorrhage, and haematologic changes affect tolerance of blood loss and coagulation processes. Additionally, 'anaesthesia management is complicated by the acute and/or chronic use of alcohol' and the synergistic effect of alcohol and some drugs can complicate pharmacologic management. The authors note the negative effects of alcohol on resistance to infection and complications induced by withdrawal from alcohol. Vitek and Lans (1982) note that 'after trauma, the metabolic clearance of alcohol is probably decreased'. The alcohol effect may be a factor, therefore, many hours after injury. The extensive range and expense of tests suggested to improve the medical management of drinking trauma victims significantly increases the cost of treatment.

This review concentrates on emergency room studies published in English and more thoroughly reviews US work than that of other countries. However, studies from a large number of developed countries are reviewed. It is important, therefore, for the reader to keep in mind cross-national variations in patterns of consumption of alcoholic beverages and in amounts consumed. Patterns of drinking vary as well as levels of consumption. For example, Finnish drinking occurs most often on weekends, does not generally accompany meals, and is often carried out for the purpose of getting 'high' or 'drunk'. French drinking most frequently accompanies meals and is very much a part of the rhythm of everyday life. Polish drinking, unlike drinking in France or Finland, is often reserved for festive occasions with typically high levels of consumption. Countries differ in the proportion of the population which consumes beverage alcohol, the ages at which drinking begins and especially in the proportions of women who drink. These differences will account for some of the variation in rates of alcohol presence in traumatic events. In particular, temporal variations in rates — time of day and day of week — must be accounted for in comparing data cross-nationally.

Emergency Room Clientele

Trauma centres and emergency rooms in the United States no longer deal only or even primarily with injury. They provide medical care when other departments of the hospital are closed or staff are unavailable and they provide primary care to families of the urban poor (Torrens and Vedvab 1970, Gibson *et al.* 1970, Satin and Duhl 1972). Studies in several urban areas show emergency rooms to be handling a population which is poor, made up disproportionately of ethnic minorities, the poorly educated and those with multiple social problems (Bergman 1976). Between 1950 and 1980, the use of emergency rooms increased by nearly 950 per cent in the United States. Clement and Klingbeil (1981) note a number of reasons for this increase. Emergency rooms deal with a large number of victims of violence; as the level of violence increases, so too does the number of victims seen in emergency rooms. Additionally, changes in funding medical care and cutbacks in social services force the poor and those who are state-supported to seek care on an acute or emergency basis. In a recent study carried out in a large, urban emergency room, Stephens Cherpitel (1989) estimates that 60 per cent of patients presented with non-traumatic problems, sometimes seeking a meal or place to sleep (*see* Chapter 16).

Countries with fuller provision of medical services than the United States may also have experienced a substantial increase in emergency care. An indirect indicator of the demand for primary care from casualty centres in Great Britain is the ever-present sign asking patients to see their general practitioner for problems which are not acute. An exploratory Swedish study to investigate the unexpected heavy use of a relatively new accident and emergency department (Magnusson 1979) showed that half of the patients attending had not attempted to obtain medical care elsewhere prior to the visit, that 62 per cent of the cases were considered acute but only 10 per cent were the result of traumatic events. In all countries, the clientele of emergency room will vary as a function of the location of the hospital, its catchment and referral system.

Alcohol Measurement in Emergency Rooms

The measurement of blood or breath alcohol is the most common measure of alcohol consumption in emergency room studies. Few studies use more than one measure and few look at drinking history or alcohol dependence. Emergency room personnel are concerned with the patient after the traumatic event has occurred and alcohol measurement is primarily directed toward medical management. The measurement of alcohol use in emergency rooms presents a number of clinical and social problems. Clinical observation of such factors as unsteady gait or slurring words have long been considered unreliable (Jetter 1938, Aarens *et al.* 1977). Questioning of the patient in the emergency room is often impossible and in many cases unreliable. Blood- and breath-alcohol testing are not always possible and are often not a high priority for a seriously injured patient. However, the importance of alcohol in medical management has been more keenly felt in recent years and with this change of perception has come an interest in the reliability of alcohol measures.

A recent US military emergency room study (James *et al.* 1984) of serum- and breath-alcohol measurement supports the view that 'breath alcohol levels as measured are a reliable and valid proxy of blood levels'. This study involved 659 patients where blood tests were taken and, of these, 434 patients also had a breath test. The correlation between the two tests was 0.94; 7 per cent of the patients were positive on only one test, but the false negatives did not exceed 4 per cent for either test.

Emergency room medical staff often rely on the smell of alcohol on the breath when deciding which patients to test for alcohol use. In a study by Rutherford (1977), 35 of 37 patients with a positive BAC had an alcohol odour. Of the eleven patients who were clinically diagnosed as negative, but who had positive BACs, seven had no alcohol odour and five of these had BACs below 100 mg/100 ml.

A 1980 study carried out in Edinburgh (Holt *et al.* 1980), exploring the intercorrelations of breath alcohol, clinical signs and level of consciousness, concludes that:

> ... almost all the patients who were scored as possessing clinical features of intoxication had positive breath-alcohol tests, but there were false-negative diagnoses in 19% of patients who had been drinking. Smell on the breath was the most useful criterion, and slurred speech and abnormal co-ordination the least useful. (p. 639)

Brismar *et al.* (1983), in a Swedish study of head injury, examined blood alcohol, blood gamma-glutamyl transpeptidase (G-GT) and the mean blood corpuscular volume (MCV). Alcohol history and alcohol consumption per day were also taken. BACs were taken in 64 of the 100 patients, of which half were positive. Elevated G-GT was noted in 35 per cent of the patients, and a history of alcoholism treatment was reported for 37 per cent. Unfortunately, no intercorrelation of alcohol measures is presented.

An ambitious French study (Papoz *et al.* 1986) also included the same three measures on a sample of 4,796 cases (*see* Chapter 15). A quarter of the men and one in ten overall showed BACs greater than or equal to 80 mg/100 ml. γ-Glutamyltransferase and mean corpuscular volume were markedly higher in the sample of cases when compared to a reference population.

Recent work with the dipstick technique suggests that it will be a reliable and inexpensive diagnostic tool for the management of trauma patients. Kapur (1989) compares the dipstick favourably with breathalyzer, gas chromatography and spectrophotometry techniques on cost, sample and technical requirements (*see* Chapter 8).

Serum osmolality has been suggested by a number of investigators as an alternative to measuring blood alcohol (Champion *et al.* 1975, Rutherford 1977). Although the correlation with blood alcohol level is adequate and the test can be performed within two to three minutes, other factors can cause an elevation in serum osmolality.

Poikolainen (1988) has called for a high priority on work testing the reliability of the 'ethyl sign' — a semi-quantitative clinical measure of the degree of intoxication (*see* Chapter 9). Until a simple, fast and inexpensive test for blood alcohol is available (e.g. the dipstick), medical management in many circumstances may have to depend on clinical evaluation.

A majority of the studies reviewed here call for more comprehensive measurement of alcohol in the emergency room. In the absence of resources for laboratory tests, clinical observation has been shown to give a reasonable estimate of patients who 'have been drinking'.

Magnitude of the Problem

Trauma is a social and medical problem of great proportion in both developed and developing countries, yet it has received relatively little research attention, except for traffic crashes. In most developed countries, trauma is the leading cause of death between the ages of one and about forty. Trauma, in these countries, is the fourth or fifth leading cause of death in the general population, after heart disease, stroke and cancer. In the US in 1982, there were approximately 165,000 deaths from trauma, more than twice that many cases of permanent injury from trauma and an estimated 70 million injuries of all types (Baker *et al.* 1984, Lowenfels and Miller 1984). It is estimated that trauma patients take up a 'total of 19 million hospital days per year in the US, more than the number needed by all cancer patients' (Trunkey 1983). While the death rate from heart disease and stroke has fallen dramatically in the past decade in the US, it is estimated that the death rate from trauma has increased by about 1 per cent per year.

Of the deaths from injury in 1982, two-thirds were classified as 'unintentional' and one-third were 'intentional'. About half of the unintentional injuries were motor vehicle crashes. Of the approximately 51,000 intentional injury deaths, slightly more than half were classified as suicides and the remaining were classified as 'homicide and legal intervention'. In 2 per cent of cases, intent could not be determined. The overall US death rate for men is two to three times greater than that for women both for intentional and unintentional injury (Baker *et al.* 1984).

The incidence of injury is more difficult to estimate than the death rate. It has been estimated that between one-fifth and one-quarter of the US population sustains an injury each year. The best estimates of serious injury (injury serious enough to result in a visit to an emergency room) are those of the Northeastern Ohio Trauma Study (NEOTS). An annual rate of an estimated 244 injuries per 1,000 males and 148 per 1,000 females, suggests that the rate of serious injury for men is nearly 250 times the death rate and for women is about 400 times the death rate. In 1977, nearly 500,000 injury cases were treated in hospital emergency rooms in Northeastern Ohio's 42 hospitals, an estimated one emergency room visit for every five residents of the area. From 41 of the 42 acute care hospitals participating in the study, a sample of 17,720 emergency room visits was drawn from 28 randomly selected days. The sampling frame was stratified by day of the week and quarter of the year. Of these visits 11,099 cases were for 'emergent conditions', including any diagnosis of trauma, heart attack or stroke, emergency visits for psychiatric reasons, hospital admissions from the emergency room and cases dead on or after arrival regardless of cause. These incidence trauma cases are presented in Table 1.1; the US external trauma mortality data are presented in Table 1.2. The investigators note:

> The rank ordering of traumatic causes of death and traumatic causes of injury are distinctly different ... Suicide and homicide rank second and third, respectively, as causes of death, but, as a cause of injury, assault (purposely inflicted) accounts for twenty times as many cases as attempted suicide. Motor vehicle crashes rank higher than assault as a cause of injury and as a cause of death, being responsible for over twice as many hospital-reported cases of each. Only falls and motor vehicle collisions rank within the five leading causes of both traumatic injury and traumatic death. (Barancik *et al.* 1983: p. 748-9)

A number of possible sources of bias identified by these investigators can also be expected to bias most injury investigations based on emergency room data. Persons treated by a private physician, in an industrial clinic, not treated or self-treated will not be included. Patients who died without coming to the hospital will be missed. However, there is evidence suggesting that emergency room data are a better source of trauma estimates than some official statistics.

Table 1.1: *Number and percentage of cases in sample and incidence of external cause-specific trauma (E800-E999) reported to hospital emergency departments in five northeastern Ohio Counties, 1977*

	ICDA 8th revision external cause category[a]		Cases in sample[a]			Estimated no. of cases in five counties[b]
Rank	Description	E Code	No.	%	SE%	
1	Falls	880-887	2,136	24.1	0.45	111,377
2	Cutting/piercing	920	1,265	14.3	0.37	65,961
3	Striking against/struck by object or caught in/between objects	916-918	1,226	13.9	0.37	63,927
4	Motor vehicle	810-823	1,029	11.6	0.34	53,655
5	Overexertion/strenuous movements	919	721	8.1	0.29	37,595
6	Insect/animal bite/sting	905-906	372	4.2	0.21	19,397
7	Purposely inflicted by other person	960-968	367	4.1	0.21	19,136
8	Foreign body entering eye or other orifice	914-915	280	3.2	0.19	14,600
9	Other road vehicle	825-827	168	1.9	0.15	8,760
10	Contact with hot or corrosive substance	924	140	1.6	0.13	7,300
11	Poisoning, unintentional	850-877	93	1.1	0.11	4,849
12	Fire and flames	890-899	71	0.8	0.09	3,702
13	Surgical & medical complications & misadventures	930-936	37	0.4	0.07	1,929
14	Excessive heat/cold	900-901	34	0.4	0.07	1,773
15	Self-inflicted	950-958	17	0.2	0.05	886
16	Rail, water & air transport	800-807	11	0.1	0.04	574
	All other or unspecified unintentional	c	677	7.6	0.28	35,301
	Undeterminable intent	980-988	206	2.3	0.16	10,741
	TOTAL	800-999	8,850	100.0	--	461,463

Note SE: Standard Error of the proportion

[a] Excludes: Late Effects (E940-E949.31, 31 cases, E959, E969, E989, E999, two cases), legal intervention (E970-E978, three cases) and cases with previous hospital treatment for the same incident

[b] Rounded to nearest case

[c] Includes 87 cases in the categories E904, E910, E913, E921, E923, E925-E928 and 590 cases in the Other and Unspecified category E929

Source: Barancik *et al.* 1983

General Emergency Room Studies

Several studies in the last decade report the blood or breath alcohol of patients attending an emergency room. In six studies from four countries, 20 to 37 per cent of the trauma patients had positive BAC's whereas only 10 to 12 per cent of the non-trauma patients tested positive for blood alcohol (Honkanen 1976 [Finland], Ward *et al.* 1982 [Texas], Haut Comité d'Etude sur l'Alcoolisme 1985 [France], Wechsler *et al.* 1969 [Massachusetts], Stephens Cherpitel 1989 [California], Walsh and Macleod 1983 [Scotland]). All are relatively well-designed and take care with the measurement of the alcohol variable; however, they differ in analytic power and in intent. For example, Ward *et al.* (1982) are primarily interested in the relationship between severity of injury and alcohol and in alcohol's exacerbation of underlying medical problems. Honkanen (1976) focuses on the role of alcohol in causing traumatic events. All of these studies attempt breath- or blood-alcohol measurement on the full series or sample of patients; however, proportions achieved vary. The

Table 1.2: *Number, percentage and rank of the 10 leading causes of death from external trauma (E800-E999), United States, 1977*

	ICDA 8th revision external cause category		Fatalities	
Rank	Description	E Code	Number	Per Cent
1	Motor vehicle collision	810-823	49,510	31.7
2	Suicide	950-959	28,681	18.3
3	Homicide	960-978	19,968	12.8
4	Falls	880-887	13,773	8.8
5	Fire/flames	890-899	6,357	4.1
6	Drowning/submersion	910	5,961	3.8
7	Accidents, mainly of industrial type	916-921 923-928	5,271	3.4
8	Poisoning	850-877	4,970	3.2
9	Surgical or medical complications & misadventures	930-936	3,107	2.0
10	Inhalation, ingestion of food or other substance	911-912	3,037	1.9
	All other and unspecified		15,573	10.0
	ALL EXTERNAL TRAUMA	800-999	156,208	100.0

Source: *Vital Statistics of the United States*, Volume II—*Mortality* Part A, 1977
Printed in Barancik *et al.* 1983

series and samples are made up of different proportions of types of traumatic events. Because types of events differ with respect to the likelihood of victims having been drinking, it would be expected that overall rates of alcohol presence in these series would also differ. The studies reviewed here also differ in the attention given to analysis of the type of injury contrasted with the type of traumatic event.

The 1969 work of Wechsler *et al.* describes the difficulties in obtaining an unbiased sample of emergency room patients and an adequate measure of blood or breath alcohol. For example, of 11,644 adults 73 per cent were interviewed, 74 per cent were breathalyzed and 40 per cent of those who were not breathalyzed had no test for alcohol presence, others had a blood test or were observed clinically. Of the 8,461 eligible adult patients, only 67 per cent were included in the final analysis (Table 1.3).

Nonetheless, this remains an important study. Since it includes all types of emergency room patients, it is possible to compare those presenting with an injury with those with a medical or surgical emergency. Overall, 17 per cent of the emergency room patients gave a positive breath test; 24 per cent of trauma patients had positive BACs, compared to 10 per cent of non-trauma patients. As in most emergency room series, assaults were the events most likely to be alcohol-involved, work-re-

Table 1.3:   *Breathalyzer alcohol level by reason for admission of patient*

Reason for admission	Number of patients	Percent negative readings	Percent positive readings	
			0.01 to 0.04	0.05 and over
Total	5,589	83.2	9.0	7.7
Accidents	2,801	78.5	11.0	10.5
Home	620	77.7	11.0	11.3
Transportation	404	70.5	12.4	17.1
Occupation	969	84.4	10.6	4.9
Other	808	75.9	10.9	13.2
Nonaccidents	2,633	81.2	6.3	2.6
Circulatory	255	92.2	6.3	1.6
Digestive	481	92.1	5.2	2.7
Sympton	551	90.9	5.8	3.3
Other	1,346	90.7	6.8	2.5
Fights or assaults	155	43.6	17.6	32.8

Source: Wechsler *et al.* 1969

31

lated accidents least likely (38.8 per cent with a BAC of 50 mg/100 ml or higher for the former, 4.9 per cent for the latter). Home and transportation accidents lay somewhere in between, depending on country and emergency room catchment. Among home accidents, head injuries and lacerations showed the greatest alcohol presence and sprains the least. Some of these injuries were, no doubt, related to intra-family violence but this was not analysed in this series.

Honkanen's 1976 study of Finnish emergency room patients presents one of the most thorough analyses of alcohol and injury and is a model for later analyses. The study is made up of four different series:

1. Helsinki 1972/3. A series of 1,012 seriously injured adults attending an emergency room in Helsinki. Alcohol use was measured by BAC and hospital records.

2. Helsinki 1973. A series of all adults who attended the same hospital emergency room. BACs were coded from hospital records.

3. Jyväskylä 1974. A series of 182 consecutive adult injury victims who had a blood sample taken and were interviewed.

4. Helsinki 1975. A case control study of pedestrians. Patients and controls were interviewed and had either a blood sample taken or were breathalyzed.

Table 1.4: *Percentages of alcohol involvement and cases with BACs above 1.0 g/l by main accident types in the Helsinki (Hki) 1972-73 and Jyväskylä (Jkyl) 1974 series, and positive ethyl sign rates in the Helsinki 1973 series*

	Hki 1972-73 AI[a]	CF[b]	Jkyl 1974 AI[a]	CF[b]	Hki 1973 Ethyl[c]
Industrial	19	9	9	4	2
Traffic	38	25	17	17	13
Home	36	25	40	27	19[d]
Other freetime	45	28	29	17	
Fights, assaults	71	54	86	71	49
Suicide attempts	56	28			35
Total	37	24	30	20	13.5

[a] AI: alcohol involvement

[b] CF: BACs above 1.0 g/l

[c] Ethyl: positive ethyl sign rates

[d] Rate in freetime falls

Source: Honkanen 1976

A high rate of alcohol-positive tests was found in the two injury series and a much lower rate for the larger, general emergency room series. The proportions for the three series are 37, 30 and 13 per cent, respectively. Those between 35 and 44 years of age in the first Helsinki series and between 25 and 34 in the Jyväskylä series had the highest proportion of positive BACs. Accidents occurred disproportionately on Saturdays and in the evenings. Head injuries were the most frequent alcohol-related injury. No clear picture emerged relating positive BAC and severity of injury. These series show the greatest degree of alcohol involvement in fights, assaults, and suicide attempts (56 to 86 per cent), and a low alcohol presence in work-related accidents (9 to 19 per cent) (Table 1.4). No analysis is carried out linking injury with type of traumatic event and both with alcohol involvement.

Walsh and Macleod (1983) (Scotland) analyse both diagnosis and place/type of accident by BAC (Tables 1.5 and 1.6). In this prospective study of 1,044 consecutive patients aged 15 years and over, 16.5 per cent had positive BACs. This varied by type of presenting problem. Almost half of the head injured patients had a positive BAC, compared with only 3 per cent of those presenting with medical and surgical emergencies. A larger number of accidents were work-related than is found in a typical emergency room series; however, the hospital serves a rural area and may see disproportionate numbers of patients in relatively hazardous types of

Table 1.5: *Alcohol consumption by diagnosis*

Diagnosis	Number of patients	Positive Alcometer no.	Positive Alcometer (%)	Alcometer ≥ 80 mg/100 ml no.	Alcometer ≥ 80 mg/100 ml (%)
Major head injury	17	7	(41.2)	6	(35.3)
Minor head injury	52	25	(48.1)	20	(38.5)
Major other trauma	52	6	(11.5)	4	(7.7)
Minor other trauma	618	97	(15.7)	53	(8.6)
Drunk	4	4		3	
Self-poisoning	25	18	(72.0)	13	(52.0)
Psychiatric	6	2		1	
Surgical (non-traumatic)	189	8	(4.2)	3	(1.6)
Medical	66	2	(3.0)	2	(3.0)
No diagnosis	15	3	(20.0)	2	(13.3)
Totals	1044	172	(16.5)	107	(10.2)

Source: Walsh and Macleod 1983

work. In this series, only assaults show a large proportion of intoxicated patients—nearly 40 had sustained head injuries. Drinking patients were more likely to visit the emergency room in the evenings and on weekends. Fewer than 10 per cent of those attending during the day had been drinking, compared with nearly 65 per cent of those attending between midnight and 3 a.m. Alcohol presence was positively related to a depressed level of consciousness; and 68 per cent of patients in this condition had BACs greater than or equal to 80 mg/100 ml.

The effect of catchment on the overall proportion of patients showing signs of drinking is demonstrated by comparing Walsh and Macleod (1983) to Holt *et al.* (1980). A sample of 702 patients examined on 17 different evenings in an accident and emergency department of an Edinburgh teaching hospital was tested for alcohol; 40 per cent of the sample was positive for alcohol; 32 per cent had BACs in excess of 80 mg/100 ml.

Ward *et al.* (1982) carried out a study of 1,198 patients admitted to the trauma service of a Texas hospital over a 14-month period. All patients had blood drawn for a serum-alcohol test within one hour after admission to the emergency room. They found that 32 per cent of patients had positive BACs, with a mean BAC of 150 mg/100 ml for the positive group and of the alcohol-positive group, 74 per cent had BACs of 100 mg/100 ml or greater. Of all types of injuries, only head injuries were disproportionately represented in the alcohol-present group.

The most comprehensive and well-designed published study of alcohol and accidents is a recent French study carried out by Haut Comité

Table 1.6:   *Place and type of incident*

Incident	Number of patients	no.	Positive Alcometer (%)	Alcometer 80 mg/100 ml no.	(%)
Assault	56	39	(69.6)	28	(50.0)
Home	192	25	(13.0)	12	(6.3)
RTA[a]	74	8	(10.8)	6	(8.1)
Work	242	19	(7.9)	9	(3.7)
Sport	79	4	(5.0)	1	(1.3)
Other	101	41	(40.6)	27	(26.7)
Not known	10	2		2	
Totals	754	138	(18.3)	85	(11.3)

[a] RTA = Road Traffic Accident

Source: Walsh and Macleod 1983

d'Etude et d'Information sur l'Alcoolisme (1985). The study included 4,796 accident cases admitted to 21 French hospitals over a period of four months. Only patients 15 years old and older were included, but all types of accidents were investigated. The sample controlled for time of day and day of the week. Blood samples were analysed for alcohol content, mean corpuscular volume and gamma-glutamyl transferase. All key variables are co-varied with each drinking-related measure. The blood-alcohol analysis is reviewed here: 21 per cent of the patients presented with BACs of 80 mg/100 ml or higher, the limit for drunk driving in France. A quarter of the men exceeded this limit compared to 11 per cent of the women. As in all emergency room studies, men were disproportionately represented (nM = 3,427, nF = 1,369); and 12 per cent of the men had BACs of 200 mg/100 ml or higher. BACs were related to family situation, especially for men; for example, 40 per cent of men widowed and divorced had BACs greater than or equal to 120 mg/100 ml. Among men, those who were unemployed and those who were professional drivers were most likely to be intoxicated; among women, housewives and 'patrons'. Type of accident by gender and BAC is given in Table 1.7. Blood alcohol levels are highest in road traffic accidents and in assaults. Women injured in assaults (some, no doubt, as a result of battering) showed surprisingly high BACs; however, a breakdown by type of incident is not presented. It is noteworthy that many patients had a previous accident history: 36 per cent of men with three previous accidents had BACs greater than or equal to 80 mg/100 ml compared to 19 per cent of those with none. Nearly three times as many men who had had 3 previous accidents had BACs greater than or equal to 200 mg/100 ml when compared to those with 0. Intoxication was also positively related to the severity of the accident: 35 per cent of men who were hospitalised were intoxicated, compared to 20 per cent of those who were not hospitalised. Proportions for women were 38 per cent and 18 per cent, respectively. A typical accident pattern of time of day and day of week showed an increasing rate of intoxicated patients from 1600 to 2400 hours, with a sharp peak at 0300. There was very little variation throughout the week except for a sharp increase on Saturday. No control groups were defined and the investigators acknowledge the difficulty in assessing the causal role of alcohol in traumatic events.

However, in work by some of the same investigators, a comparison of GGT and MCV levels in a reference population showed markedly elevated levels in the patient population compared with the 'healthy population' (Papoz *et al.* 1981). Papoz *et al.* (1986) suggest that a substantial proportion of casualty victims in France are chronic drinkers; indeed, it is asserted that 'most of the intoxicated subjects were probably chronic drinkers'.

Table 1.7: *Distribution par nature d'accident [Distribution by the nature of the accident]*

	V.pub	Trajet	Circ/tr	Travail	Domest.	Sport	Rixe
			Hommes				
N =	959	247	109	880	579	229	421
Alc. (g/l)			**Pourcentages**				
0.00 - 0.09	49.4	71.9	64.7	72.9	59.3	83.9	30.0
0.10 - 0.29	6.1	6.9	10.2	11.0	8.3	9.6	7.1
0.30 - 0.49	4.3	3.7	5.6	4.3	4.1	1.7	2.9
0.50 - 0.79	3.7	2.0	2.8	3.9	3.3	1.7	3.6
0.80 - 1.19	4.0	1.2	7.4	2.1	4.7	1.7	7.9
1.20 - 1.99	13.0	5.7	6.5	4.0	8.1	0.9	19.5
2.00	19.5	8.6	2.8	2.1	12.2	0.5	29.0
	100.0	100.0	100.0	100.0	100.0	100.0	100.0
			Femmes				
N =	448	120	10	112	482	70	123
Alc. (g/l)			**Pourcentages**				
0.00 - 0.09	82.8	85.0	--	84.7	76.2	95.7	58.5
0.10-0.29	5.1	8.4	--	10.8	6.8	2.9	6.5
0.30 - 0.49	0.9	2.5	--	2.7	2.5	0.0	4.1
0.50-0.79	1.1	1.7	--	0.9	2.1	0.0	2.4
0.80 - 1.19	2.5	0.8	--	0.0	1.6	0.0	4.1
1.20 - 1.99	4.0	0.8	--	0.9	5.0	0.0	8.1
2.00	3.6	0.8	--	0.0	5.8	1.4	16.3
	100.0	100.0	100.0	100.0	100.0	100.0	100.0
			Ensemble				
N =	1,407	367	119	992	1,061	299	544
Alc. (g/l)			**Pourcentages**				
0.00 - 0.29	0.0	76.2	67.0	73.9	67.0	86.7	36.4
0.10 - 0.29	5.8	7.4	9.3	11.0	7.6	8.0	7.1
0.30 - 0.49	3.2	3.3	5.1	4.1	3.4	1.3	3.2
0.50 - 0.79	2.9	1.9	2.5	3.5	2.7	1.3	3.3
0.80 - 1.19	3.5	1.1	6.8	1.9	3.3	1.3	7.0
1.20 - 1.99	10.2	4.1	5.9	3.7	6.7	0.7	16.9
2.00	14.4	6.0	3.4	1.9	9.3	0.7	26.1
	100.0	100.0	100.0	100.0	100.0	100.0	100.0

V. pub: Motor vehicle, public highway   Travail: Work
Trajet: Motor vehicle, to and from work   Domest.:   Home
Circ/trav.: Motor vehicle, while working   Sport: Sport
Rixe: Fights/assaults

Source: Haute Comité d'Etude et d'Information sur l'Alcoolisme 1985

The analysis of a U.S. study (Stephens Cherpitel 1989, *see* Chapter 16) offers a similar picture; 15 per cent of the sample had positive BACs, 23 per cent of those injured had positive BACs. Positive BACs were associated with both type of injury and cause of injury.

Although few studies investigate drinking histories of trauma patients, those that do show a considerable proportion of heavy or dependent drinkers in each series. In addition to the studies cited above, two studies, one Australian (Saunders 1987) and the other Spanish (Rodes *et al.* 1987) add evidence to the hypothesis that many of those with high BACs who present to the emergency room are regular drinkers. In a Spanish sample of 850 patients visiting a trauma ward, 80 per cent had consumed alcohol the day of the hospital visit, half of all patients in the series drank daily, and nearly one-fifth drank more than 50 grams of pure ethanol a day. In the Australian sample (daytime patients only), 18 per cent of 351 patients attending a casualty department were labelled 'alcoholics' on the basis of a previously diagnosed alcohol problem, 14 per cent had a weekly pure ethanol intake of 300 grams or more; one-quarter of the 'non-alcoholics' had had an alcohol-related problem in the past year and substantial proportions indicated a variety of dependency symptoms 'over the last year'.

A much earlier Swedish study of alcohol in a surgical emergency unit (Rydberg *et al.* 1975) shows an interesting association between BAC and problem drinking. In this series, 28 per cent of the patients were registered with the Swedish Board of Excise for an alcohol-related offence or 'alcohol abuse'. Half of the registered 'problem-drinking' group was found to have alcohol in the blood. Of those not registered, only 12 per cent had positive BACs. A significant association emerged between problem drinking and BAC: 'In the alcohol-free group (i.e. BAC = 0) 18 per cent were known for alcohol abuse, against 89 per cent of the patients in the group with more than 250 mg alcohol per 100 g blood'.

Alcohol-positive patients in the trauma-only series of the studies reviewed here range from 20 per cent (Scotland) to 37 per cent (Finland). The Scottish emergency room series also shows a lower proportion of intoxicated patients; 10 per cent of patients presenting to the emergency room in rural Scotland were intoxicated compared to 24 per cent of those in the Finnish series. These results are not unexpected. Event types vary across studies and alcohol positive tests vary as a function of event type. Only 11 per cent of injuries resulting from motor vehicle trauma in the Scottish study show positive BAC's compared to 50 per cent in the French study. This may be explained by proximity to casualty care as much as by cross-cultural differences in drinking-driving.

Studies reviewed here show assaults and fights, without exception, to be the most alcohol-involved traumatic events. The proportion of alcohol present cases in assaults and fights ranges from 36 to 70 per cent; intoxication ranges from 26 to 58 per cent; and the proportion of assault cases in these studies ranges from 6 to 27 per cent.

Alcohol and Head Injuries

The best estimate of the annual incidence of head injuries in the US comes from the National Head and Spinal Cord Injury Survey (Kalsbeek *et al.* 1980). This study shows an incidence rate of about 200 cases per 100,000 population. Another US estimate from a smaller study carried out in Rhode Island (Fife *et al.* 1984b) shows an incidence rate 25 per cent lower. Since the single most important cause of head injury accidents is traffic crashes, the estimated incidence will vary cross-nationally and from emergency room to emergency room, depending on the types of accidents seen. Estimated incidence will also vary in relation to different methods of coding types of injury.

Walsh and Macleod (1983) report a relatively low proportion of head injuries among a series of trauma patients in Scotland. This study, which gave each patient a single injury diagnosis, found 9 per cent of the cases to have a major or minor head injury, while a US study which coded multiple injuries for each patient found nearly a quarter of trauma patients had some head injury (Ward *et al.* 1982).

A major concern of medical personnel treating patients with head injuries is differentiating both minor and major injuries from the alcohol intoxication, which is often present. Rutherford (1977) notes:

> Alcoholic intoxication and concussion have many features in common....Failure to diagnose alcohol intoxication where it exists may be serious in some cases. To diagnose it where it does not exist is always bad medicine. (p. 1021)

Intracranial haemorrhage, trauma-induced brain damage and alcohol intoxication can produce many of the same symptoms, such as blurring of consciousness and loss of memory. Monitoring the level of consciousness is essential in the early stages of the treatment of head injury. Rutherford (1977) argues that coma should not be attributed to alcohol when a BAC less than 300 mg/100 ml is present, nor confusion attributed to alcohol in a patient with a BAC of less than 200 mg/100 ml. Alcohol presence may additionally affect the length of the period of coma or loss of memory and thereby inappropriately affect the prognosis in cases in which this time period is used to determine the severity of injury. The diagnostic problems created by alcohol are highlighted by Murray (1976) in a series of nearly 1,000 head-injured patients in a large casualty department in Scotland. Higher BACs were found in all of the patients with coma or disorientation when compared to those who were fully conscious.

Emergency rooms which are aware of the probability of alcohol intoxication in head-injured patients use both physical observation and blood and/or urine tests to assess alcohol presence and level; some rely only on clinical observation for initial treatment. One study (Rutherford 1977), which compared clinical signs with the presence of a positive BAC, shows a surprising degree of correspondence; in a sample of 114 patients with head injuries, only 14 errors were recorded.

Most of the studies reviewed here attempted a BAC for the full series of patients investigated; the others used laboratory tests only for those with clinical signs. Most studies had substantial BAC non-response due to the severity of the injury or oversight on the part of the receiving medical personnel.

Among the studies reviewed, several are noteworthy. They are relatively well-executed, have large numbers of cases, raise interesting analytic questions or show up the methodological problems in studies of this type. Rimel *et al.* (1982) conducted a 20-month prospective study of head injury patients admitted to the University of Virginia Medical Center. Assessment took place within two to four hours after injury. All patients were evaluated with the Glasgow Coma Scale (GCS)[2]. Those with moderate injuries were more likely to have a BAC taken, less likely to have a negative BAC and significantly more likely to have a BAC which indicated legal intoxication. Alcohol presence was not correlated with either age or gender, although 77 per cent of the moderately injured group were men and 29 per cent under 21 years of age. The importance of motor vehicle crashes in causing head injuries is noteworthy. Sports injuries figure fairly prominently in minor head injuries.

A similar Swedish study (Edna 1982), carried out over a two-year period, included patients admitted within twelve hours after injury and omitted children under twelve years. Alcohol was present in 41 per cent of the men and 11 per cent of the women. The level of consciousness was lower and duration of coma was longer in the BAC-positive patients in contrast with the BAC-negative group. Brismar *et al.* (1983), in another Swedish study, investigated both acute intoxication and alcohol dependence in a three-month series of head injury patients. Of the patients tested, 52 per cent had BACs of 50 mg/100 ml or greater; 36 per cent had BACs over 250 mg/100 ml. This study shows a high rate of alcohol dependence, with 35 of the 100 patients drinking over 140 grams per day, 38 indicating loss of control and 37 with a treatment of alcoholism (not necessarily discrete criteria). The highest proportion of injuries involving intoxication was for violence (81 per cent) and falls (63 per cent). The relatively large proportion of patients injured in an assault (32 per cent)

---

2.   Refer to notes following the text of this chapter.

is noteworthy. The investigators note the youth of the patients and the fact that 'the social structure within the catchment area of the hospital includes a considerable number of socially maladjusted'.

Murray (1976) also reports the effect of the catchment on the presenting injuries and their causes. In this study only 23 per cent of men and 28 per cent of women received their injuries as a result of motor vehicle crashes whereas 56 per cent of the injuries to men were a result of assaults or falls. The investigators report that the hospital 'is situated in a high density tenement area with numerous public houses'. Rimel *et al.* (1982) report that 66 per cent of the moderate head injuries presenting in their US study are caused by motor vehicle crashes. However, the study hospital provides the only neurological coverage for a 14-county area. Selection bias is likely to be less in this case than in emergency rooms with a large local catchment where there is a greater likelihood of having to provide routine medical care as well as acute care, and where the social characteristics of local residents may well be related to the types of accidents seen.

The studies above and other studies do not present a clear picture of the relationship between the cause of the head injury and alcohol presence. In general, it can be argued that a very substantial proportion of head-injured patients, where assault is the cause of injury, will be intoxicated; but the evidence is inconsistent and limited for other causes.

Head injuries are not a homogeneous category of injury and a large proportion of patients present with additional, often severe, injuries. However, two types of head injury have received particular attention in relation to alcohol. Among a group of serious facial injuries, McDade (1982) found a high degree of alcohol use. Of 20 patients, eleven had been drinking on the day of the injury and nine were judged moderately or severely 'alcohol dependent'. In addition, eleven of the injuries were caused by assault. A Swedish study of jaw fractures found that 63 per cent were caused by assault (Heimdahl and Nordenram 1977). Fatal subarachnoid haemorrhages present another category of head injury which shows substantial alcohol presence and serious post-trauma alcohol-related complications. These injuries most often occur as the result of fights. In a series of 20 cases investigated by Simonsen (1984) in Denmark, only two were thought to be unrelated to drinking. The investigator notes, 'It should be underlined that alcohol intoxication was present in all cases where the haemorrhage occurred from a ruptured vertebral artery.'

The evidence relating *severity* of head injury with BAC is limited and inconsistent. No investigators analyse their data by co-varying cause of injury, BAC, and severity of injury. In many studies the small series size precludes this. Also, it is unclear whether children are included in some analyses. For example, with regard to Rimel *et al.* (1982), if the analyses had been carried out on patients 15 years of age or older, the relationship between drinking and severity of injury may well have been mitigated. Vicario *et al.* (1983) show no relationship between the severity of trauma (evaluated by GCS) and BAC in 63 patients. Luna *et al.* (1984), in a series of 139 motorcycle accidents, report a significantly greater incidence of severe head injury among those intoxicated compared with those who were not. The incidence of critical head injury was higher as was subsequent mortality among the critically injured. This analysis suggests the need for detailed multivariate analysis which is cause-specific.

Several studies report the time of day and day of week in which head-injured patients are received in the emergency room. These times are consistent with what is known from previous work on alcohol-related injuries (Aarens *et al.* 1977). As expected, more positive BACs are found on weekends and in the hours from 8 p.m. to 8 a.m. (Edna 1982). This is not surprising, given the significant role that road traffic accidents play in causing the injuries. As Edna and other investigators note, 'The increase of alcohol-influenced head trauma patients in the night and in the weekend may cause a considerable strain on the hospital staff, which during nights and weekends are minimal.' The demands on staff of head-injured patients can be particularly great when a large proportion of cases are due to assaults and are often 'obstreperous' (Murray 1976).

Other Injuries

Injuries, other than head injuries, have received limited attention in relation to alcohol involvement. A Wisconsin study of spinal cord injuries, over an 18-month period reports half the patients as 'drinking just before the accident' and five of the 15 patients who had been drinking, as drunk. Nearly a quarter of the injured report a previous history of alcoholism (Fullerton *et al.* 1981). A Finnish study of abdominal trauma compares alcohol presence and outcome in a series of patients with blunt or penetrating wounds (Hockerstedt *et al.* 1982). Most (95 per cent) of those with penetrating wounds had been stabbed and an estimated 70-80 per cent were judged intoxicated at the time of the injury. Of patients with blunt wounds, 28 per cent showed signs of intoxication. The majority of blunt trauma victims had suffered a fall or had been in a major motor vehicle accident. Despite the fact that the presence of alcohol was significantly greater in the penetrating wound group, those who had a blunt trauma had more serious injuries and poorer outcomes. The fact that organ injuries after blunt trauma may take a considerable time to show significant symptons, often means a delay in seeking treatment. This delay may bias alcohol measurement considerably and give the impression that stabbing is more often the result of drinking when compared with other abdominal injuries.

Motor Vehicle-Related Trauma

Although motor vehicle-related accidents are responsible for nearly half of all injury-related deaths in the United States, they account for only one in eight of all emergency room visits. The Northeastern Ohio Trauma Study estimates an incidence rate of about 23 cases per 1,000 population. This varies substantially by sex and age. Men and women between the ages of 15 and 24 and 25 and 34 are most at risk of injuries serious enough to be seen in an emergency room (Fife *et al.* 1984a). As with all trauma, motor vehicle deaths have been much more rigorously investigated than injuries, despite the fact that motor vehicle crashes are responsible for some of the most severe injuries seen in an emergency room. Motor vehicle crashes cause more than half of all spinal cord injuries (Kraus *et al.* 1975), and half of all head injuries (Kalsbeek *et al.* 1980). A study of facial injuries treated in an emergency room indicates that almost half of the severe injuries are related to car crashes (Karlson 1982). A Rhode Island study of hospital discharge data (Fife *et al.* 1984b) investigated the role of motor vehicle crashes in causing other injuries. These investigators report:

> Motor vehicle crashes cause approximately two-thirds of all injuries to the chest organs (heart or lung), liver and spleen, and approximately one-third of kidney injuries, traumatic pneumothorax or hemothorax, femoral shaft fractures, pelvic fractures, intestinal injuries, patellar fractures. (p. 1263)

Alcohol is more frequently present in fatal than non-fatal crashes and in those which result in more serious rather than less serious injuries. In addition, alcohol is more frequently present in single-vehicle than multiple-vehicle crashes, irrespective of the severity of the resulting injury. Alcohol-related traffic crashes occur more frequently on weekends and in the evenings (Farris *et al.* 1975). It is estimated that one-quarter to one-third of drivers requiring emergency room care after a non-fatal accident have BACs of 100 mg/100 ml or higher (Perrine 1975, Carlson 1973).

A Canadian study of non-fatal motor vehicle crashes offers one of the best pictures of alcohol presence in these events (Warren *et al.* 1982). Of the 1,148 crash victims tested for blood or breath alcohol in four New Brunswick emergency rooms, 713 were drivers. The age distributions of these drivers are similar to the age distributions of fatally injured drivers: 45 per cent of the drivers were between the ages of 16 and 25 years of age.

Also 75 per cent were men. Injured drivers had a 28 per cent positive testing for alcohol whereas this finding was reported in 46 per cent of those fatally injured (Simpson *et al.* 1982). Not only were alcohol levels lower among the non-fatally injured than those fatally injured, but an analysis of the severity of injury shows a positive relationship with BAC. However, fatal crash victims show BAC levels considerably higher than even those who are seriously injured.

Studies in several countries have shown the relationships between seatbelt use and severity of injury sustained in a traffic accident. An Australian study (Christian 1984) agrees with previous reports from Sweden (Edna 1982) and the US (Rimel *et al.* 1982) that severity of injury is clearly related to seat belt use, which in turn is related to alcohol use — that is, positive BAC is inversely related to using a seatbelt. Canadian research has shown that as BACs increase, fewer drivers are restrained (Ontario 1980).

Motorcycle deaths in the US continue to increase as a result of the repeal or weakening of laws requiring cyclists to wear helmets. Per mile travelled, motorcyclists have a risk of death seven times that for automobile occupants. Luna *et al.* (1984) report evidence of alcohol in motorcycle accidents in studies carried out in California, Maryland, Minnesota and Arizona. These studies show ranges in alcohol use of 26 to 50 per cent. In their own study of acute intoxication and motorcycle crashes, these investigators examined 139 seriously injured victims of crashes who were admitted to hospital from the emergency room over an 18-month period. The incidence of 'acute intoxication' was 25 per cent in this group. Intoxicated victims suffered more severe injuries, most commonly a severe head injury. Only 11 per cent of the intoxicated victims had been wearing helmets compared to 38 per cent of the others. Intoxicated victims, whether helmeted or not, appear to have sustained more severe injuries and had double the mortality rate of the other group. It is noteworthy that none of the helmeted, non-intoxicated patients who sustained severe head injuries succumbed to their injuries.

A North Carolina study of moped accidents reported 30 per cent of the victims had been drinking (Hunter and Stutts 1979). An audit of moped registration cards found that one-fifth of the drivers had a recent suspension of their driver's license, the cause of the suspension in two-thirds of the cases being driving under the influence of alcohol. However, in an eight-month prospective study of moped crashes in South Carolina (McHugh and Stinson 1984), 14 per cent, including an unknown number of children, were noted to be intoxicated.

Pedestrian Trauma

In the USA approximately 8,000 pedestrians are killed and 100,000 injured each year. Studies of the incidence of trauma in emergency rooms do not typically separate pedestrian accidents from other road traffic accidents, making it difficult to estimate the burden on emergency rooms which comes from pedestrian trauma. Both the very young and the elderly are disproportionately victims of pedestrian accidents. Nearly one-quarter of all pedestrian deaths and injuries occur to children under the age of ten. It is estimated that 14 per cent of fatal pedestrian accidents involve an intoxicated driver, while 24 per cent involve an intoxicated pedestrian. This overall figure of 37 per cent varies with the time of day and day of the week. From a daytime low of 18 per cent of fatal accidents involving one intoxicated party, the figure rises to 62 per cent for night-time accidents (National Center for Statistics and Analysis 1983).

Atypically for research on traumatic events, several studies of pedestrian accidents have made use of control groups. A Belfast study (Irwin *et al.* 1983) found that of 50 consecutive pedestrian accidents, 18 had BACs of 80 mg/100 ml contrasted with seven of the controls. The relative risk of a pedestrian with a BAC at this level being involved in an accident was estimated at 3.6, based on unmatched pairs; a significant positive association between BAC and severity was noted.

A comprehensive US study (Blomberg and Fell 1979) investigated the accidents of all pedestrians requiring or seeking treatment at a New Orleans emergency room following non-fatal pedestrian accidents, as well as fatal pedestrian accidents in the same period. It is noteworthy that the distributions of BACs for those fatally and non-fatally injured were quite similar: half of the pedestrians in both groups had BACs of zero; 46 per cent of those fatally injured and 36 per cent of those with non-fatal injuries had BACs of 100 mg/100 ml or higher. Three risk calculations were made using site-matched controls (N = 559); using age/sex site-matched controls (N = 193); using random site controls (N = 80). Overall, 14 per cent of the accident site controls, 8 per cent of the random site controls and 43 per cent of the (tested) accident victims were found to have BACs equal to or greater than 50 mg/100 ml. The age/sex matched controls give the most conservative estimate.

In one of the most careful analyses of situational variables in these studies, Blomberg and Fell (1979) investigate both behavioural errors and accident types. They conclude:

> Pedestrian errors as compared to driver errors, are more prevalent in those accidents where the pedestrian had been drinking ... [further] these figures imply that location of crossing or loca-

tion in the road is more relevant to the alcohol than the non-alcohol accident. (Blomberg and Fell 1979)

The evidence shows the driver to have been culpable in about 23 per cent of accidents involving a non-drinking victim and in only 7 per cent of those in which the pedestrian was intoxicated.

Falls

Falls, by a good measure, are the leading cause of trauma leading to an emergency room visit, yet little research attention has been devoted to alcohol involvement in such accidents. Falls are the primary cause of hip injuries, and second only to motor vehicle crashes in causing spinal cord and brain injuries. Hip injuries account for the largest number of injury-related hospital admissions in the US — an annual estimate of 3.6 million hospital days per annum for those over 65 years of age (Baker *et al.* 1982).

Waller, in his 1973 study of falls among the elderly, found a relatively low rate of alcohol involvement; 13 per cent were self-reported to have been drinking prior to the fall. Only Honkanen *et al.* (1983) have seriously analysed alcohol involvement and risk in falls; although only pedestrian falls are included in the series. Of 313 adults who attended a Finnish emergency room over a period of five weeks as a result of falls in public places, 53 per cent had BACs above 20 mg/100 ml. Twenty six per cent of the cases had an incomplete record — often because of extreme intoxication. In a control group made up of randomly selected adult pedestrians of the same sex as the patients, interviewed exactly one week after the accident at the same site, only 15 per cent had BACs above 20 mg/100 ml. A number of demographic characteristics were analysed: patients were older than the controls, more often divorced or widowed, more often from working class backgrounds, and were more likely to have a disease which hampered walking. Road conditions and shoe factors were controlled. Several different risk estimates are presented. The investigators conclude:

> The relative risk (of a fall), if 1.0 at zero BAC, did not increase at BACs below 50 mg/ml, was about 3 at BACs of 50-100 mg/ml, about 10 at BACs of 100-150 mg/ml, and about 60 at BACs of 160 mg/ml and higher ... Alcohol is a common cause of accidental falls. (Honkanen *et al.* 1983: p. 244)

Fires and Burns

Fires and burns account for 5 to 7 per cent of deaths in the US each year (depending on how these are categorised) but only slightly more than one in 1,000 emergency room visits. These deaths and injuries occur most frequently in winter months and in rural areas. Although the elderly and very young are more likely than others to die in fires, burn injuries occur in all age groups. A 1977 review of fires (Levine and Radford) in one metropolitan area reported that 59 per cent of fire victims suffered minor injuries, 25 per cent required hospitalisation and 16 per cent died. Fires resulting in casualties were most often the result of careless smoking. A recent study of burn injuries reviewed the medical records of 70 consecutive burn patients (Vogtsberger, 1984). The study revealed that 36 of burn patients had been drinking at the time of injury, 7 per cent had used an illicit drug and 10 per cent had used both. Younger patients were more likely to have been drinking than older patients. More than half of the men had been drinking prior to the injury, compared with fewer than one-third of the women. Men were often injured while driving or working around motor vehicles, while women were often injured in the kitchen. Women were more likely than men to have psychiatric problems, or physical disorders. MacArthur and Moore (1975) investigated several predisposing factors in a consecutive series of 155 hospitalised, burned adults. Factors included were alcohol and drug dependence, degenerative disease, mental illness and any other factors which would affect arousal and escape. Half of the 50 women and 38 per cent of the men had one or more predisposing factors in his history, and 36 per cent of the series were described as 'under the immediate or long term influence of alcohol'. Severity of injury and mortality was greater among those with predisposing factors.

The effects of drinking and smoking on burn injuries have not yet been investigated, although the association is well known in studies of fatalities.

Work-Related Trauma

Work-related injuries have received little attention in emergency room studies. Baker *et al.* (1984) in a review which suggests the lack of attention to work-related injury and death, show certain categories of workers are shown to be at particular risk of injury and death from injury: these include farmers, people who drive on the job, those who operate heavy machinery and those who operate shops and are at risk of robbery.

A recent telephone survey of households in New England shows that a significant proportion of accidents among adults occur at work. Of the

2,565 adults surveyed, 17 per cent reported an injury requiring medical attention in the previous year. Of these, 41 per cent occurred at work. However, the reported drinking on the job was low. Only 4% reported drinking on the job in the 'previous month'. However, 18 per cent acknowledged having drunk at lunch, during breaks or during the hour prior to arriving at work (Hingson *et al.* 1985).

The difficulty in obtaining accurate reporting of alcohol-involved accidents at work is underscored in a Polish paper (Morawski and Moskalewicz 1989, *see* Chapter 13). Official statistics show only 0.5 per cent of accidents to have involved alcohol use, though labour surveys show between 8 and 15 per cent of accidents to be alcohol-involved. The authors point out that intoxicated workers are not entitled to accident allowance:

> This law which the public opinion regards as too severe and harmful when injury itself is enough punishment illustrates how legal norms that are not reconciled with a social sense of justice are not respected. It happens sometimes that friends of a labour accident victim help conceal the role of alcohol in the accident by giving their own blood for alcohol measurement tests. (p. 254)

Trauma Related to Fights and Assaults

Fights and assaults are the most likely traumatic events to result from a drinking occasion. Although assaults have received considerable attention in research on crime, little emergency room research has focussed on them. As Pittman and Handy (1964) have observed, a large proportion of assaults are not serious enough to need emergency room attention. Within the emergency room an unknown proportion of injuries, which are thought to be inflicted by others, are labelled as 'falls', 'lacerations', or 'fractures'. Typically, it is the presence of and types of multiple trauma that lead medical personnel to suspect assault. Because many victims do not want police involvement, many assaults go unrecorded. Emergency rooms vary in the proportion of presenting injuries that are the result of fights. One Alaskan emergency room series shows over half of the traumas to be the result of fighting, whether provoked or unprovoked. The most frequent injuries were lacerations (Nighswander 1982).

The studies reported in the section 'Magnitude of the Problem' (p. 27) describe a very large proportion of fighting-related injuries presenting with an elevated BAC. These proportions are especially large in the French and Finnish studies. A Danish study (Hedeboe *et al.* 1985) covered a 12-month period in the Accident Analysis Center in Aarhous. Of the 1,639 assault cases seen during that period, 43 per cent showed a positive BAC or were clinically judged to be under the influence of alcohol. The investigators point out that the majority (of cases) were young men and 30 per cent of the assaults were committed in or around bars and restaurants where male victims constituted the largest clientele. Almost 80 per cent of the assaults were committed between 6 p.m. and 6 a.m. In 16 per cent of the cases, the assault happened in the home; 64 per cent of the these victims were women.

However, studies are surprisingly silent on the difficulties of treating those injured as a result of fights who are often intoxicated and difficult to treat. Kirkpatrick and Taubenhaus (1967) note that interns and residents anticipated a higher proportion with elevated blood-alcohol levels than actually appeared in their series. The drunk and angry patient may wear disproportionately on medical staff who must, at the same time, treat the catastrophically injured and seemingly innocent victims.

The problem of battered women is one area of assaultive traumatic injury that is receiving increasing research attention. However, research shows that only a very small percentage of women attending an emergency room, with injuries suggestive of battering are identified as such by medical personnel (Stark *et al.* 1981). In an analysis of the trauma histories of 2,676 women treated in an urban emergency room, 6 per cent presented with injuries during the sample year 'that were attributed to a male intimate'. A further 8 per cent were judged by investigators to be likely victims of battering; 21 per cent of all women attending had a history of abuse. The 'at risk' women (those at risk in the most recent visit or the previous five years) were compared to those who had no history of battering. Battered women had a significantly greater number of emergency room visits than the controls; the mean number of visits for the former group was 5.88 and for the latter 1.96. Battered women show levels of alcohol use and dependence no higher than controls before their first reported battering incident, but significantly higher dependence after. After the first reported incidence, 15 per cent of battered women report 'alcohol abuse' compared to 2 per cent of the controls.

In a similar study, Appleton (1980) found no clear differences in the drinking patterns of battered and non-battered women presenting to an emergency room. However, those with a history of battering thought their partners were more likely to be heavy drinkers and two-thirds reported their partners had been drinking prior to the 'usual battery'. The author found that battered women and their partners had 'interacted with the judicial system' considerably more often than controls, were considerably more likely to have had an incidence of psychiatric hospitalisation and were more likely to be divorced.

In a retrospective study in a Swedish hospital covering a period of two years, 1,444 patients were admitted to hospital for injuries. Battering was the cause of 33 per cent of the injuries to men and 29 per cent of the injuries to women. Half of the battered women were under the influence of alcohol on admission to hospital, nearly half were undergoing treatment for alcoholism or drug abuse. The investigators note, 'One reason for the very high frequency of woman beating in this study compared with findings among out-patients may be that most women do not seek help until the battering has caused such severe injuries as to require hospitalization....' (Brismar and Tuner 1982).

Battered women make considerable demands on emergency rooms, are often not identified as battered and the evidence suggests that alcohol is frequently implicated in these battering events. There is little investigation of the dynamics of the battering event, the victim's drinking in the event or her drinking history.

Self-Harm

It is estimated that fewer than 0.4 cases of self-harm are seen per 1,000 emergency room cases (Northeastern Ohio Trauma Study—Barancik *et al.* 1983) however, but estimates of suicide attempts vary widely. In part, the problem is jurisdictional; some 'attempts' will be labelled psychiatric problems, and in some settings patients will go through a special psychiatric emergency service (Jacobs 1982/3).

M. Aarens and R. Roizen observe:

The literature on suicide has tended to consider the suicidal act as representing an end to a stream of events, situations, and predispositions in the life of the person; thus the studies of alcohol and suicide have most often looked at the victim's life patterns in using alcohol instead of drinking done at the time of the act. (Aarens *et al.* 1977: p. 477)

However, even emergency room settings cause investigators to look beyond the event to the patient's drinking history. Bogard (1970) reported that 3 per cent of 138 attempted suicides seen in a six-month period had a history of 'alcoholism'. More recently, Murphy and Wetzel (1982) report a history of 'alcoholism' in 10 per cent of a sample of 127 patients having attempted suicide.

An English study (Hawton *et al.* 1982) of self-poisoning and self-injury presents a substantial alcohol presence. In this review of suicide attempts in the Oxford area, 28 per cent of men and 18 per cent of women had been drinking at the time of the event, 49 per cent of men and 29 per cent of women had been drinking within six hours of the traumatic event, and 7 per cent were diagnosed as suffering from 'alcoholism'.

Alcoholism and Trauma

Problem drinkers and labelled alcoholics have a considerably greater risk of traumatic injury and violent death than members of the general population (Aarens *et al.* 1977, Choi 1975, Combs-Orme *et al.* 1983). A full review of the use of emergency rooms by alcoholics is beyond the scope of this paper. It has been noted that the recent cut-backs in social services for the medically disadvantaged in the US have resulted in the over-use of emergency services, and thus not the least, by alcoholics. The proportion varied significantly by the time of day: 11 per cent of the daytime group were alcoholics, contrasted with 29 per cent of the night-time patients. Rund *et al.* (1981) found the overall prevalence of 'alcoholism' in a randomly selected population of daytime and night-time emergency room patients to be 20 per cent. Several hospital studies have shown an above average use of emergency services by alcoholics (Lewis and Gordon 1983, Magnusson 1979). In the Magnusson study male alcoholics had an average of 3.9 visits in the study period compared to 0.5 for males in the control population. Female alcoholics had an average of 2.1 visits compared to 0.7.

The proportion of patients labelled as 'alcoholics' who visit for acute care and trauma needs further consideration. Some studies suggest that the need is for a bed and a meal while others (Rund *et al.* 1981) suggest that a significant proportion visit because of injury. Whitney (1983) identifies two discrete populations: namely, those with multiple emergency room visits and prior alcoholism treatment, and those with few or no prior visits. While the former is considered to comprise only 20 per cent of the total population, this group was more readily identified and the latter poorly identified as alcohol dependent. Many alcoholic patients who present to emergency rooms with traumatic injury leave undiagnosed as drug or alcohol abusers, due to oversight or lack of time on the part of medical personnel. It is suggested that large emergency rooms are in need of methods of screening for alcoholism, via laboratory tests and drinking histories, as well as links to appropriate treatment facilities.

Discussion

In contrast to earlier work on casualties reviewed elsewhere (Aarens *et al.* 1977, Roizen 1982), the work reviewed here is, by a good measure, considerably better science. Most of these studies occur by design rather than happenstance; the alcohol variable is relatively accurately measured; most are either a consecutive series of all cases over many months or are a sample of cases from different time periods and on different days, thus controlling for known temporal variation in drinking patterns; some use control groups or quasi-control groups (e.g. non-injured emergency room patients). Numbers of cases are large; many make use of appropriate statistical tests; there is no evidence of problem enhancement in relation to alcohol nor is there evidence of problem minimisation. Many of these studies are concerned, at least in part, with the medical management of the drinking patient – and to this they make a valuable contribution. However, the reader is left less than satisfied with the contribution this body of work makes to understanding alcohol's role in *causing* serious events. In particular, the proximate determinants of accidents are rarely investigated. The work of the French Haut Comité, the best of the studies to date, offers excellent coverage of a large geographical area, excellent measurement of the alcohol variable and a useful analysis of the social background of patients. Severity of injury and temporal variations are analysed. However, except for alcohol presence by external cause of events, the analysis is carried out in aggregation on all injuries, in all types of events. Thus, for example, we cannot discover the ages of drinking victims of falls in relation to those who were not drinking. While the general analysis offered in this report is useful in giving a global estimate of drinking prior to traumatic injury and is useful in estimating the demands drinking patients make on emergency rooms, we cannot learn much about the events as they happened; and, therefore, we cannot learn much about proximate determinants of trauma.

An example comes from the various analyses of temporal variations in accidents. The temporal variations in motor vehicle accidents and the disproportionate numbers of drinking-involved accidents in different time periods is well known. However, studies which do not disaggregate the analyses by types of accidents weight the analyses by the characteristics of motor vehicle accidents since these are always a large proportion of traumatic events. Arriving at a satisfying explanation of the causes of traumatic events is in part particular, in part epistemological and in part social. First, the necessary data must be available to analyse in the various ways necessary to fit into a causal explanation. But, as important, there must be some agreement as to what constitutes a causal explanation that implicates drinking. As Simpson *et al.* write:

> It is often bewildering, if not unbelievable, for many individuals to learn that there is no direct causal proof ... that alcohol-induced impairment causes road crashes. The *indictment* for such a causal relationship has been achieved inferentially, and has required years of painstaking research, bringing to bear a variety of strategies that collectively produced the necessary compelling evidence ... As a consequence, a critical and fundamental question in road safety remains unanswered to this day: 'How many collisions would be prevented if alcohol were not involved?' (Simpson *et al.* 1982: p. 46)

We must ask of the work on trauma if it is possible that it will succeed where the work on motor vehicle crashes has failed.

Let us begin with what we know. The variability in estimates of alcohol presence in accidents is significantly reduced by the studies of the last decade. Careful attention to obtaining blood and breath tests allows the conclusion with some certainty that a large proportion of events resulting in physical trauma are preceded by drinking. For most of these events, a significant proportion of those drinking are intoxicated or seriously impaired. There is considerable variation in the alcohol presence in events of different types. In all the countries with studies represented here, assaults and fights are, in most series, the traumatic events most likely to be preceded by drinking and by heavy drinking. We know, as well, that the proportions of those drinking and drunk who are involved in non-fatal accidents are—in general—considerably smaller than those who are involved in fatal accidents. There is by now considerable evidence that there is a positive relationship between severity of injury and drinking. Patients who have been drinking, especially those who have been drinking heavily, are more likely to be seriously injured than others. However, it is by no means the case that all or most severely injured patients have been drinking. Only one of a number of recent studies suggests that alcohol has a protective effect in serious injury.

Ward *et al.* (1982), in a series of trauma patients over a 14 month period (N = 1,198), did not find the expected relationship of severity of injury and drinking. These investigators point out that the total mortality in the group found to have been drinking was significantly less than in those with no detectable alcohol (10.9 versus 16.5 per cent). Although there was no significant difference between the severity of injury in the two groups, those surviving in the ethanol group tended to be more severely injured (injury severity score 19.9 versus 17.5). A protective effect of ethanol in releasing catecholamines which mediate the metabolic response to injury is suggested. However, further information on the co-variation of specific types and causes of injury, ethanol level and severity of injury, as well as data on the time between the alcohol test and injury, are required to support this argument.

Huth *et al.* (1983) tested this 'protective' effect hypothesis in a study of 182 patients admitted to hospital following traffic crashes. Acute alcohol intoxication had no apparent protective or detrimental effect on response to injury. The patients were divided into two groups for analysis—those intoxicated at the time of injury and those not intoxicated. An Injury Severity Score[3] was calculated for each patient. No relationship was found between severity of injury and BAC or mortality and BAC.

---

3.   Refer to notes following the text of this chapter.

Work on pedestrian accidents and falls which have used control groups show a substantially increased risk of accidents, especially at elevated blood alcohol levels. Only three studies reviewed here use this analytic technique; several argue that it is uneconomic or unreasonable as a method of analysing risk or cause.

Let me now turn to the practical, epistemological and social difficulties which stand in the way of knowing more than we know. The practical difficulties arise from the need to gather a substantial amount of information in a setting where it is expensive and often impractical to do so.

Measurement of the Alcohol Variable

As many as a third of the patients attending emergency rooms do not receive a blood- or breath-alcohol test due to severity of injury or oversight on the part of medical personnel, even during periods when a concerted effort to test is made. It is questionable whether the results of the most rigorous study would be acceptable to the severe critic if this proportion were not substantially reduced.

Further, although an event orientation is necessary for analysing the aetiology of trauma, an understanding of the victim's drinking history is equally important. Without knowing the drinking history, heavy drinking preceding trauma may simply be an indirect indicator of a life in which drink is an accompaniment to all the day's activities, in which case the question is not 'What is the role of alcohol?' but 'Why, given that this activity is routinely accompanied by drink, did an injury occur this time?'

Analysis of the Event and Injury

In only a few studies presented here are events (i.e. 'external causes') and the nature of the injuries analysed. It is noteworthy that where this does occur (Wechsler *et al.* 1969 and Stephens Cherpitel 1989 *see* Chapter 16), alcohol presence in injuries of different types was comparable in the two studies, as was alcohol presence in different events. No analyses present type of injury by type of event analysed by amount of drinking. Indeed, to do so would require a very large sample. However, it is questionable what analytic power we have without such an analysis. For example, a laceration in the kitchen is a different event in the presence of a heap of vegetables than an angry husband. Medical personnel and the eventual analyst of data gathered in an emergency room will need to make a judgement of 'external cause' in light of the situational variables which are known and the nature of the injuries. As McDade *et al.* (1982) note, 'Many falls were in fact assaults. Patients are often unwilling or unable to discuss the cause of their injuries in any depth....'

53

Severity of Injury

Most injuries are not severe and only a small minority are fatal. However, the cost of severe injuries to the individual and to society is considerable. A test for severity of injury is important in attempting to assess a dose-response relationship between drinking and subsequent injury. A number of studies suggest that the risk of severe injury is greater as BACs increase. However, more work is needed in obtaining a reliable judgement of injury severity.

Trauma History

A number of studies have shown a significant proportion of patients presenting to an emergency room to have had a previous history of traumatic injury. This proportion appears to be higher for those who test positive for alcohol. The seemingly acute alcohol-related injury may, in fact, be one in a long series of related events. There is considerable evidence in these studies to indicate that those who come to an emergency room as a result of trauma, suffer from multiple social problems. Brismar *et al.* (1983) noted that 40 per cent of those with head injuries had been treated for alcoholism. Further work is needed on the trauma history and social and demographic characteristics of victims of trauma.

Intention

Perceptions of the degree of chance or risk involved in a traumatic event will affect both society's perception of the event and the analyst's method of investigating causal relationships. Room (1978) has argued this point well:

> Controlled studies have been done for accidents rather than crime or suicide. This partly reflects the different training of workers in the different fields: the controlled study is an epidemiological rather than criminological stock-in-trade ... the concept of a controlled study seems to break down for ... studies of events such as suicide and crime where intention enters in. It does not seem to make much sense to measure the alcohol of a customer in the store at the same time and place that a hold up occurred on a previous day, or of a pedestrian on a bridge where a suicide occurred. Where intention is explicitly a part of our definition of the situation, we assume that alcohol affects intentions, and the choice of the context for the event is in turn affected by intentions. Of course, these assumptions are not necessarily true: many crimes are crimes of opportunity. But the seeming incongruity of a case-control study of

alcohol in the criminal event should sensitize us to potential problems in the use of such studies for accidents, since in these situations too intentions and a voluntary choice of the context of behaviour are potentially involved. (Room 1978: p. 14)

In order to fit an analytic framework to a series of events, especially if that analytic framework involves using controls, the degree of intention or perceived risk on the part of the victim needs to be assessed. Accidents like suicide attempts may be the result of a need for more personal or societal attention and taking known risks may facilitate injuries which will cause the victim to receive this attention.

Two questions need to be asked in relation to the form of causal explanation of alcohol's roles in trauma: is the case-control method adequate for use in traumatic events (e.g. pedestrian accidents) and what form of explanation is adequate for use in events in which a control group is inadequate or impossible? In relation to the first question a number of additional questions can be raised. Honkanen and some others take the view that although the case-control method does not show a causal relationship but only a statistical association, 'the strength of the association, the existence of a dose-response relationship and consonance with existing knowledge ... indicate that causality can be considered certain'. If we are to take this view, then the evidence on pedestrian falls and other pedestrian accidents, without doubt, shows that alcohol is the 'cause of' some proportion of these traumatic events.

With the development of techniques for multivariate analysis of case-control studies, potentially confounding variables can be analysed and controlled (Schesselman 1982, Holford *et al.* 1978). However, as these analyses become more complicated and the number of variables increases, the underlying logic of the case-control method is called into question. Ideally the case and control groups should be drawn from the same population and characteristics of individuals should be similar. However, as the Honkanen work demonstrates – except for the variables on which cases and controls were matched – it appears that the two groups represent different populations, who just happened to have been walking down the same street at approximately the same time. The assumption that those walking in the same place at the same time are one population except, perhaps, for drinking, ignores purposive action in the actors – intentionality. The assumption is made that the reasons for walking from one place to another are roughly similar in the two groups. If we were to find that most of the controls were walking to and from work and most of the cases were walking to and from their favourite pubs, the logic of the case-control method would break down. The fact that nearly eight times as many cases as controls were drunk (46 versus 6) might suggest that their purposes were different, that drinking might well be linked closely with the purposes of the walk and that a good many of the drunken walkers may have been aware of their increased risk. It can then be argued that the greater relative risk of falls among cases may be caused by the type of lives they lead rather than the alcohol on the occasion.

Schlesselman (1982) in his authoritative book on case-control research acknowledges that 'control of extraneous variables may be incomplete; selection of an appropriate comparison group may be difficult; detailed study of mechanism is rarely possible'. Indeed these are linked. Without knowledge of the 'mechanism' or 'mechanisms' involved, it is impossible to know which variables to control for.

Let us take the second case: traumatic events for which it is difficult to imagine a control group—e.g. assaults. Here the question becomes, when is an explanation sufficient to show that alcohol was causally implicated in the event? It is worth asking whether it would be more satisfying, for explanatory purposes, to have case histories of the events rather than abstracted information about the event. Formal, statistical, explanation would be replaced by a more historical form of explanation. The advantage of case histories is that they allow the investigator to stay very close to the event, and also allow the multiple factors that cause events to emerge. An illustration follows from a study of self-inflicted gunshot wounds among Alaskan natives (Kost-Grant 1983).

Case D

A 16-year old Eskimo male shot himself in the abdomen with a low-caliber pistol. He had been drinking at the time and used this fact to explain the shooting; 'It was an accident ... I was drinking.' The motive given was remorse following a fight with a girl he described as disliked by the majority of villagers; 'I just couldn't get the bad feeling inside of me away ... I wanted to get that feeling out.' Twelve months earlier a brother of the patient shot himself in the abdomen and died. The patient was close to this brother. The patient had recently expressed to friends that he felt alone and lonely. He had told someone at school that he had a pocketful of bullets and would be dead by the next day. (p. 74)

One cannot review case histories such as this without the realisation both that alcohol plays only a small part in such events and that the actions themselves by no means follow a 'normal' or 'usual' chain of events.

In conclusion, it must be noted that although more recent studies of alcohol's involvement in traumatic events are very much better than earlier research, many studies are rendered relatively useless by some simple methodological flaw. There is a need for agencies concerned with work on alcohol and trauma to offer assistance and create guidelines for researchers who are often trained as medical doctors. The interest within the medical community is obvious in the large number of studies carried out in hospitals throughout the world. Unfortunately, these researchers and their work are often not known to one another. The work often lacks the full methodological rigour that it could have had and the area as a whole is not cumulative in the sense that later studies build on earlier ones.

The guidelines that follow emerge from what are the most common problems found in current research. In short, empirical studies of traumatic events carried out in the future will need:

1. More than one measure of the alcohol variable; preferably a measure of blood or breath alcohol and drinking history. It must be recognised that measuring blood and breath alcohol on only a small proportion of the sample is useless, given the differences between rates of alcohol presence in evenings compared to days, weekends compared to weekdays and differences in rates related to many other factors.

2. To be either a consecutive series of all cases over a period of time long enough to control for temporal variation in incidence and alcohol presence, or a sample which controls for temporal variation.

3. To exclude children from either the sample or the analysis. Lack of attention to this makes many published studies unusable.

4. Numbers large enough to control for age, sex, and injury.

5. A greater number of demographic variables.

6. More extensive analyses, especially intercorrelation of alcohol variables; more attention to relationships between the alcohol and demographic variables; more extensive analysis of types of injury within types of event.

7. More attention to situational variables.

Moreover, if alcohol reporting systems are to yield much more than alcohol presence in traumatic events, they will need to be linked to a form of explanation that is agreed to be adequate. The question of the nature of these explanations is a first order priority.

© 1989 Judy Roizen

Notes

BAC: Blood-alcohol concentration 'measures in percentages the weight of the alcohol in a fixed volume of blood. In certain countries, including the US, BAC for 7 parts of alcohol per 10,000 parts of blood, for example, is expressed as .07 per cent. In Canada and some other nations the equivalent would be 70 milligrams per 100 millilitres of blood, expressed as 70 mg per cent. In Sweden, it would be recorded as 0.7 promille. Each system records the same percentage of alcohol.' (O'Brian and Chafetz 1982, p. 49)

GCS: The Glasgow Coma Scale is 'a 13-point scale ranging from 3 through 15 and is divided into three categories of neurological responsiveness: eye opening, verbal responses, and motor responses. The scale has become a standardized method of grading the severity of brain injury, and good reproducibility among observers has been demonstrated. A score of 8 or less on the examination constitutes coma and is defined as severe head injury.' (Rimel *et al.* 1982, p. 344)

ISS: 'In 1974 a system was introduced by Baker *et al.* in the US quantifying severity of injury (abbreviated injuries scale 76). In that system seven body regions are defined and injuries in each scored according to the code. These range from a score of 1, for the most minor, to 6, defined as injuries currently unsurvivable in the light of present knowledge. From that information is derived the injury severity score, which is the sum of the square of the highest totals obtained in three separate regions. The scoring system was amended in 1980 and it is necessarily a prognostic index. Since 1966 the abbreviated injuries scale 76 and latterly the abbreviated injuries scale 80 have been widely used and internationally accepted as a means of assessing the severity of injury and, although primarily designed for use in injuries sustained in road traffic accidents, have been used effectively in circumstances. The use of injury severity scoring combined with clinical assessment probably provides the most accurate method at the moment of clarifying severity of injuries.' (Christian 1984, p. 1525)

RTA: Road Traffic Accident

Acknowledgements

I am grateful to Andee Mitchell and her staff at the Alcohol Research Group for helping to assemble the material reviewed. The preparation of this paper was supported, in part, by the US National Institute of Alcohol Abuse and Alcoholism.

References

Aarens, M., T. Cameron, R. Roizen, R. Room, D. Schneberk and D. Wingard (eds) (1977) *Alcohol, casualties and crime*. Alcohol, Casualties and Crime Project Final Report, Report No. C-18, Social Research Group, University of California, Berkeley

Appleton, W. (1980) The battered woman syndrome. *Annals of Emergency Medicine, 9*, 84-90

Armyr G., A. Elmer and U. Herz (1982) *Alcohol in the world of the 80's.* Sober Forlags Ab, Stockholm

Baker, S.P., J.S. Samkoff, R.S. Fisher and Carol (1982) Fatal occupational injuries. *Journal of the American Medical Association, 248,* 6, 692-7

Baker, S.P., B. O'Neill and R.S. Karpf (1984) *The injury fact book.* Lexington Books, D.C. Health and Company, Lexington, Massachusetts; Toronto

Barancik, J., B. Chatterjee, Y.C. Greene, E. Michenzi and D. Fife (1983) Northeastern Ohio Trauma Study: 1. Magnitude of the problem. *American Journal of Public Health, 73,* 7, 746-51

Bergman, A.S. (1976) Emergency room: a role for social workers. *Health and Social Work, 1,* 33-45

Blomberg, R.D. and J.C. Fell (1979) A comparison of alcohol involvement in pedestrians and pedestrian casualties. American Association for Automotive Medicine, *Proceedings,* October 3-6, Louisville, Kentucky, pp. 1-17

Bogard, H.M. (1970) Follow-up study of suicidal patients seen in emergency room consultation. *American Journal of Psychiatry, 126,* 7, 141-44

Brickley, W.J. (1915) The relation of alcohol to accidents. *Boston Medical and Surgical Journal, 172,* 2, 744-7

Brismar, B., A. Engstrom and U. Rydberg (1983) Head injury and intoxication. *Acta Chirurgica Scandinavica, 149,* 11-4

Brismar B., and K. Tuner (1982) Battered women: A surgical problem. *Acta Chirurgica Scandinavica, 148,* 103-5

Carlson, W.L. (1973) Age, exposure and alcohol involvement in night crashes. *Journal of Safety Research, 5,* 4, 247-59

Champion, H.R., S.P. Baker, C. Benner, *et al.* (1975) Alcohol intoxication and serum osmolality. *Lancet, 1,* 1402

Choi, S.Y. (1975) Death in young alcoholics. *Journal of Studies on Alcohol, 36,* 1224-9

Christian, M.S. (1984) Morbidity and mortality of car occupants: Comparative survey over 24 months. *Journal of the American Medical Association, 252,* 6, 796-7

Clement, J., and K.S. Klingbeil (1981) The emergency room. *Health and Social Work, 6,* 4, 83-90

Combs-Orme, T., J.R. Taylor, E.B. Scott and S.J. Holmes (1983) Violent deaths among alcoholics. *Journal of Studies on Alcohol, 44,* 6, 938-49

Edna, T.-H. (1982) Alcohol influence and head injury. *Acta Chirurgica Scandinavica, 148,* 209-12

Farris, R., T.B. Malone and H. Liliefors (1975) 'A comparison of alcohol involvement in exposed and injured drivers', Report by the Essex Corporation, Alexandria, Virginia, prepared for National Highway Traffic Safety Administration, U.S. Department of Transportation under contract L DOT HS-4-00954

Fife, D., J. Barancik and B. Chatterjee (1984a) Northeastern Ohio Trauma Study: 11. Injury rates by age, sex and cause. *American Journal of Public Health, 74,* 5, 473-8

Fife, D., M. Ginsburg and W. Boynton (1984b) The role of motor vehicle crashes in causing certain injuries. *American Journal of Public Health, 74,* 2, 1263-4

Fullerton, D.T., R.F. Harvey, M.H. Klein and T. Howell (1981) Psychiatric disorders in patients with spinal cord injuries. *Archives of General Psychiatry, 38,* 12, 1369-71

Gibson, G., O. Anderson and G. Bugbee (1970) *Emergency medical service in the Chicago area.* Chicago Center for Health Studies, University of Chicago, Chicago

Giesbrecht, N., and H. Fisher (eds) (1987) *Alcohol-related casualties.* Addiction Research Foundation, Toronto

Haut Comité d'Etude et d'Information sur l'Alcoolisme (1985) *Alcool et accidents: Etude de 4,796 cas d'accidents admis dans 21 Hospitaux Français, entre Octobre 1982 et Mars 1983,* La Documentation Française, Paris

Hawton, K., J. Fagg, P. Marsack and P. Wells (1982) Deliberate self-poisoning and self-injury in the Oxford area: 1972-1980. *Social Psychiatry, 17,* 175-9

Hedeboe, J., A.V. Charles, J. Nielsen, F. Grymer, B.N. Moller, B. Moller-Madson, and S.E.T. Jensen (1985) Interpersonal violence: Patterns in a Danish community. *American Journal of Public Health, 75,* 6, 651-3

Heimdahl, A., and A. Nordendram (1977) The first 100 patients with jaw fractures at the Department of Oral Surgery Dental School, Hunninge. *Swedish Dental Journal, 1*, 177-82

Hingson, R.W., R. Lederman and D.C. Walsh (1985) Employee drinking patterns and accidental injury: A study of four New England states. *Journal of Studies on Alcohol, 46*, 4, 298-303

Hockerstedt, K., I. Airo, E. Karahaju and A. Sundin (1982) Abdominal trauma and laparotomy in 158 patients. *Acta Chirurgica Scandinavica, 148*, 1, 9-14

Holford, T.R., C. White and J.L. Kelsey (1978) Multivariate analysis for matched case-control studies. *American Journal of Epidemiology, 107*, 3, 245-56

Holt, S., I.C. Stewart, J.M.J. Dixon, R.A. Elton, T.V. Taylor, and K. Little (1980) Alcohol and the emergency service patient. *British Medical Journal*, 281, 638-640

Honkanen, R. (1976) Alcohol involvement in accidents: The role of alcohol in injuries treated at emergency stations. PhD dissertation, Department of Public Health Science, University of Helsinki

Honkanen, R., L. Ertama, P. Kuosmanen, M. Linnoila, A. Alha and T. Visuri (1983) The role of alcohol in accidental falls. *Journal of Studies on Alcohol, 44*, 2, 231-45

Hunter, W.W., and J.C. Stutts (1979) *Mopeds — An analysis of 1976-1978 North Carolina accidents.* University of Carolina Highway Safety Research Center, Chapel Hill, North Carolina

Huth, J.F., R.V. Maier, D.A. Simonowetz and C.M. Herman (1983) Effect of acute ethanolism on the hospital cause and outcome of injured automobile drivers. *Journal of Trauma, 23*, 494-8

The Insurance Institute for Highway Safety (1981) *The year's work 1981-1982.* Watergate Six Hundred, Washington, DC

Irwin, S.T., C.C. Patterson and W.H. Rutherford (1983) Association between alcohol consumption and adult pedestrians who sustain injuries in road traffic accidents. *British Medical Journal, 286*, 522

Jacobs, D. (1982/3) Evaluation and care of suicidal behaviour in emergency settings. *International Journal of Psychiatry in Medicine, 12*, 4, 295-311

James, J.J., D. Dargon and R.G. Day (1984) Serum vs breath alcohol levels and accidental injury: Analysis among US Army personnel in an emergency room setting. *Military Medicine, 149*, 369-74

Jetter, W.W. (1938) Studies in alcohol: I. The diagnosis of acute alcoholic intoxication by a correlation of clinical and chemical findings. *American Journal of Medical Sciences, 196*, 475-487

Kalsbeek, W.D., R.L. McLauren, B.S.H. Harris and J.D. Miller (1980) The national head and spinal cord injury survey: Major findings. *Journal of Neurosurgery, 53*, 19-31

Kapur, B.M. (1989) Alcohol: Pharmacology, methods of analysis and its presence in the casualty room. In N. Giesbrecht, R. González, M. Grant, E. Österberg, R. Room, I. Rootman and L. Towle (eds), *Drinking and casualties: Accidents, poisonings and violence in an international perspective*. Routledge, London, pp. 172-87

Karlson, T. (1982) The incidence of hospital-treated facial injuries from vehicles. *The Journal of Trauma, 22, 4, 734-7*

Kirkpatrick, J.R., and L.J. Taubenhaus (1967) Blood alcohol levels of home accident patients. *Quarterly Journal of Studies on Alcohol, 78*, 4, 734-7

Kost-Grant, B.L. (1983) Self-inflicted gunshot wounds among Alaska natives. *Public Health Reports, 98*,1, 72-78

Kraus, J.F., C.E. Franti, R.S. Riggins, D. Richards and N.O. Borhani (1975) Incidence of traumatic spinal cord lesions. *Journal of Chronic Diseases, 28*, 471-92

Levine, H.G. (1983) *The good creature of God and the demon rum: Colonial American and 19th century ideas about alcohol, crime and accidents*. U.S. Department of Health and Human Services, NIAAA Research Monograph, No. 12, Rockville, Maryland

Levine, M.S., and E.P. Radford (1977) Fire victims: Medical outcomes and demographic characteristics. *American Journal of Public Health, 67*, 11, 1077-80

Lewis, D.C., and A.J. Gordon (1983) Alcoholism and the general hospital: The Roger Williams Intervention Program. *Bulletin of the New York Academy of Medicine, 59*, 2, 181-97

Lowenfels, A.B., and T.T. Miller (1984) Alcohol and trauma. *Annals of Emergency Medicine, 13*, 11, 1056-60

Luna, G.K., R.V. Maier, L. Sowder, M.K. Copass and M.R. Oneskovich (1984) The influence of ethanol intoxication on outcome of injured motorcyclists. *Journal of Trauma, 24*, 8, 695-700

MacArthur, J.D., and F.D. Moore (1975) Epidemiology of burns: The burn-prone patient. *Journal of the American Medical Association, 231*, 3, 259-63

Magnusson, D. (1979) The use and abuse of accident and emergency service patient. *British Medical Journal, 281*, 638-40

Maris, R.W., and B. Lazwerwitz (1981) Physical context of suicide: Alcohol, drug use, and physical illness. In A. Richter (ed) *Pathways to suicide: A survey of self-destructive behaviours*, John Hopkins University Press, Baltimore, Maryland, pp. 170-204

McDade, A.M., R.D. McNicol, R.Ward-Booth, J. Chesworth and K.F. Moos (1982) The aetiology of maxillo-facial injuries, with special reference to the abuse of alcohol. *International Journal of Oral Surgery, 2*, 152-5

McHugh, T.P., and E.C. Stinson (1984) Moped injuries. *Annals of Emergency Medicine, 13*, 1, 63-7

Metropolitan Life Insurance Company (1979) Mortality from accidents. *Statistical Report, July-September, 60*, 3, 668-71

Morawski, J., and J. Moskalewicz (1989) Casualties in Poland: focus on alcohol. In N. Giesbrecht, R. González, M. Grant, E. Österberg, R. Room, I. Rootman and L. Towle (eds), *Drinking and casualties: Accidents, poisonings and violence in an international perspective.* Routledge, London, pp. 245-59

Murphy, G., and R.D. Wetzel (1982) Family history of suicidal behavior among suicide attempters. *Journal of Nervous and Mental Disease, 170*, 2, 86-90

Murray, W.R. (1976) Head injuries and alcohol. In G. Edwards and M. Grant (eds), *Alcoholics: New knowledge and new responses.* University Park Press, Baltimore, pp. 228-33

National Center for Statistics and Analysis (1983) Alcohol in fatal accidents: National estimates — USA. US Department of Transportation DOT HS-806 371, Washington, DC

National Safety Council (1984) *Accidents Facts.*

Nighswander, T.S. (1982) The demography and health consequences of violence in an emergency room setting. *Alaska Medicine, January/February*, 7-10

O'Brian, R., and M. Chafetz (1982) *The Encyclopedia of Alcoholism.* Facts on File Publications, New York, pp. 49-51

Ontario Interministerial Committee on Drinking Driving (1980) *The 1979 Ontario Roadside BAC Survey: Summary Report.* Government of Ontario, Toronto

Papoz, L., J.M. Wainet, G. Pequignot, E. Eschwege, J.R. Claude, D. Schwartz (1981) Alcohol consumption in a healthy population. *Journal of the American Medical Association, 245*, 17, 1748-51

Papoz, L., J. Weill, C. Got, J. L'Hoste, C. Yvon and Y. Goehrs (1986) Biological markers of alcohol intake among 4,796 subjects injured in accidents. *British Medical Journal, 292*, May 10, 1986, 1234-7. Reprinted in N. Giesbrecht, R. González, M. Grant, E. Österberg, R. Room, I. Rootman and L. Towle (eds)(1989), *Drinking and casualties: Accidents, poisonings and violence in an international perspective.* Routledge, London, pp. 277-88

Perrine, M.W. (1975) Alcohol involvement in highway crashes: A review of the epidemiologic evidence. *Clinics in Plastic Surgery, 2*, 1, 11-34

Phelps, E.B. (1911) *The mortality of alcohol.* Thrift Publishing Co., New York. Reprint from *The American Underwriter Magazine and Insurance Review, 36*

Pittmann, D.J., and W. Handy (1964) Patterns in criminal aggravated assault. *Journal of Criminal Law, Criminology, and Police Science, 55*, 4, 462-70

Poikolainen, K. (1989) Research into and registration of alcohol-related non-fatal casualties in Finland: The need for improved classification. In N. Giesbrecht, R. González, M. Grant, E. Österberg, R. Room, I. Rootman and L. Towle (eds), *Drinking and casualties: Accidents, poisonings and violence in an international perspective.* Routledge, London, pp. 188-94

Rimel, R.W., B. Giordan, J.T. Barth and J.A. Jane (1982) Moderate head injury: Completing the clinical spectrum of brain trauma. *Neurosurgery, 11*, 3, 344-55

Rodes, J., A. Pares, J. Caballeria, M. Rodcmilans, A. Urbano and L. Back (1987) Alcohol consumption, casualties and traffic accidents in Spain (abstract). In N. Giesbrecht and H. Fisher (eds), *Alcohol-related casualties.* Addiction Research Foundation, Toronto, pp. 73-4.

Roizen, J. (1982) Estimating alcohol involvement in serious events. In *Alcohol and health monograph.* Lexington Books, Lexington, MA, pp. 129-219

Room, R. (1978) 'Alcohol in casualties and crime: The current state of research and future directions', prepared for the 24th International Institute on the Prevention and Treatment of Alcoholism, Zurich

Rund, D.A., W.K. Summers and M. Levin (1981) Alcohol use and psychiatric illness in emergency patients. *Journal of the American Medical Association, 245*,12, 1240-1

Rutherford, W.H. (1977) Diagnosis of alcohol ingestion in mild head injuries. *Lancet, 1*, 8020, 1021-3

Rydberg, U., K. Bjerver and L. Goldberg (1975) The alcohol factor in a surgical emergency unit. *Acta Medicine Legalis et Socialis (Liege), 22*, 71-82

Satin, D.G. and F.J. Duhl (1972) Help?: The hospital emergency unit as community physician. *Medical Care, 10*, 257

Saunders, J.B. (1987) Alcohol intake and related morbidity among patients attending the Casualty Department at Royal Prince Alfred Hospital, Sydney (abstract). In N. Giesbrecht and H. Fisher (eds), *Alcohol-related casualties.* Addiction Research Foundation, Toronto, pp. 79-80.

Schesselmann, J. (1982) *Case control studies: Design, conduct, analysis.* Oxford University Press, Oxford

Senay, E.C., and R. Wettstein (1983) Drugs and homicide: A theory. *Drug and Alcohol Dependence, 12*, 152-66

Simonsen, J. (1984) Fatal subarachnoid haemorrhages in relation to minor injuries in Denmark from 1967 to 1981. *Forensic Science International, 24*, 57-63

Simpson, H.M., D.R. Mayhew and R.A. Warren (1982) Epidemiology of road accidents involving young adults: Alcohol, drugs and other factors. *Drug and Alcohol Dependence, 10*, 35-63

Soderstrom, C.A., R.W. Du Priest, C. Benner, K. Maekawa and R.A. Cowley (1979) Alcohol and roadway trauma: Problems of diagnosis and management. *The American Surgeon, 45*, 129-36

Stark, E., A. Flitcraft, D. Zuckerman, A. Grey, J. Robinson and W. Frazier (1981) Wife abuse in the medical setting. *National Clearing House on Domestic Violence, 7*

Stephens Cherpitel, C.J. (1989) A study of alcohol use and injuries among emergency room patients. In N. Giesbrecht, R. González, M. Grant, E. Österberg, R. Room, I. Rootman and L. Towle (eds), *Drinking and casualties: Accidents, poisonings and violence in an international perspective.* Routledge, London, pp. 289-301

Torrens, P.R., and D. Vedvab (1970) Variations among emergency room populations: A comparison of four hospitals in New York City. *Medical Care, 8*, 60-75

Trunkey, D.D. (1983) Trauma. *Scientific American, 249*, 2, 28-35

Vicario, S.J., R. Coleman, M.A. Cooper and R.M. Thomas (1983) Ventilatory status early after head injury. *Annals of Energy Medicine, 12*, 3, 145-148

Vitek, V., and D.J. Lans (1982) Aggravating effect of alcohol on admission serum insulin patterns of patients with trauma and in a state of shock. *Surgery, Gynaecology and Obstetrics, 154*, 326-32

Vogtsberger, K. (1984) Psychosocial factors in burn injury. *Texas Medicine, 80*, 43-6

Waller, J.A. (1973) Falls among the elderly – Human end environmental factors. Department of Epidemiology and Environmental Health, University of Vermont

Walsh, M.E. and D.A.D. Macleod (1983) Breath alcohol analysis in the accident and emergency department. *Injury: The British Journal of Accident Surgery, 15*, 1, 62-6

Ward, R.E., T.C. Flynn, P.W. Miller and W.F. Blaisdell (1982) Effects of ethanol ingestion on the severity and outcome of trauma. *American Journal of Surgery, 144*, 1, 153-7

Warren, R.A., M.A. Buhlman, L.A. Bourgeois and L.S. Chattaway (1982) *The New Brunswick Study: A survey of the blood alcohol levels of motor vehicle trauma patients.* Traffic Injury Research Foundation, Ottawa

Wechsler, H., E.H. Kasey, D.T. Demone and H.W. Demone (1969) Alcohol level and home accidents. *Public Health Reports, 84*, 12, 1043-50

Whitney, R.B. (1983) Alcoholics in emergency rooms. *Bulletin of the New York Academy of Medicine, 59*, 2, 216-21

Wilson, R., H. Malin and C. Lawman (1983) Facts for planning 9: Uses of mortality rates and mortality indexes in planning alcohol programs. *Alcohol Health and Research World, 8,* 1, 41-53

2

Alcohol-Related Casualties in Latin America: A Review of the Literature

Maria Elena Medina-Mora and Laura González

Casualties related to alcohol abuse represent a major public health problem. Casualties resulting from intoxication or from the intake of high quantities of alcohol in circumstances involving risk contribute to accidents and violence and this pattern is common to many Latin American countries. The purpose of this paper is to review the existing literature in Latin American and to make an indepth analysis of the registration system and extent of the problem in Mexico.

The relevant published literature in Latin America is scarce and in many cases difficult to obtain. Apart from reviewing publication indexes, personal correspondence was established with people who work in the alcohol field. Another major source was Caetano's (1984) review on epidemiology of alcohol-related problems in Latin America. The articles reviewed in this paper are not representative of the problems in each country. Concern with casualties and registration of alcohol-related casualties varies from country to country. Furthermore, the specific justice system determines which casualties are the point of focus, which cases are represented and how reliably the role of alcohol is assessed. These factors, in turn, are related to the existence or absence of a registration system and, if there is such a system, the type of events that are reported and the proportion registered of the total that occur.

Culture also plays an important role in that the same behaviour will have different consequences depending on the culture. For instance, being intoxicated when one is expected to be sober can lead to violence, whereas in contexts where one is expected to drink, the outcome may be otherwise. As indicated in studies reviewed by the Alcohol Research Group (Berkeley) (Aarens *et al.* 1977), the role of culture in alcohol-related casualties is important; for example, cultural expectations may be as relevant as pharmacology in the link between drinking and violence.

The registration of a problem is also related to culture. Assaults on women associated with drinking are expected to be higher in contexts where this behaviour is not highly restricted, and thus drinking can facilitate this behaviour. At the same, time its registration may depend more on the interest of health authorities to deal with the problem than with its frequency of occurrence. Quite often the interest in studying a problem is higher when it is not expected to happen.

After reviewing the existing literature on alcohol-related casualties in the United States, Roizen (1982) has concluded that few studies outside those of traffic accidents are purposely designed to examine the role of alcohol in the event. Most studies only report the presence of alcohol in casualties and thus they do not lead to conclusions on the causal role of alcohol. The authors of this paper, and Aarens *et al.* (1977) in a previous review, divide the type of studies into three major groups:

1. Alcohol use at the time of the event.

2. Drinking history and drinking problems of persons involved in serious events.

3. The proportion of alcoholics who experience serious events.

In this paper, we will follow the scheme of analysis proposed by these authors and add a fourth category:

4. The estimation of the presence of alcohol in populations at risk (i.e. drivers).

The main data from the reviewed articles are summarised in Table 2.1. In order to compare the data, rates due to alcohol cirrhosis are shown in Table 2.2.

Argentina

Of the four studies available, two report the proportion of persons who were intoxicated or under the influence of alcohol at the time of a violent event (homicide in particular and crimes against persons in general). In the first case, a variation from 2 to 10 per cent was reported between 1960 and 1969 (Vidal 1967 cited in Caetano 1984). Negrete (1967) reports that in 28 per cent of the crimes against persons the individual admitted having been under the influence of alcohol (cited in Caetano 1984). Two other authors report estimations on the presence of alcohol from population at risk. Calderon (Caetano 1984) reports that in 1961, 67 per cent of the people arrested in shanty towns were alcoholics and Mardones re-

Table 2.1: *Casualties associated with alcohol in selected countries from Latin America*

Country/ Author	Year	Percentage	Type of casualty	Study
Argentina Vidal, 1967[1]	1960-1969	2 - 10	Homicides	Alcohol use on the time of the event.
Calderón[1] (Saavedra et al, 1970)	1961	67	Arrests in shanty towns were alcoholics	Estimations from populations at risk.
Mardones[1]	1980	20	Drivers examined with alcohol test	Estimations from populations at risk.
Negrete[1] 1976		28	Crime against persons	Alcohol use on the time of the event.
Chile Marconi[1] 1967	1965	25	Suicide	Alcohol use on the time of the event.
		52	Crimes against persons	Alcohol use on the time of the event.
Vargas[1] (Moser 1974)		70	Traffic accidents	Alcohol use on the time of the event.
Viel et al 1970[1]	1960-64	41 males 5 females (heavy drinkers)	Autopsies	History of drinking of persons involved in the event.
		46	Deaths due to traffic accidents	Alcohol use on the time of the event.
Mena et al. (1984)		8.8	Fetal alcohol syndrome in schools of special education	Estimation from population at risk.
Naveillan and Vargas (1984b)		52	Homicide	Proportion of heavy drinkers who experience serious events.
Naveillan and Vargas (1984b)		2.52 12.40	Accidents Males Females	Proportion of heavy drinkers who experience serious events.
		7.8 8.7	Suicide males Suicide females	
Honduras Zavala 1984	1980-1982	1.14	Percentage of hospitalizations due to accidents, poisoning and violence related to alcohol from all alcohol-related hospitalizations.	Alcohol use on the time of the event

Table 2.1: *Continued*

Country/ Author	Year	Percentage	Type of casualty	Study
Costa Rica Morales[1] Chassuol	1961	17/100 000	Road accidents	Alcohol use on the time of the event.
(Moser 1974)	1965	26/100 000		
Adis Castro and Flores[1] (1967)	1965	9166/13370	Arrests	Alcohol use on the time of the event.
Instituto[1] National sobre alcoholismo (Moser 1974)	1977	59	Arrests	Alcohol use on the time of the event.
Mexico Mas C. *et al* (1985) Information System G.D. of Statistics	1977-1983	Males 2-.85 Females 6.6-8.0 Total 5	All suicide	Alcohol use on the time of the event.
	1975-1981	Males 2.5 - 3.5 Females .44 - .61	All mortality	Alcohol use on the time of the event and mortality due to alcohol related diseases.
	1976-1983	Males 4.14 Females .61 Total 2.03	All suicide attempts	Alcohol use on the time of the event.
	1976-1982	.12 - .06	All divorces	Alcohol use on the time of the event.
Terroba (1985)	1979	27.5	Suicide in Mexico city	Case study in a representative sample. Alcohol use on the time of the event.
	1979	13.7	Suicide in Mexico City	History of drinking of persons involved in the event.
Heman (1984)	1980	37.1	Suicide attempt	Case study. History of drinking.
Rosovsky and Lopez (1986)	1982	4	Accidents in Federal roads	Alcohol use on the time of the event.
DDF intoxication reporting system	1985	37	Intoxication at emergency rooms	Alcohol use on the time of the event.
Silva (1972)		7	All traffic accidents	Alcohol use on the time of the event.

Table 2.1:   *Continued*

Country/ Author	Year	Percentage	Type of casualty	Study
Mexico (cont'd) Rosovsky and Lopez (1986)	1983	16	All traffic accidents in Mexico city	Alcohol use on the time of the event.
Justice information system	1983	85	Traffic accidents, in particular against the property of the nation in Mexico city	Alcohol use on the the time of the event.
Lopez and Rosovsky (1986)	1984	38.61	Arrests	Alcohol use on the time of the event.
Lopez and Rosovsky (1986)	1973	19	Crime	Alcohol use on the time of the event.
Justice infor- mation system	1981	24	Crime	Alcohol use on the time of the event.
Medina- Mora *et al.* (1985)	1984	23	Autopsies of all violent deaths in Mexico city	Alcohol use on the time of the event.
Manterola (1985)	1985	19.82	Child abuse	Alcohol use on the time of the event.
Prevention program on injured minors				
Guatemala Rivera-Lima[1] (1973)	1967-71	9	Traffic accidents	Alcohol use on the time of the event.
Venezuela Boada[1] (1976)	1961-63	66	Arrests	Alcohol use on the time of the event.
Alvarez (1983)	1980	26	Crime	Alcohol use on the time of the event.
	1977	18.4	Crime	Alcohol use on the time of the event.
	1977-78-79	56	Homicides	Alcohol use on the time of the event.
		22	Crime against property	Alcohol use on the time of the event.
		4.5	Crime against persons	Alcohol use on the time of the event.

[1] quoted from Caetano, 1984

Table 2.2: *Age-adjusted death rates per 100,000 population for cirrhosis of liver in selected countries of the Americas*

Country	Year	Male	Female	Total
		Rates		
Argentina	69-70	17.5	5.7	11.4
Chile	74-75	33.9	12.4	22.6
Colombia	74-75	4.7	2.4	3.5
Costa Rica	74-75	8.0	3.3	5.6
Ecuador	73-74	9.2	4.1	6.6
El Salvador	73-74	10.5	3.1	6.7
Guatemala	75	13.2	6.8	10.0
Honduras	74-75	7.9	4.2	6.0
Mexico	73-74	35.0	10.8	22.7
Nicaragua	73	7.1	3.4	5.1
Panama	73-74	4.1	2.5	3.3
Paraguay	74-75	7.5	2.6	4.9
Peru	71-72	9.1	4.9	6.9
Uruguay	75-76	8.0	2.0	4.9
Venezuela	74-75	10.9	4.3	7.5
Canada	74-75	10.3	4.4	7.3
United States	74-75	10.9	5.8	9.0

Source: PAHO (1978)

ports that in 1980, 20 per cent of a group of drivers examined had blood-alcohol levels considered dangerous (Caetano, 1984).

Chile

Naveillan and Perez (cited in Naveillan and Vargas 1984b) reported that in 52 per cent of the homicides the victim was an excessive drinker. No important differences were observed by sex. Naveillan and Vargas (1984a, 1984b) report causes of death of excessive drinkers by sex due to accidents (2.52 and 12.4 per cent for males and females, respectively and suicide (7.8 and 8.7 per cent, respectively). In the case of the female population, proportions were higher than the rates of death due to diabetes, oral and respiratory cancer, arteriosclerosis, ulcers and cardiovascular complications. In the case of the male population, the proportion of death by accidents was similar to the one reported by other causes.

As can be seen in Table 2.1, high rates of alcohol involvement are reported for several types of casualties in Chile: 25 per cent of suicides, 52 per cent of crimes against persons, 70 per cent of traffic accidents and 46 per cent of deaths through traffic accidents (Marconi 1967, Vargas cited in Moser 1974, Viel *et al.* 1970 cited in Caetano 1984).

Mena *et al.* (1984) studied the prevalence of fetal alcohol syndrome in three schools of special education in a province of Chile and found the syndrome present in 8.8 per cent of the sample studied (n = 380). Excessive alcohol intake also had been present in 70 per cent of the parents and one-fifth of had died of hepatic cirrhosis. The rate of excessive intake of this group was considerably higher than the one found in the general population (15 per cent).

Honduras

Zavala (1984) analyses the high burden that alcohol represents to the country; he reports an increase of 1.7 per cent over two years in the number of hospitalisations due to accidents, poisoning and violence related to alcohol (from 12,994 in 1980 to 13,864 in 1982). The rate of admissions due to these causes is considerably higher than the one related to other complications such as alcoholic psychosis (185 cases), alcoholism (1,428 cases) and hepatic cirrhosis (350 cases).

Costa Rica

Of the three reports available, one reports on road accidents associated with alcohol and two focus on arrests for drunkenness. The rate of alcohol involvement in accidents increased in the period between 1961 and 1965, but it is considerably lower than the rates reported from other countries. The rates of arrests due to drunkenness – 7 per cent in 1965 and 59 per cent in 1977 – are similar to ones reported in other countries (Adis Castro and Flokes, 1967, I.N. sobre Alcoholismo 1980 cited in Caetano 1984).

Guatemala

The rate of accidents (9 per cent) and arrests due to drunkenness (66 per cent) are comparable to other countries (River-Lima 1973 cited in Caetano 1984).

Venezuela

As in most countries in the region, alcohol involvement in events is only determined by police officers when the state of intoxication is extreme, when witnesses offer information or when empty bottles of alcohol are found in automobiles. The total rate of accidents shows a continuous increase in Venezuela. It has been reported that between 1961 and 1964 at least 50 per cent of accidents occurred under the influence of alcohol (Boad 1976 cited in Caetano 1984).

In 1980, 25.7 per cent of 'crime' was considered to occur under the influence of alcohol; whereas in 1977 only 18.4 per cent of events were reported to have occurred under the influence of this drug. These percentages were obtained from the total population convicted in the year. When this type of offence is considered, very interesting variations are observed. The offender was considered intoxicated in 56 per cent of the homicides in 1977, 1978 and 1979. For crimes against property, the proportion was 22 per cent and for crimes against persons, only 4.5 per cent of the offenders were said to be under the influence of alcohol.

Mexico

Several reporting systems are available in Mexico (see Table 2.3). Although some allow for recording the presence of alcohol in events, it is not always considered a priority. Thus the alcohol component is not always stated and when it is stated, it is not always analysed. The main systems are: Disease Reporting System (SSA); General Direction of Statistics, Social and Demographic Reporting System (SPP); and Intoxication Reporting System, Mexico City (DDF).

The first two systems report on a national scale while the third one is operational only in Mexico City. The disease and intoxication reporting systems are administered by the Ministry of Health and thus the information is restricted to the health area. The disease reporting system does not include information on alcohol. The social and demography reporting system obtains by-law information from all institutions.

Other health institutions such as the Mexican Institute of Social Security and the Health Institute for State Workers are included with the reporting systems, but the involvement of alcohol is not usually reported except when a related complication such as cirrhosis or alcoholic psychosis is the main diagnosis. The same is true for the Mental Health Surveillance System from the Ministry of Health.

The toxicology attention programme of the Department of the Federal District was created in 1985 in order to reduce mortality due to intoxication. It functions 24 hours a day every day of the year in four

Table 2.3: *Reporting systems in Mexico*

Reporting system	Sources of information	Coverage	General Information	Information on alcohol
Disease reporting system. SSA	All health institutions in the country	National	Contagious diseases and intoxications	Not included
Intoxication reporting system DDF	Cases attended at four public emergency hospitals within Mexico City	Local limited	Intoxication by causes	Proportion of intoxications due to alcohol
Mexican Institute of Social Security Reporting System IMSS	Cases attended at the Institute	National: 36% of the population	Health consultations	Not considered except when main diagnosis
Mental Health Epidemiological Surveyance SSA	Specializes inpatient and outpatient facilities	National	Consultations Alcohol psychosis	Main diagnosis
Information on general directions of social and demographic characteristics within the health system	All health institutions in the country	National	Mortality and morbidity Hepatic cirrhosis Alcoholism Acute hepatitis Alcohol dependence Suicide Attempted suicide	Cause of death due to alcohol abuse place in relation to other causes
Justice system	Courts	National	Accidents Crimes Divorces	Presence of alcohol at the time of the event Proportion events related

emergency hospitals in Mexico City. The programme is also linked with an emergency telephone service. The latter is open to the general public but is used mainly by people from a low socio-economic stratum, except in the event of an accident in the street. In these cases the ambulance service delivers cases either to these hospitals or to the Red Cross. Most cases in attendance in the first four months of the year in the toxicology programme were between 15 and 44 years of age and 56 per cent were males. The main presenting symptom was etilic intoxication (37 per cent) followed by intoxication with medicines (19.6 per cent) (Departamento del Distrito Federal 1985).

Suicide

There are two sources of information on suicides in Mexico: official statistics from the National Information System (General Direction of Statistics) and special studies of a sample drawn from the total cases that committed suicide in 1979.

In Mexico, the law requires that all persons who die through violence must be autopsied. Blood-alcohol level is determined by the coroner with the use of a chromatograph and then registered in the national information system. According to this source, 5 per cent of suicides in 1983 were under the influence of alcohol. In 1979, in the Federal District, the proportion was 2.2 per cent (Mas *et al.*, 1985).

Terroba (1985) conducted a review of all files in the coroner's office, which maintains a record of all cases occurring within the Federal District. A sample of cases was selected and a psychological autopsy was obtained through interviewing a qualified informant. Reliability was adequately tested for both informant and interviewer.

Among other information, Jackson's (1957) indicators of alcohol preoccupation were applied. In 27.5 per cent of the cases, the blood-alcohol test was positive (more than 10 mg/100 ml) but in only 14 per cent of the cases were the results positive according to Jackson's test. Thus, only one-half of the persons that committed suicide under the influence of alcohol had problems related to their drinking patterns; official statistics report a little less than one-fifth of the cases.

In the case of suicide attempts, the official system reports a considerably lower rate: 2.6 per cent in 1983 in rural areas and none in the Federal District. This information is not reliable because of the limited coverage. These rates are considerably different than the ones reported by Heman (1984) from a study conducted in 1981. Heman interviewed all cases involving a suicide attempt, intoxications and injuries seen in emergency rooms over four months. The interviews took place at the subjects' homes. The response rate was 51.2 per cent. No suicide attempt had occurred in another 23.2 per cent; in 37 per cent of the suicide attempts the subject reported having alcohol problems according to Jackson's indicators. Unfortunately, no information on alcohol use at the time of the event is available.

Traffic Accidents and Crime

Information on traffic accidents shows a similar picture. According to official statistics, alcohol was involved in 7 per cent of the accidents occurring in rural areas. In the Federal District the proportion is slightly more than two times higher (16 per cent). The proportion is considerably higher only when accidents that involve damage to public property are considered: for example, 85 per cent in Mexico City for 1983. To the authors' knowledge, only one comparable study has been conducted. Rosovsky and Lopez (1986) interviewed a sample of cases who had been arrested and detained at a police station, or who had attended an emergency room for different casualties. Doctors reported the presence of alcohol in 15 per cent of the cases in the police headquarters and in 7 per cent of the emergency room. In the interviews, another 24 and 10 per cent of the cases respectively, reported being under the influence of alcohol. In these cases, the medical doctor had not performed the examination either because the physician had been absent or had not considered it necessary. Of this study's traffic accidents, 40 per cent of drivers reported being under the influence of alcohol. This percentage is higher than the one reported by the official information system (Mas *et al.*, 1985). Neither source (emergency room or police) shows a complete picture as the reporting agencies only note cases where there has been damage to public property, injury or lack of agreement between the persons involved.

Police regulations state that when alcohol is involved the person should be taken to the corresponding authorities. The information is registered and reported but, unfortunately, only the most severe cases are detected and, even then, they are not always reported to the authorities.

Though the estimates of alcohol involvement have preoccupied both authorities and researchers working in the field, other casualties deserve more consideration. In Mexico City in 1984, 23 per cent of all autopsies performed (n = 5,543) involved a blood-alcohol level that was higher than 10 mg/100 ml. From the total cases involving alcohol (n = 1,259), only 24 per cent (307) died in accidents and 62 per cent (188) were pedestrians (see Table 2.4).

Crime related to alcohol has increased in the past years from 19 per cent in 1973 to 24 per cent in 1981. Alcohol involvement in this event is ascertained by the physician or person in charge and is registered and reported according to two criteria: alcohol on the breath and partial inebriation. No other tests are performed. On the other hand, in 28 per cent

Table 2.4: *Cause of death, alcohol use at time of the event. Autopsies performed in Mexico City. 1984*

Cause of Death	Males % (n = 1,202)	Females % (n = 57)	Total % (n = 1,259)
Traffic accidents (automobile)	9.32	12.28	9.45
Traffic accidents (pedestrian)	15.06	12.28	14.93
Homicide	28.78	14.03	28.11
Injuries	4.74	3.50	4.66
Suicide	7.32	- -	7.22
Burns	0.75	- -	0.87
Drowning	7.65	8.77	7.70
Alcohol congestion	1.58	3.50	0.71
13 TCE	4.40	- -	4.28
Hepatic cirrhosis	0.25	- -	0.23
Other medical complications	22.3	38.6	23.03
Not determined	16.0	- -	0.23
Total	95.0	5.0	100.0

In 23% of the total cases, alcohol was present.
In 3 cases the cause of death was not determined.

of the autopsies with positive BAC in Mexico City in 1984, the cause of death was homicide, where it occupied first place as a single cause, and another 5 per cent of deaths were caused by injuries (see Table 2.4).

Family Burden

Two indicators are available in relation to family burden: divorce and child abuse. Information on the first indicator is not reliable as official statistics include only those cases where alcoholism is the reason for divorce. While alcoholism is among the most common grounds for divorce, the first, common agreement, represents more than two-thirds of all divorces and alcohol involvement is not stated. As a motive for divorce, alcoholism has decreased in the last eight years, from 0.12 per cent in 1976 to 0.06 per cent in 1982 (Mas *et al.* 1985). However, in 19 per cent of the cases of child abuse reported in a case study, one of the parents had been intoxicated. This motive occupied second place after socio-culture and economic causes (Manterola 1985).

Accidents

Though other accidents related with alcohol consumption have been considered important indicators of alcohol abuse, very little information is available: 13 per cent of the persons with positive BAC autopsied in 1984 died due to accidents such as cranial encephalic traumatisms (TCE), drowning (7.7 per cent) and burns (0.87 per cent).

Medical complications were responsible for 23 per cent of the cases. Hepatic cirrhosis occupied the last place in frequency as a single cause (0.2 per cent).

Discussion and Conclusions

It may be said that, in general, the Mexican information system is acceptable in relation to the type of data gathered and institutions included in the system. Unfortunately, in only a few events is the presence of alcohol registered. Other limitations are related to the loss of information in a

Table 2.5:   *Casualty reported by country and type of study*

	Argen-tina	Chile	Hon-duras	Costa Rica	Guate-mala	Vene-zuela	Mexico	Total
Casualty Reported								
Traffic accidents	1	2		1	1	1	4	10
Other or undetermined accidents		1						1
Crime	2	2				5	2	11
Arrests	1			2	1		1	5
Suicide		2					6	8
Family violence		1					1	2
Autopsies or hospitalizations		1	1				1	3
Divorces							1	1
Type of Study								
Alcohol use on the time of the event	2	4	1	3	2	6	15	33
Drinking history of persons in the events		1					2	3
Estimations from populations at risk	2	1					3	6
Proportion of heavy drinkers who experienced serious events		2						2

system that centralises the national data and to the methods of determining the involvement of alcohol. In spite of these drawbacks, registration of alcohol-related casualties is possible through improvements in the existing information system. Unfortunately, information is available from only a few countries and, furthermore, when information is available it is not always presented in terms of rates *per capita*.

As alcohol-related casualties are not reliably reported, it is quite difficult to compare these rates with those of cirrhosis of the liver. The two countries with the highest rates of deaths due to the latter cause also have considerably higher rates of alcohol-related casualties.

References

Aarens, M., T. Cameron, J. Roizen, R. Roizen, R. Room, D. Schneberk and D. Wingard (1977) *Alcohol, casualties and crime*, Report C-18, Social Research Group, Berkeley, California

Adis Castro G., and I. Flores (1967) Estado actual de la epidemiología del alcoholismo y problemas del alcohol en algunos países de América Latina; Costa Rica. In J. Horwitz, J. Marconi and G. Adis Castro (eds), *Epidemiologia del alcoholismo en América Latina*, Acta, Buenos Aires, pp. 86-91

Alvarez, C.N. (1983) Epidemiología del alcoholismo en Venezuela. Centro de Investigaciones Neuro Psiquiátricas. Fundación CINEPSI

Boada, J.M. (1976) Drogas y accidentes de tránsito. *Revista Venezolana de Sanidad y Asistencia Social, 41*, 54-66

Cabildo, H.M. (1967) Estado actual de la investigación epidemiológica en América Latina: Mexico. In J. Mariategui and G. Adís Castro (eds), *Epidemiológica psiquiátrica en América Latina*, Acta, Buenos Aires, pp. 126-139

Caetano, R. (1984) Manifestations of alcohol-related problems in Latin America: a review. *PAHO Bulletin 18*, 3

Departamento del Distrito Federal (1985) *Estadísticas de la dirección general de servicios médicos: México*

Heman, C.A. (1984) Deseo de morir y realidad del acto en sujetos con intento suicidio. *Salud Pùblica de México No. 1, 36*, 39-49

Jackson, J.K. (1957) The definition and measurement of alcoholism. *Quarterly Journal of Studies on Alcohol, 18*, 240-62

Lopez, J.L. and H. Rosovsky (1986) Estudio epidemiologico sobre los accidentes y delitos relacionados con el consumo de alcohol. *Salud Publica, 28*, 5, 515-20

Manterola, M. (1985) Investigación del programa de prevención sobre el menor maltratado. DIF, Mexico

Marconi, J. (1967) Estado actual de la epidemiología del alcoholismo y problemas del alcohol en algunos paises de America Latina; Chile. In J. Horwitz, J. Marconi and G.A. Castro (eds), *Eidemiología del alcoholismo en América Latina*, Acta, Buenos Aires, pp. 92-7

Mardones, J. (1980) El alcoholismo en América Latina. *Revista de Associacao Brasileira de Psiquiatría*, *2*, 88-92

Mas, C., C. Varela and A. Manrique (1985) 'Indicadores médicos y no médicos del problema del alcohol en México', *Instituto Mexicano de Psiquiatría (En prensa)*

Medina-Mora, M.E., L. Gonzáles, A. Manrique and C. Varela (1985) 'Muertes relacionadas con el consumo de alcohol: análisis de expedientes'. Reporte Interno

Mena, R.M. *et al.* (1984) Prevalencia del síndrome alcohólico fetal en escuelas de educación diferenciada de concepción (Chile). *Boletín de la Oficina Sanitaria Panamericana,97*, 423-33

Miguez, L.H.A. (1983) Prevalencia de niveles de ingestión de alcohol en Costa Rica. *Boletín de la Oficina Sanitaria Panamericana, 95*, 451-8

Ministerio de Salud Pública (1984) Características de la morbi-mortalidad, gastos de tránsito y disponibilidad de pago: Un estudio de caso sobre 1,017 hogares en Honduras. *Salud para Todos, 3*, 9-14

Moser, J. (1974) Problems and programs related to alcohol and drug dependence in 33 countries. *Offset Publications No. 6*, World Health Organization, Geneva

Navarro, R.J. (1975) Muertes en hechos de tránsito. *Salud Pública de México, 17*, 777-92

Naveillan, F.P., and L.S. Vargas (1984a) Expectativa de la vida del bebedor problema en Santiago de Chile: I Aspectos metodológicos y de población. *Boletín de la Oficina Sanitaria Panamericana, 96*, 160-7

— (1984b) Expectativa de la vida del bebedor problema en Santiago de Chile: II Estimación de defunciones. *Boletín de la Oficina Sanitaria Panamericana, 96*, 222-8

— (1984c) Expectativa de la vida del bebedor problema en Santiago de Chile, III Estimación de tasas especificas de mortalidad, *Boletín de la Oficina Sanitaria Panamericana, 96*, 334-341

Negrete, J.C. (1976) Alcoholism in Latin America. *Annals of the New York Academy of Sciences, 273*, 9-23

Pan American Health Organization (1978) Health conditions in the Americas: 1973-1976. *PAHO Scientific Publication No. 364*

Ripstein, H.R. (1981) Panorama del impacto del consumo de alcohol en México. Paper presented at the International Meeting on las Estrategias preventivas ante los problemas relacionados con el alcohol, June 6-7, Mexico, DF

Rivera-Lima, J. (1973) El alcoholismo como un problema médico social en Guatemala. In E. Tongue, R.T. Lamlee and B. Blair (eds), *Proceedings of the International Conference on Alcoholism and Drug Abuse*. ICAA, San Juan, Puerto Rico

Roizen, J., and D. Schneberk (1977) Alcohol and crime. In M. Aarens, T. Cameron, J. Roizen, R. Roizen, R. Room, D. Schneberk and D. Wingard (eds), *Alcohol casualties and crime*, Report C-18, Social Research Group, Berkeley, California, pp. 265-90

Roizen, J. (1982) Estimating alcohol involvement in serious events. In *Alcohol consumption and related problems: alcohol and health monograph, 1*, DHHS; Publication (ADM) 82-1190, United States Government Printing Office, Washington

Room, R. (1982) Alcohol and crime: alcohol and criminal behavior and events. In *Encyclopaedia of Crime and Justice*, MacMillan, New York

Rosovsky, H. and J.L. Lopez (1986) Accidentes y violencias relacionadas con el consumo de alcohol revista. *Salud Mental, 9*, 3, 72-76

Saavedra, A. and J. Mariategui (1970) The epidemiology of alcoholism in Latin America. In R.E. Popham (ed), *Alcohol and alcoholism*, University of Toronto Press, Toronto, pp. 307-18

Silva, M. (1972) Alcoholismo y accidentes de tránsito. *Revista de Salud Pública de México, 14*, 6, 809-25

Terroba, G.G. (1985) El consumo de alcohol y su relación con la conducta suicida, *En proceso de publicación, Instituto Mexicano de Psiquiatriá*

Terroba, G.G., and M.T. Saltijeral (1983) La autopsia psicológica como método para el estudio del suicidio. *Salud Publica de Mexico 25*, 285-93

Vidal, G. (1967) Estado actual de la epidemiología del alcoholismo y problemas del alcohol en algunos países de America Latina: Argentina. In J. Horwitz, J. Marconi and G.A. Castro (eds), *Epidemiología del Alcoholismo en América Latina*, Acta, Buenos Aires, pp. 61-71

Viel, B., D. Salcedo and S. Donoso (1970) Alcoholism, accidents, atherosclerosis, and hepatic damage. In R.E. Popham (ed), *Alcohol and alcoholism*, University of Toronto Press, Toronto, pp. 319-37

Zavala, C. (1984) Diagnóstico de la situación actual del alcoholismo en Honduras. *Salud para Todos, 3*, 23-30

3

Alcohol-Related Casualties in Africa

Alan Haworth

Introduction

Public health problems in the developing world are changing although it seems likely that the importance of alcohol-related problems has not yet been recognised. The number of persons injured in accidents is frequently ignored. It was reported recently (WHO 1981) that in 1973 the ratio of the number of cases of cholera, smallpox and road traffic casualties was 1.09:1.36:8.0, this figure not taking into account the under-reporting of road traffic casualties. In one very limited survey (WHO 1981) conducted in six of nine developing countries, accidents were recorded as the primary cause of death among children between the ages of 10 and 14, and two other countries reported accidents as the second most frequent cause. In a recent report (1980), the Zambian Ministry of Health stated that accidents account for nearly 8 per cent of all hospital admissions, 3.6 per cent of deaths and 9 per cent of total new out-patients. In children aged 14 and under, falls and burns constitute the main type of accident, ranking tenth in hospital admissions, eighth in health centre admissions and accounting for just under 4 per cent of all admissions. Accidents are not recorded as a significant cause of mortality in adults but injuries due to road traffic accidents are listed as ranking ninth in the causes of admissions to hospital. Injuries rank second as a cause for out-patient treatment (9.2 per cent) — the first being upper respiratory tract infections — and also rank high among child out-patients, being third and making up 9.2 per cent of the total. There is a marked tendency, when describing the medical consequences of drinking, to think only of 'alcoholism' thus:

We do not refer here to the weekend load of drunks and stab-wounds arriving in casualty, but to the decent solid middle class and middle income Blacks (mainly male) with jobs, home and families who now, nearly 20 years after liquor was made freely available to them, are presenting with the white man's problem. (McCabe 1982)

This paper will focus on a wide range of alcohol-related problems, particularly as they are reflected in official statistics and in studies of the work of accident and casualty departments and admission wards. There is a lack of information from Africa on alcohol-related problems generally and in order to set the scene the paper first reviews some general reports on drinking and alcoholism, and then focuses upon statistics relating to alcohol-related injuries and accidents. An examination of road traffic statistics in particular will allow exploration of the problems to be met in relying upon official data. Other studies will then be reviewed which help to show how the quality of data might be improved, followed by a consideration of the methodology of data collection (both in specific projects and in improvements in official statistics), starting with a more detailed examination of the types of alcohol-related problems which might be significant in any such studies. Finally, there will be a summing up in which policy issues are examined and recommendations made. Literature from sub-Saharan Africa is reviewed and while South Africa is not examined, the paper mainly concentrates upon problems of the majority, namely the developing nations of that continent.

Alcohol-Related Problems in Africa: Some General Reviews

The literature on drinking in Africa is sparse although it has been possible to compile a bibliography of some 140 items (Haworth and Freund 1985), referring mainly to anthropological and sociological studies of drinking practices and problems. However, most early accounts of drinking problems are to be found as more or less incidental references in anthropological works, the following being fairly typical:

In general the factor of beer drinking...seems to represent a lowering of inhibitions, which permits violence to result from pre-existing differences not otherwise sufficient to cause it...but it must be stressed here too that most of the cases which can be attributed to drunkenness took place away from home in the context of beer parties of the modern commercial type...Formerly...beer was either drunk quietly or at various ritual occasions the solemnity of which precluded quarrelling. (Southall 1960)

A search of the archives in most former colonial territories reaps a rich harvest of sometimes vivid descriptions of the ill-effects of drinking, written by administrators in various official reports. Chaplin (1961) quotes a 1933 annual report from Zambia:

> The harvest in several parts of the country was exceptionally good and greater quantities than usual of native beer have been brewed. Assaults and affrays have been exceptionally numerous and in almost every case it has been shown that the persons concerned were incited by drink.

Ambler (1984) has given a detailed account of the attitudes of colonial administrators to changing patterns of drinking in Kenya from 1900 to 1939. These accounts of alcohol-related problems are in the main anecdotal as are the more recent medically oriented descriptions. Tongue (1976) reviewed materials from seven countries including reports presented at a workshop of the Association of Psychiatrists in Africa, held in Kenya in 1974, on Alcohol and Drug-Related Problems. She was not able to quote any statistical data from the Ivory Coast, Ghana, Nigeria, Kenya or Tanzania. From Mauritius, it was reported that although alcoholism seemed to have a high prevalence, statistics were sparse. It had been said that in recent years 25 to 30 per cent of patients admitted to mental hospitals were being treated for alcoholism. In 1977 there were 336 admissions for alcoholism and delirium tremens and in 1978, 287 admissions — to the only hospital serving a population of 900,000. From Ghana, Adomakoh (1974) presented a report to the workshop on 'Who seeks treatment for alcoholism in Ghana', and found a total of 26 cases admitted to the psychiatric hospital and 15 to the general hospital in Accra in 1973, numbers which, as he remarked, 'were small when compared with the total admissions to the hospitals'. Not one of the general hospital admissions was because of a need for the treatment of alcoholism, but for conditions such as haematemesis, coma, polyneuropathy and pneumonia. From Nigeria, Marinho mentioned that 'driving under the influence of alcohol is also common but only a moderate number of cases come to the attention of the law enforcement officers. There appears to be a preponderance of psychogenic over sociogenic alcoholism.'

Further information from Nigeria was provided in response to an invitation from the World Health Organization to submit profiles of policy and programmes for prevention of alcohol-related problems in 1978. It was reported that 60 patients with a diagnosis of alcoholism had been admitted to a neuro-psychiatric hospital in Abeokuta between 1964 and 1973 (Asuni 1974), 34 cases had been admitted in Lagos over a ten-year period (Anumonye *et al.* 1977) and in Benin City only two cases had been admitted and four treated as out-patients between 1973 and 1978.

Tongue (1976) reported no systematic research from Kenya and was able to quote only one study by a psychiatrist (Otsyula 1974) on the categorisation of patients with drinking problems. There have been a few recent papers from Kenya including one by Bittah *et al.* (1979) on a study of alcoholism in a rural setting. These authors, using the 1952 WHO definition of 'alcoholism' found that 27 per cent of males, 24 per cent of females and up to 7 per cent of secondary school students could be classified as alcoholic.

In a review of alcohol- and drug-related problems in Kenya, Acuda (1982) cited a study of Mathare Valley, Nairobi, a notorious 'shantytown' area of Nairobi in which up to 46 per cent of males and 24 per cent of females were alcoholic according to these same criteria. He also reported that in the year 1978, 50 patients were admitted to a large general hospital with acute alcoholic gastritis and 168 were treated in the emergency department of the hospital for severe alcoholic intoxication. In the same year, 17 per cent of 86 new psychiatric out-patients were reported, during a three-month period, as alcoholics. Unfortunately, the total number of admissions to the general hospital are not given, so that these figures cannot be put into perspective but it may be noted that the hospital serves a population of at least 800,000.

Between 1974 and 1980, between 20 and 25 per cent of patients admitted to a mental hospital in Swaziland were given a diagnosis of alcohol- or drug-related psychosis, this corresponding to a rate of about three or four cases per 10,000 population per annum (Haworth 1982). From Botswana, Finlay and Jones (1984) reported that possible alcohol-related diagnoses accounted for only 1.1 per cent of all general hospital diagnoses for the 15 year-and-over age group in 1979. (These did not include any forms of trauma, but did include alcohol dependence.) Data from a mental hospital listed alcoholic psychosis and alcoholism for 12.6 per cent of all discharges and 18 per cent of all male discharges. Of 6,697 out-patient visits to mental health clinics in 1979, 5.9 per cent were for alcohol-related conditions (all patients), 9 per cent among males.

In Zambia in 1973, 1974 and 1975, there were respectively 551, 408 and 487 diagnoses of 'alcoholism' reported by the Ministry of Health. About 8 per cent of patients admitted to a mental hospital serving a population of about half a million in the same period were given this diagnosis — a rate of about 19 per 100,000. In a later study of patients admitted to the same hospital (Haworth *et al.* 1981), one-quarter of all male patients were found to be suffering from an alcohol-related condition. It was noted in this study that, not surprisingly, diagnoses on discharge were more likely to mention the alcohol factor than initial diagnoses, since a number of patients were unable to give a detailed history at the time of their admission. It was also noted that few of the doctors interviewing these patients had been able (or perhaps had taken the trouble) to take a detailed drinking history, noting types of beverage, quantities and frequency of drinking.

It appears from the figures given that there are either massive differences in the drinking habits of various African countries (Nigeria, for example, has a substantial Muslim population) or that the means of collecting data are so disparate that no comparisons can be made. It also seems, however, that when a reasonably accessible mental health service is provided (in three countries in the southern part of the continent) and similar criteria are used for making diagnoses, there is some similarity in the rates of occurrence of alcohol-related psychoses.

Accidents and Injuries

Just as there is very little reliable statistical information on 'alcoholism' in Africa, so is there a lack of data on accidents and injuries. The review by Tongue (1976) noted above made no mention of such alcohol-related problems. Only four countries responded to the World Health Organization request to provide country profiles on alcohol-related problems. In the WHO compendium (Moser 1980), Mauritius reported that the road traffic accident rate rose from 254 per 100,000 population in 1971 to 418 in 1975, but the influence of alcohol was not known. Kenya provided similar imprecise information, stating that traffic accidents due to drunken driving were common and in 1978 over 1,500 people died in road accidents, 'most of which were reported to result from drunken driving'. Kenya also mentioned crimes of violence resulting in drunken brawls, sometimes ending in homicide and aggravated assault; rape, attempted rape and child molestation; and endemic quarrels, spouse beating and child neglect within families. The report from Nigeria stated that there were no police statistics nor any on the number of industrial or domestic accidents due to alcohol. In addition, there were very few case reports of public disorder and nothing was available on injuries resulting from problems within families. Subsequent information on road traffic accidents and casualties as supplied by the police was published in a report prepared for a conference on traffic accidents in developing countries (Owosina 1981). In commenting upon information systems in Nigeria, Owosina remarked that the Nigerian police had the best organised system for data collection but even though individual hospitals kept records with varying degrees of seriousness and accuracy, the figures from the federal Ministry of Health were much higher and most likely more accurate than figures from the police. He gave the main causes of accidents as motor vehicles and accidental falls with the remaining possible causes accounting for no more than 5 per cent at any age. For those aged 45 or more, motor vehicle accidents accounted for about 52 per cent of all accidents.

Although stating that up to 80 per cent of highway drivers indulge in drinking alcoholic beverages (which they offer freely also to their young apprentices), he gives no data on the alcohol component in causation of accidents.

The Zambian Ministry of Health issues annual reports which use the ICD-8 Classification and a summary for the years 1973 to 1977 is given in Table 3.1. Overall, 8.8 per cent of all males and 1.7 per cent of all female admissions were the result of road traffic accidents or assaults. During this period, 45 per cent of all injuries were reported as resulting from these two causes. But there is no indication in these statistics of the role played by alcohol. A major problem in many countries is that police statistics often refer to the alcohol component, but inaccurately, while the health statistics make no mention of alcohol as a factor.

Table 3.1: *Sample statistics on injuries from assaults and road traffic accidents as reported from all hospitals in Zambia: 1975-1977*

| | | (in-patients aged 15+) | | | | | | | |
| | 1975 | | | 1976 | | | 1977 | | |
	Male	Female	Total	Male	Female	Total	Male	Female	Total
Due to RTAs as % of all injuries	16.9	10.3	15.0	18.7	10.9	16.4	17.3	10.6	15.3
Due to RTAs as % of all diseases	3.49	0.4	1.36	3.88	0.42	1.49	3.65	0.4	1.39
Due to assaults as % of all injuries	22.2	28.7	26.4	22.2	28.5	24.0	22.5	27.9	24.1
Due to assaults as % of all diseases	4.59	1.1	2.19	4.61	1.1	2.19	4.76	1.06	2.18
Total injuries	15,691	6,414	22,105	16,221	6,733	22,954	16,195	6,677	22,872

Source: Ministry of Health Annual Reports, 1985-77

From police statistics on road accidents over a ten-year period in Swaziland (Haworth 1982), alcohol was given as the primary cause when drivers were involved in 4.3 per cent of cases, in about 5.4 per cent where cyclists were involved and in 8 per cent where pedestrians were involved. There were, however, no general hospital statistics. At a recent workshop on alcohol-related problems in Swaziland, a police officer stated that in 24.1 per cent of 871 urban and 30.8 per cent of 967 rural accidents occurring in 1983, alcohol had been a contributing factor. Finlay and Jones (1984) have recently reviewed the situation in Botswana. According to official transport statistics, the category 'intoxication' accounted for 154 of 2,253 motor vehicle accidents in 1980 − 6.8 per cent of all traffic accidents (Botswana has a population of about 810,000). This was down slightly from 1979 when this cause was given for 9.1 per cent of 1800 accidents. The 154 alcohol-related traffic accidents in 1980 accounted for 24 per cent of the 116 deaths. Table 3.2 gives figures taken from a report on alcohol-related problems in Zimbabwe presented to the recent workshop in Swaziland. The authors of this report also stated that the percentages of accidents attributed to alcohol in the three years were 38, 47 and 50 respectively but they do not discuss the disparity between these and the percentages reported by the police.

Table 3.2: *Number of road traffic accidents, fatalities and whether caused by drink*

Year	Total accident	No. accidents caused by drink or alcohol	Fatalities	Accident caused by drink or drugs as % of total
1981	18,035	638	1,047	3.54
1982	15,738	783	1,990	4.98
1983	13,566	661	1,038	4.87

Source: Zimbabwe Police

Kobus (1980) has described the use of 'Breathalyzer Model 1000' in Zimbabwe and reports that in 1978 a total of 595 cases were tested, of which only 4 per cent had a blood-alcohol concentration of less than 80 mg/100 ml. These are probably the cases where intoxication was listed as a cause in the following years.

Problems with Regard to Police Statistics on Accidents, Injuries and the Alcohol Component

Although road traffic accidents are not numerically as important as accidents from other causes, more information tends to be available concerning them. This is perhaps partly because the car is such a potentially lethal weapon that fatalities are more numerous and injuries tend to be much more serious than in, for example, drunken brawls. This is an example of a factor which influences the accuracy of reports concerning the incidence of various types of injuries and their causes. Owosina (1981), in reviewing the situation in Nigeria, notes that some accidents are not reported to the police and fear of prosecution leads to:

a) only about 5 per cent of accidents causing no injury being reported;

b) only 55 per cent of accidents causing injuries which may require hospitalisation for six days or more are reported;

c) of accidents causing death on the spot, 'a good number' are still hidden from the police;

d) of deaths occurring at home or in hospital ten or more days after the accident, over 40 per cent are not reported as deaths related to accidents. Factors such as these indicate that the picture of alcohol-related injuries found from sources other than police records will be very different.

The under-reporting of injuries by the police has been noted in a number of countries (WHO 1976). One survey found that only 42 per cent of 770 victims at a large hospital (Sweden) appeared in the national returns. In one UK survey, only 44 per cent of accidents involving injuries to cyclists were found to have been reported. Misreporting also occurs. In one UK survey, only 34 per cent of victims detained in hospital and recorded by the police as seriously ill were considered to be so from the medical point of view. Injuries to protected users were likely to be more accurately reported than to unprotected users. In Sweden, official statistics indicated that twice as many protected road users were injured as unprotected users, whereas the numbers were about equal in hospital surveys. Moreover, the unprotected make up almost two-thirds of those killed and seriously injured.

Although there may be little difference in death rates as given in Table 3.3, the differences in distribution of population and in the level of risk must be kept in mind. For instance, of 36,212 km of roads in Zambia, only 5,565 km were paved roads in 1980. Since its area is four times that of England, with a population of only about 6.5 million and 45 per cent of the population living in towns, the rural density is very low, at about 7 persons per square kilometre. It appears that the danger in travelling further in unpopulated areas on unpaved roads is greater than that of travelling shorter distances in densely populated areas on paved roads.

'The Copperbelt', the industrial region of Zambia — which contains its mining industry, its main urban area and Lusaka, the capital city — accounted for on average two-thirds (67.2 per cent) of all reported accidents in a ten-year period, and for just over half the deaths (51.8 per cent). The mainly rural remainder of Zambia and its two other major towns accounted for only 24.4 per cent of accidents but 37 per cent of deaths.

Table 3.3:   *Death rates and various parameters in five countries*

	Canada	France	United Kingdom	Zambia	Nigeria
Per 10,000 population	2.52	2.29	1.5	1.57	2.69
Per 10,000 vehicles	7.37	7.11	6.42	60.0	17.5
Per casualty	0.04	0.09	0.03	0.146	-

Source: World Health Organization, various sources

Table 3.4:   *Mean numbers of accidents (with standard deviations) for the years 1971-80 in selected areas of Zambia*

	Selected areas in Zambia				Ratio Accidents/Killed	
	Accidents		Killed			
	Mean	S.D.	Mean	S.D.		
Copperbelt	3,279	448	1,559	268	2.103	0.476
Lusaka	3,679	617	1,181	119	3.115	0.321
Kabwe	553	123	317	47	1.744	0.573
Livingstone	317	127	286	10	1.148	0.871
Other areas	2,523	771	1,958	329	1.288	0.776

Source: Central Statistical Office, Lusaka

It would appear that although road traffic accidents are not as common in rural areas, fewer persons are likely to survive. But as compared with developed countries, the risk of death is greater for all areas, as is shown in Table 3.4. Primarily in rural areas, but also in urban areas, the risk of dying before reaching hospital is higher because of poor communications, the lack of efficient mobile resuscitation services and so forth.

Korsah (1969) demonstrated the problem in a study of mortality rates in the accident service in Accra, Ghana in relation to the mode of transport to hospital and he drew attention particularly to the danger of asphyxia in an unconscious person. The danger is even greater in the case of those consuming large quantities of alcoholic beverages who may easily vomit and inhale the vomitus. Death is more likely to ensue in victims of violence in Africa because often in rural areas they are in poor physical condition (heavy drinkers may already be vitamin deficient) and in areas where malaria is endemic, many people have enlarged and fragile spleens — a blow to the abdomen, which would otherwise be innocuous, can result in a fatal internal hemorrhage. Thus a higher proportion of drunken fights in these areas are likely to result in charges of manslaughter.

One other aspect of communication difficulties must be taken into account. In the case of injuries, the likelihood of a person seeking medical help depends upon the distance from a medical facility and the relative 'gain' to be had from attendance, seen not only in terms of possibility of receiving treatment but also in terms of certification of the extent of injury should there be a 'case' to settle — for ideas concerning compensation for injuries are highly developed in many parts of traditional Africa (Gluckman 1955). Persons living near medical facilities will be more likely to attend with much less severe injuries than those living some distance away — a point discussed in relation to illness generally by King (1966), and to psychiatric illness by Haworth (1981b).

In Africa, injuries to unprotected road users (pedestrians and cyclists) are particularly important, though they are often the least likely to be recorded in statistics from the police. Ferguson (1974) found that in a series of 10,000 *post mortem* examinations on persons dying from unnatural causes in Durban, South Africa, 17 per cent were due to traffic accidents of whom 21.5 per cent were whites (mainly motorists) and 55.5 per cent were blacks — mainly pedestrians. Ferguson noted that more black pedestrian commuters were killed during the hours of darkness. Likewise, Patel and Bhagwat (1977) in a similar study in Zambia noted that pedestrians formed 50.2 per cent of road accident fatalities and cyclists a further 5.5 per cent. Nair and Khan (1977) reported similar statistics from a large hospital in the main industrial and mining area of Zambia. Of over 300 autopsies performed on accident victims in a one-year period, 41 per cent were on pedestrians, 9 per cent on cyclists hit by a motor vehicle and 3.5 per cent on people who had fallen off moving vehicles. Twenty-two per cent were on victims of vehicles colliding with each other and a further 15.6 per cent on those killed when vehicles overturned.

In a World Health Organization paper (1981), it was reported that in developing countries there was a preponderance of crashes involving a pedestrian and a vehicle. The highest proportion of crashes was observed among unprotected road users in one country in Africa where 87 per cent of the fatally injured died before any medical help could be rendered.

Not only do the police tend to under-report various types of road traffic accidents and to under-estimate the severity of injuries, they also often avoid action on (and reporting of) certain types of incidents where the accident component may be very important. Hall (1980) remarked upon the reluctance of the police in Lusaka to get involved in incidents of domestic violence involving spouses. However, the wife often requires police help in these situations to obtain a certificate for use in court at a later date. Thus, in two studies of a casualty department in Lusaka (Haworth *et al.* 1981, Haworth 1983a), the police were involved in sending patients to hospital in 34.5 per cent and 18.6 per cent of cases respectively. Apart from a small number of road traffic accidents, the majority of these cases involved fights between people and often between spouses.

Even when there is a statutory requirement, as in road traffic accidents, the police appear officially to attribute a very small proportion to alcohol. Figures from Swaziland and Zimbabwe have already been cited where careful evaluations of the use of a Breathalyzer Model 1000 were carried out before bringing it into use (Kobus 1980). In Zambia, over a period of ten years, the percentages of accidents attributed by the police to alcohol when the driver of a vehicle was involved average just less than 1.0 and when a pedestrian was involved 0.42. In reference to this situation in Lusaka, a group of mathematicians remarked:

> In our preliminary reading of existing police reports, depending entirely upon subjective judgement, we have found the proportion of accidents caused by alcohol incredibly low...there is great need for an objective procedure aimed at detecting dangerous quantities of alcohol in the blood... (Ciampi *et al.* 1985)

Apparent confirmation of this comes from Nigeria (Aguwa *et al.* 1982). They examined 32 drivers who had been admitted to an accident ward and found that there was detectable blood alcohol in 28, but that only one person had a concentration higher than 50 mg/100 ml. This led the authors to speculate that 'Probably Black Africans may have a higher risk of accidents than other races under the influence of the same alcohol concentration.' *Post-mortem* studies of accident victims give a very different picture. From information provided by the public analyst, it appears that 53 per cent of deceased accident victims in Lusaka (mainly cyclists and pedestrians) in the period 1958 to 1965 had blood-alcohol levels of over 150 mg/100 ml, 14 per cent had a BAC of between 50 and 150 mg/100 ml, and 33 per cent had less than 50 mg/100 ml (Haworth *et al.* 1981). Patel and Bhagwat (1977), in a similar study, found that 36 per cent of 588 autopsies carried out in 1974/5 involved road traffic accidents. Fifty-eight of the victims (26.7 per cent) had detectable blood-alcohol levels – about one-third of all types of road users. Only one BAC of less than 80 mg/100 ml was recorded and 42 (72 per cent) were over 200 mg/100 ml.

Kobus (1980) was able to report on breathalyzer tests on drivers either involved in accidents or suspected for some other reason of being under the influence of alcohol or drugs. The law in Zimbabwe mentions two levels – above 80 mg/100 ml is referred to as 'driving above the limit' and above 140 mg/100 ml as 'drunk while driving'. In 1978, out of 595 analyses only 15 were in the range 80 to 100 mg/100 ml and 77 per cent were greater than 150 mg/100 ml. The average was 202 mg/100 ml. 'The average drunk driver is not someone who has had one or two drinks on the way home from work.' Similar results were reported in 1979.

It seems that, given the right tool and the correct training, the police are capable of confirming that at least the highly intoxicated have been taking alcohol. But in general, the ordinary constable seems to be disinclined to even note alcohol as a factor, especially if there is no legal requirement for him to do so. In a study by Haworth *et al.* (1981), it was noted at one Lusaka police station that the official diary (the 'Occurrence Book') made reference to alcohol in 13.5 per cent of incidents. In a later study of two very similar police stations, however, in which special (separate) note was taken of whether alcohol had been a factor in incidents dealt with at the stations, it was mentioned in about one-third of all cases. The fact that the police do not regularly report the alcohol component in many offences does not mean that this may not emerge if the case comes to trial. Studies of court records have been carried out in both Zambia and Zimbabwe. In Zambia (Okada 1967), data were collected from 1,866 cases heard in two urban 'local' courts (courts of first instance) representing all cases heard in 1965/6. A criminal offence such as rioting, assault or unlawful wounding was involved in 41.3 per cent of the cases, and these made up 71 per cent of offences, the remainder being 'drunk and disorderly'. At least a proportion of those who had been injured might have been taken to hospitals or health centres but there would have been no record of alcohol involvement. Gelfand (1971) found that alcohol could have been a factor in between one-half and two-thirds of cases of homicide tried in the higher courts, but was hardly ever mentioned in cases of assault tried at a number of courts, similar to the 'local' ones studied by Okada.

Alcohol and Patients Dealt with in Accident or Casualty Departments and Wards

As has been suggested already, there must be a process of selection in determining the kinds of patients dealt with in any particular accident or casualty department. This will be discussed further in the section on methodological issues. In a large city there are likely to be alternative facilities and persons with only minor injuries may well attend at the local health centre rather than the main hospital department, which for many may mean a long journey and a feeling of bewilderment in unfamiliar surroundings. That patients with minor trauma do attend local health centres in Lusaka is confirmed by two studies (Noak 1967, Haworth 1983a). Noak found that 13 per cent of all patients attending a large municipal clinic or health centre complained of some form of injury and a further 0.7 per cent (of a total of 769 patients of all ages) were suffering from burns or scalds. Haworth was able to report on those aged 15 or more separately and of these, 17.9 per cent were injuries and a further 1.9 per cent burns or scalds. Noak did not give any further breakdown but Haworth noted that there were no cases of fracture or of voluntary overdose with drugs.

In some cities with large industrial concerns, there are well-equipped accident departments or there are private clinics to serve the more affluent. In a city like Lusaka, however, facilities are very limited and for the majority of the population the only alternative to the local clinic is the casualty department of the teaching hospital or the 'filter clinic'. The latter is mentioned because its functions overlap with the casualty department. It accepts patients with a variety of mainly medical conditions but patients may be reclassified on being seen by a doctor and sent to the surgically oriented channel of the hospital. Certainly a proportion of patients seen there are likely to have attended on account of alcohol-related conditions — patients with severe attacks of gastritis, for example. Bittah and Acuda (1979) noted that 50 patients with severe alcoholic gastritis were admitted to the University of Teaching Hospital in Nairobi in 1978 — a number, however, perhaps most remarkable for its small size. Most patients in Zambia would more likely attend as out-patients at their local health centre. The overlap in types of client was also shown in two studies of the casualty department at the teaching hospital in Lusaka (Haworth 1981a, Haworth 1983a).

Table 3.5 shows the pattern reported in the first study. Since the main focus of interest was upon patients with alcohol-related problems, there was some over-sampling at times when these problems were more likely to be seen. Therefore, the actual number of 'general illnesses' was likely to have been somewhat higher than the 25 per cent reported. In the second study in the casualty department, 15.4 per cent of first attenders had general medical or surgical, non-traumatic complaints. An examination of the types of trauma requiring hospital admission has been reported from Zimbabwe (Castle *et al.* 1978).

Table 3.6 gives some instructive insights both into the types of causes of injuries and into the vagaries of classification systems. The admissions reported represented 14 per cent of all African admissions and 8 per cent of all white admissions but very different proportions of the populations from which they were drawn (being 1:1.8/Africans:Europeans as based upon the race-specific rates). For Africans, assaults, fights and so on made up 25.3 per cent of the causes — just the type to be frequently associated with an alcohol component. Curiously, the authors state that road accidents made up the largest group overall but this is not confirmed by these figures.

The authors speculate about the relatively lower rate of admissions for Africans (the race-specific rate is only 40 per cent that of the rate for Europeans) and suggest that there may be greater tolerance for injuries, not enough beds in the African hospital or, since this is a teaching hospi-

Table 3.5: *Tables of patients attending casualty department and at two urban clinics in Lusaka, Zambia*

	Casualty department			Health centres		
	Male	Female	Total	Male	Female	Total
General illness	21	41	25	89	96	92
Assault	43	25	40	2	1	2
Accidents	29	31	29	8	3	6
RTAs	7	2	6	1	0	1
	(350)	(87)	(441)	(301)	(219)	(521)

Table 3.6: *The ten most common causes of admissions in Africans and Europeans*

Africans	% of Number	Total	Europeans	% of Number	Total
Assault means (NK)	345	12.9	Tripping/ stumbling	225	16.95
Motor vehicle hits pedestrian	289	10.81	Motor vehicle hitting motor vehicle	108	8.24
Fight/brawl/ rape	195	7.29	Fall furniture/tree	103	7.86
Scale	141	5.27	Loss control motor vehicle	77	5.88
Accidental cut/stab	140	5.23	Over-strenuous movement	69	5.27
Deliberate cut/stab	136	5.09	Motor vehicle accident (NK)	54	4.12
Tripping	127	4.75	Attempt suicide poison	51	3.89
Loss control Motor vehicle	110	4.11	Pushed (e.g. sports)	46	3.51
Fall furniture/ tree	102	3.81	Struck by object	41	3.13
Cycle accident	70	2.62	Accidentally cut/stabbed	32	2.44
Total for race	2,674	61.88		1,310	61.29

Source: *Central African Journal of Medicine*

tal, out-patient facilities may be better than at the European hospital. While all these may be true, some of the other factors discussed earlier may have been important (for example, that some Africans may have gone first to their local clinic, from which admission is somewhat less easy to organise than from an accident department in the same hospital).

Alcohol-Related Causes Bringing Patients to Casualty Departments

Table 3.6 gives some impression of the range of possible reasons why patients may have to attend at accident or casualty departments. The following are the more important causes — and it will be noted that what may be termed a 'high index of suspicion' will often be necessary, especially where the injured person was not the person who had been drinking.

Road Traffic Accidents

These form a relatively small proportion of all cases dealt with at accident departments in Zambia and this is almost certainly the case in other countries too. In the two studies carried out in Zambia, 6 and 8 per cent of the attendences were because of road traffic accidents, that is, whether alcohol-related or not; and it must be remembered that, as the only major medical facility in Lusaka, this casualty department would deal with all major incidents.

Assaults and Fights

Studies at police stations in Zambia (Hall 1980, Haworth 1981b) have shown how frequently alcohol is involved in violent behaviour. Hall (1980) collected data from dockets opened at three police stations over a three-month period on 99 sexual offences, 171 robberies and 739 assaults. The most common time of occurrence for all three types of crime was between eight and ten p.m. and 65 per cent of robberies and assaults occurred between seven p.m. and midnight. A third of robberies took place in bars and a quarter of assaults in bars or liquor stores. There was some evidence from the police records that either the complainant or the aggressor or both had been drinking in 40 per cent of cases of assault and 30 per cent of cases of robbery; one-sixth of victims of sexual offences had been drinking. In the study by Haworth *et al.* at two police stations in Lusaka, alcohol was mentioned by the complainant in 30 per cent of cases and was noted to be a factor by the police (being prompted by having to fill in the study questionnaires) in 35 per cent. Overall, the police thought that alcohol was a factor in 55 per cent of cases of assault and in at least 48 per cent of cases the complainant himself had been drinking.

There were some differences in rates of reporting of various types of offences between the two police stations, which suggested that police attitudes and decisions on how to label behaviours affected the rates at which alcohol was being reported as a cause by these police officers.

What of the situation at the casualty department to which patients from the areas served by these police stations would have gone? In one study (Haworth 1983a), conditions leading to attendance included assaults (39%), road traffic accidents (8%), work accidents (7%), home accidents (6%), and sporting injuries, foreign bodies in the eye and so forth make up the remaining 11 per cent. Of the 73 cases of assault, 19 per cent were by a spouse, 11 per cent by other relatives, 19 per cent by friends and 45 per cent by strangers. Four patients did not mention the type of assault. Alcohol was involved in only two cases of fighting between spouses. Of the 59 other cases of assault, 30 involved alcohol but not all the assaulted had themselves been drinking. Twenty of 27 men had and nine admitted that their drinking had been an important factor; three of eight women had been drinking and this was considered by them to be a factor. Violent behaviour between persons then makes up an important part of casualty work where alcohol may have been an important contributory factor, but elucidating its exact relationship to any particular incident may be difficult.

Falls and Home Accidents, Including Burns

Burns and scalds are likely to be especially important in Africa (even in towns), where so much cooking is done upon open fires. Likewise, falls are more common in situations where people in rural areas have to move at night (they mostly try to avoid travelling at night over any distance) and, in addition, many urban areas are ill-lit. However, many of the injuries may well be minor and hence will not result in attendance at casualty departments. In the Castle *et al.* (1978) study in Zimbabwe (Table 3.6), 'tripping' and 'falls' accounted for 8.6 per cent of admission among Africans. Including 'sports injuries' for Europeans, this becomes the major group accounting for 28.3 per cent of admissions – 10 per cent more than road traffic accidents. Honkanen (1983) has shown that alcohol increases a pedestrian's risk of accidental fall somewhat more than it does a driver's risk of traffic accident. The relative risk of 1.0 at zero blood-alcohol concentration was about 2 at BACs of 50 to 100 mg/100 ml, about 10 at BACs of 100 to 150 mg/100 ml and about 60 at BACs of 160 mg/100 ml or higher.

Alcoholic Hypoglycemia

This is a condition which is seen with some frequency in casualty departments, at least in Southern Africa and it is neither well-known nor always recognised for what it is. It has, however, found its way into textbooks on the medical consequences of heavy drinking (Clark and Kricka 1980). Willcox and Gelfand (1976) reviewed ten cases of spontaneous hypoglycemia admitted to hospital and discussed the problems of definitely confirming the condition as alcohol-related. The study, being a retrospective one, suffered from the inherent defect of all such studies — incomplete information — and it was evident that insufficient information had been obtained on the drinking habits of seven of the ten patients. Over 250 patients had been admitted to the casualty department and they had not even had their blood glucose estimated — one characteristic of this condition is the very prompt response to treatment with glucose which would frequently be given on clinical grounds alone. Neame and Joubert (1961), reporting from South Africa, found evidence of liver disease in 50 per cent of their subjects but behavioural as well as other health problems were likely to be present. There is a need for more systematic investigations.

Some Acute Medical and Psychiatric Conditions

Because of their acute onset, these sometimes cause patients to be brought to casualty departments though the alcohol component is frequently either not recognised or ignored by the medical and nursing staff. A useful analysis (Jeffery 1979) of physicians' categorisation of patients as 'interesting,' or as the kind to be avoided, shows why these conditions get so little attention as compared with the far more interesting and challenging problems of dealing with 'stove-in' chests and such like.

A few patients may be admitted in a stupefied state as the result of acute intoxication, but this is likely to be rare unless there is a superadded condition, such as hypoglycemia. Patients in acute confused states associated with vitamin deficiencies are admitted more often, although in Zambia the police will often take them directly to a mental health unit. Acute alcoholic hallucinosis (without clouding of consciousness) appears to be more common in some African countries than *delirium tremens* and such patients may also be brought to casualty departments.

Suicide and Parasuicide

The link between alcohol and suicide and parasuicide is well established in the western world. No such link has been described in Africa. Although drinking is mentioned fairly regularly in Bohannan's book, *African Homicide and Suicide* (1960), there is no discussion of possible links between drinking behaviour and liability to commit suicide. Rittey and Castle (1972) do not mention alcohol in their discussion of suicide in Zimbabwe. Swift and Asuni (1975) do not mention alcohol as a factor in describing suicidal behaviours in their textbook of psychiatry for Africa. Chaplin (1961), in a review of the records of inquests on 1,001 suicides in Zambia, found only one case where alcohol was implicated. In Lusaka, young people are regularly admitted to hospital with drug overdose but there has so far been no investigation of a possible alcohol component and this is another area which needs more work.

Industrial Accidents

Industrial accidents are seen with some regularity in accident departments but links with drinking when reliance is placed only upon self-reports are hard to establish. The penalties for being caught drunk at work in certain occupations is so severe that workers prefer the certainty of paying a lesser penalty by staying away from work altogether. However, sporadic cases do occur and as Hirschfeld and Behan (1963) have pointed out, many industrial accidents are the culmination of a process of increased anxiety, tension and often guilt in the individual which (though he does not mention this) could well be linked to the use of alcohol as well.

Special Consideration of Children and Adolescents

Children and adolescents need consideration as special risk groups. Risks can be manifested in a number of ways:

1. Children are at risk as pedestrians in dark over-crowded streets in some African cities. It has been mentioned that, in Nigeria, girl street-hawkers are at special risk.

2. There is risk of assault from parents, guardians or others. Sarungi and Kaduri (1980), in a study of trauma in children in Dar-es-Salaam, found eleven cases of child abuse (1.5 per cent of the total) in which there were four deaths. He makes no mention of alcohol as a factor though this has been cited by other authors in their country profiles of alcohol-related problems (Moser 1980). Apart from direct abuse there is also evidence that children developing protein caloric malnutrition often come from families with other severe psycho-social problems, including those arising from drinking. While malnourished children are not likely to be brought to casualty departments themselves, they may be found being carried on the backs of women who

have perhaps been assaulted, offering another clue to an underlying domestic problem.

3. Severe intoxication and its results are sometimes seen in children or young people who are experimenting with drinking. In Zambia and neighbouring countries, a form of commercially made home-brewed beer or 'opaque' beer with an alcohol concentration of between 3 and 3.5 per cent in volume is widely available. While not supposed to be sold for consumption off the premises in Zambia, this is a frequently ignored law and many parents send their children for 'chibuku' to be taken home, in quantities of several litres. A recent survey into how children begin drinking found that the majority of informants, described as boys of twelve or thirteen years of age from many parts of Zambia, begin by stealing small amounts of their parents' chibuku and subsequently buying it for themselves at the local tavern, stating that they were buying for their parents. A surprisingly large number of informants in this recent survey were able to describe the exact prices and quantities sold of various illicit beverages — a litre of one for example, containing an average of 7 per cent alcohol by volume can be obtained for the price of a loaf of bread.

It is thus possible that such children or young people could be brought to accident departments in a stupefied condition (sometimes exhibiting the hypoglycemic syndrome), a forewarning of other alcohol-related problems in the future.

Suspecting Alcohol as a Factor

While the police regularly under-estimate the alcohol factor in their official statistics, the health authorities tend often to ignore it completely. To what extent do medical workers become aware of alcohol-related problems in their patients and what are the best means of detection of these problems? Mbaruku (1980) investigated the role of alcohol in injured patients in Dar-es-Salaam by deliberately smelling the breath and then asking for a second opinion.

In the Project on Community Response to Alcohol-related Problems (Haworth *et al.* 1981), questions were asked of both patients and physicians in order to attempt an assessment of the significance of alcohol. The physicians were asked to indicate whether there were signs of the patient having been drinking or whether he or she appeared 'drunk' (this term was not defined). One problem was that the pressure of work was often so great that some doctors were unwilling to provide the information needed and 9 per cent of cases had to be recorded as missing data. This questionnaire was obviously not always fully understood by agency staff filling in the section concerning the patient's drinking. There was a question on whether the patient appeared drunk and also one on whether there were *other* signs of drinking. But of the 41 patients for whom these were noted, 51 per cent were said to be smelling of beer, 12 per cent to have slurred speech, 2 per cent to be talkative and 2 per cent to have blood-shot eyes. Naturally some patients would have had time to recover from their drunken state by the time they were seen in the casualty department. Twenty-six per cent of those who stated that they had been drunk at the time of the incident did not appear drunk to the casualty doctor. Thirty-one per cent of those who did appear drunk stated that they had not been drunk at the time of the incident (when, presumably, the effects of drinking would have been manifest). Of those patients (N = 47) who said they were drunk at the time of the incident, the casualty medical officer thought that alcohol was a major factor in 65 per cent, a minor factor in 15 per cent and not a factor in 21 per cent.

Comparison may be made with the findings of Holt *et al.* (1980) on patients who attended the accident department at the Royal Infirmary in Edinburgh. Breath-alcohol analysis was performed on 702 patients; 40 per cent had consumed alcohol before attending and 32 per cent had a blood-alcohol concentration exceeding 80 mg/100 ml. Clinical assessment of intoxication (the doctor was asked to record four specific symptoms: alcoholic factor, slurred speech, abnormal motor coordination and red conjunctivae) resulted in a false negative diagnosis in 10 per cent of inebriated patients.

In our studies in Lusaka, a constantly recurring question arose concerning whose drinking could be 'blamed' for any incident. Of the 170 patients who had been involved in an incident with someone else before coming to casualty (19 per cent of the total) 75 reported that the other person had been drinking and, in the majority of cases, drunk. Only 34 men and one woman in the total sample admitted that their own drinking had been a principal factor in the incident bringing them to the casualty department, and of the men, three-quarters stated that the other person's drinking was also a factor. It is apparent that, with the individual incident, it may often be very difficult to apportion blame — to determine whether this incident was indicative of the patient having other problems related to drinking.

While it is, of course, important for policymakers to become aware of the total of alcohol-related problems, it is also important to know of the number at risk for further problems. Quite apart from symptom check lists and ways of determining whether a person is developing, for example, the alcohol dependence syndrome, further information may be obtained of numbers at special risk from casualty statistics alone, where note is taken of repeat attenders. In one of the studies in the Lusaka casualty department (Haworth 1983a), 14 per cent of the currently drinking patients had previously had to attend because of an alcohol-related incident. Seven patients had had a previous accident and two had had further accidents while five were attending again because of assaults. Of eight who had previously been involved in a fight, five had returned for the same reason and three had been involved in accidents. While inquiries regarding previous attendance at the casualty department were not made in this study, they were made regarding previous 'social problems'. Of 60 patients who had been assaulted, 43 per cent reported having been in a previous fight and 5 per cent had had a road accident, in the previous twelve months; of 25 who were attending because of an accident three had previously been in a fight and eight had had a road accident in the previous twelve months. There appear to be no special studies of 'accident-prone personalities' from Africa, but there have been two reviews from South Africa (Cheetham 1974, Shaw 1965). A cautious and in some ways provocative statement on the topic was made by a WHO *ad hoc* Technical Group (1981):

> Alcoholism and drunken driving are not identical and a distinction must be made for example between social or moderate drinkers, problem drinkers and alcoholics...It seems probable that persons with an instability and certain weak points in their personality structure are more inclined to consume alcohol and drugs, and they are more likely to have difficulties with themselves or others...Drunken drivers [show] in their personal life history as a group an amount of delinquency more similar to that of normal drivers. (WHO 1988)

In terms of gathering statistics, a decision will certainly need to be made as to whether the focus will be upon individuals with alcohol-related problems or upon the occurrence rates of the problems themselves — different techniques are, therefore, required.

Methodological Issues

Policymakers and planners in any country need to have regularly supplied national data which are reliable (using the same definitions from year to year, for example), easy to interpret and to use as a basis for change and which, if possible, will be in such a form as to be fairly readily compared with data from other countries. The account I have given earlier shows that this is far from the case at present and that, in many countries in Africa, there are special obstacles to the collection of complete and representative data. Even when data on accidents or injuries are collected and reported, the alcohol component is rarely if ever dealt with fully and often, especially in Ministry of Health returns, there is reference only to conditions such as 'alcoholism' or 'alcoholic psychosis'.

If changes are to be effected and the inertia of those operating current reporting systems is to be overcome, it will be necessary to demonstrate that changes are both needed and possible. This is the fundamental reason for suggesting that special studies should be undertaken in order to determine both what is needed by planners and others and what data it will be feasible to collect.

Undertaking large-scale studies in developing countries is a daunting task when there is rarely sufficient manpower to meet service commitments and where resources are very limited. There are, however, many other problems which must be faced realistically, of which the following are some of the more important.

In the event that data are collected on a continuous basis by the normal staff of a casualty department, questions of motivation, professional and 'linguistic' competence arise. With regard to the latter, in a country like Zambia, for instance, information may initially have to be obtained in three or four distinct languages, depending on the amount of detail required in interviewing. Haworth and Mambwe (1985) have recently discussed the very considerable problems in translating a standard psychiatric instrument into two Zambian languages. Fortunately, any instrument used in a casualty study would probably not present such great difficulties.

If the normal staff of a department are to collect data, the information required will have to closely approximate what they routinely require, or will have to be of a limited amount, easy to obtain, quick and simple to record. As already mentioned, in the Community Response Project, even with a very simple form, about 10 per cent of information which ought to have been gathered was lost. In the study of police stations, it was found that a visit at least once in every shift (preferably towards the end) was the only way of ensuring our forms were correctly filled in (or even filled in at all) and if there had not been a separate record book to check against the ongoing work, it would have been necessary to arrange for more regular visitation.

Problems also continuously arise in data collection when staff changes take place and when different members of staff working at different times adopt varying attitudes toward a project. Finding means of motivating participating staff members is important.

Many problems are liable to arise in obtaining suitable samples:

1. In order to determine how representative a sample of patients seen in a large casualty department is, it is preferable to explore what alternative sources of help are available to potential clients and what proportion of patients are likely to use them, and in what circumstances. Previous references to patients' use of health centres underlines the need.

2. Where there is a very heavy flow of patients in a casualty department and the majority do not have alcohol-related problems, it is likely to be necessary to over-sample the high-risk group. Various methods might be chosen, after exploratory studies, such as
   a) times of highest expectation;
   b) by mode of referral, e.g. all police cases;
   c) on the basis of blood-alcohol concentration estimates;
   d) on the basis of type of medical condition, e.g. all injuries;
   e) on the basis of certain demographic characteristics, and so forth.
   The use of rapid method for BACs seems to be particularly valuable in some circumstances and it has recently been shown, for example, that workers in health centres in Lusaka can be taught to use a simple technical (laboratory) procedure (use of RPR in antenatal clinics) with high reliability (Hira 1984).

3. Although similar problems may not arise in other settings, special difficulties encountered in Lusaka might be mentioned. It was hoped to carry out random sampling on the basis of new attendances, using the initial entries in the attendance register for selection of the sample. However, at busy times, the register was not used at all, especially if there was a shortage of clerical staff. In addition, patients referred from other departments, for example the 'filter clinic' or outlying health centres, were allowed to retain their original record cards and were not given new numbers.

   It may seem that these are exactly the kind of difficulties which can be overcome with some ingenuity and they hardly require special mention. But the over-crowding and under-staffing in some developing countries are such that special account must be taken of them.

4. Problems of the follow-up of patients who could not be interviewed on admission because they were too ill, or unconscious, or too intoxicated or unwilling to answer questions are much more amenable to suitable action except that, in a country like Zambia, things are not always as easy as they might seem. For example, in a pilot study on patients with alcohol-related medical problems, it was found that, if the ward became too crowded, the least sick patients were discharged sometimes so soon after admission that ward records were never up-to-date. It proved to be possible to monitor all patients sent to a particular ward only by having someone continuously on duty within that ward.

Conclusions and Implications

A number of facts stand out. Because of the different population structure in Africa, accidents are likely to emerge as relatively much more important causes of morbidity and mortality than in developed countries. The concept of a measure of potential years of life lost (PYLL) is of value in this regard. Meade (1980), for instance, has calculated PYLL for several countries in South East Asia and mentions that, for males in Singapore, deaths due to the circulatory system account for 32 per cent of all deaths but only 23 per cent of PYLL. Similarly, the loss of life due to motor accidents takes on much greater weight.

PYLL is easily calculated and could obviously provide significant information for planners and health and other administrators, provided that valid data were available. It is probable that statistics are issued in many African countries, often continuing a system initiated in colonial times, which are subject to the many reporting errors described here. It is not known if data are available from insurance companies (in Zambia there is only one and it has a research department, but relies upon police statistics) or from industrial injuries tribunals and so forth, but for reasons already mentioned, their statistics are unlikely to be any more accurate, particularly regarding the alcohol component. Systems of obtaining factual data are going to be required which are relevant, reliable and cost efficient and, when suitably simplified, may be operated on a continuing basis in order to be able to study (and act upon) trends.

Will casualty data provide sufficient information on trends in alcohol-related problems and will it be possible to overcome any difficulties in the collection of these data? It is only possible to conjecture about the answers to these questions at present — but it can be said that the defects in most systems operating at present in African countries are likely to be so serious that any change must be an improvement. The objective of research at this stage will be to show what can be done and with what resources and then demonstrate to the ministries and departments concerned how improvements can be made.

We have already had the experience of introducing a new system of reporting on the work of our mental health services in Zambia. 'Experimental' annual report forms were sent out to all parts of the country for two years and then a one-week workshop was organised in order to design the final version. This was attended not only by mental health workers but by those in related sectors and by experts in relevant fields, such as demographers. The 'final' version of the form appears to be performing well and will need only minor modifications next time, but it goes out with an explanation which is almost as long as the form itself and a glossary of key terms. In view of the amount of 'interaction' needed, the best systems would probably be based upon use of a micro-computer.

106

Moves have already been made towards the more systematic reporting of casualties (WHO 1978) and experience has been gained using a standard form with, for instance, the Abbreviated Injury Scale. This, then, is the time to ensure that the alcohol component is not neglected and for showing the relevance of such data for dealing with the many other types of alcohol-related problems likely to be seen, with increasing frequency, in many developing countries. There is need, however, for careful evaluation of various technical matters — for example, sampling procedures where they are used — and of means of assessing alcohol consumption and degree of intoxication (including rapid BAC assessment methods), as well as a need for operational definitions of 'alcohol-related problems' in the casualty setting.

If the challenge is great, especially in the developing countries of Africa, the effort made to improve reporting systems will surely prove to have been worthwhile.

© 1989 Alan Haworth

Acknowledgements

I would like to thank Mr. Chola Mutale, F.R.C.S., Consultant Surgeon, University Teaching Hospital, Lusaka, for the loan of a number of WHO and other reports on Road Traffic Accidents.

References

Acuda, S.W. (1982) Drug and alcohol problems in Kenya today: a review of research. Report of the Fourth World Congress for the Prevention of Alcoholism and Drug Dependency, International Commission for the Prevention of Alcoholism, Washington, pp. 187-91

Adomakoh, C.C. (1974) Who seeks treatment for alcoholism in Ghana. Proceedings of the Workshop of the Association of Psychiatrists in Africa, Alcohol and Drug Dependence, ICAA Publication, Nairobi, Kenya, pp. 89-93

Aguwa, C.N., E.O. Anosike and P.I. Akubue (1982) Road accidents in Nigeria: level of alcohol in the blood of automobile drivers. *Central African Journal of Medicine, 28*, 171-4

Ambler, C.H. (1984) Drunks, brewers and chiefs: the political economy of prohibition in rural central Kenya 1900-1939. Paper presented at a conference on the Social History of Alcohol, Berkeley, California, January, 1984

Anumonye, A., N. Ominiwa and H. Adaraniyo (1977) Excessive alcohol use and related problems in Nigeria. *Drug and Alcohol Dependence,* 2, 23-30

Asuni, T. (1974) Patterns of alcohol problem seen in the neuropsychiatric hospital, Aro, Abeokuta: 1964-73. Proceedings of a Workshop on Alcohol and Drug Dependence, ICAA Publication, Nairobi, Kenya, pp. 66-71

Bittah, O., J.A. Owola and P. Oduor (1979) A study of alcoholism in a rural setting in Kenya. *East African Medical Journal,* 56, 665-70

Bittah, O., and S.W. Acuda (1979) Alcoholic gastritis at Kenyatta National Hospital. *East African Medical Journal,* 56, 577-9

Bohannan, P. (1960) *African homicide and suicide.* Princeton University Press, Princeton

Castle, W.M., N. Ravalis and W.F. Boss (1978) A survey of trauma requiring hospital admissions in Salisbury, Rhodesia. *Central African Journal of Medicine, Supplement to 24,* 13-16

Central Statistics Office, Lusaka (1982) Transport and communication statistics, Lusaka (1980)

Chaplin, J.H. (1961) Suicide in Northern Rhodesia. *African Studies, 20,* 145-75

Clark, P.M.S., and L.J. Kricka (1980) *Medical consequences of alcohol abuse.* Ellis Horwood Limited, Chichester

Cheetham, R.W.S. (1974) Road safety and mental health in South Africa. *South African Medical Journal, 48,* 225-29

Ciampi, A., H. Emenalo, H. Joshi and M. Puustelli (1985) Analysis of road traffic accident data in Zambia. Department of Mathematics, University of Zambia

Ferguson, A.L. (1974) Epidemiology of traffic accidents. *South African Medical Journal, 48,* 599-602

Finlay, J., and R.K. Jones (1984) Alcohol consumption and the nature of alcohol-related problems in Botswana: a preliminary report. Mimeo.

Gelfand, M. (1971) The extent of alcohol consumption by Africans: the significance of the weapon at beer drinks. *Journal of Forensic Medicine, 18,* 53-64

Gluckman, M. (1955) *The judicial process among the Barotse of Northern Rhodesia.* Manchester University Press, Manchester

Hall, M. (1980) Research in violent crime in Lusaka: 1972. Mimeo, University of Zambia, Mental Health Association of Zambia, Zambia Police Force

Haworth, A., M. Mwanalushi and D. Todd (1981) Community response to alcohol-related problems in a Zambian historical and social context. Community Health Research Reports, No. 5, Institute for African Studies, Lusaka

Haworth, A. (1981a) Community response to alcohol-related problems in Zambia: drinking problems. Community Health Research Reports, Institute for African Studies, Lusaka

—(1981b) The distance factor in the use of psychiatric facilities. *Medical Journal of Zambia, 15*, 6-9

—(1982) An assessment of the magnitude and nature of changes in alcohol consumption and alcohol-related problems in Swaziland. Assignment Report, World Health Organization Regional Office for Africa, Brazzaville

—(1983a) Alcohol and patients attending the university teaching hospital casualty department, Lusaka. Paper presented to the Annual Meeting of the Association of Physicians of East and Central Africa

—(1983b) Psychiatric morbidity in patients attending general health facilities in Zambia. Paper presented to a WHO workshop on Recording Health Problems Thiaxially, Lusaka

Haworth, A., and P. Freund (1985) A bibliography of drinking in Africa. Typescript

Haworth, A., C. Mambwe and V.C Kothari (1985) Field research procedure and problems: linguistic problems as they impinge on standardised instruments in psychiatric research. Paper presented to a seminar on research, Educational Research Bureau, University of Zambia

Hira, S.K. (1984) Epidemiology of maternal and congenital syphilis in Lusaka and copperbelt provinces of Zambia. Mimeo, Ministry of Health, Lusaka

Hirschfeld, A.H., and R.C. Behan (1963) The accident process: etiological considerations of industrial injuries. *Journal of the American Medical Association, 186*, 113-19

Holt, S., I.C. Stewart, J.M.J. Dixon, R.A. Elton, T.V. Taylor and K. Little (1980) Alcohol and the emergency service patient. *British Medical Journal, 281*, 638-40

Honkanen, R. (1983) The role of alcohol in accidental falls. *Journal of Studies in Alcohol, 44*, 231-45

Jeffery, R. (1979) Deviant patients in casualty departments. *Sociology of Health and Illness, 1*, 90-107

King, M. (1966) *Medical care in developing countries*. Oxford University Press, Oxford

Kobus, H.J. (1980) Breath analysis for control of drunk driving in Zimbabwe Rhodesia. *Central African Journal of Medicine, 26*, 21-7

Korsah, K.G. (1969) A study of mortality rate in the accident service and its relation to methods of transportation to hospital. *East African Medical Journal, 18*, 192-4

Mbaruku, D.M.D. (1980) Motor traffic accidents in Dar-es-Salaam, their effects on mortality. *Dar-es-Salaam Medical Journal, 8*, 16-19

McCabe, E.M.I. (1982) Alcoholism—its emergence in the Black townships of South Africa. *South African Medical Journal, 61*, 881-2

Meade, M.S. (1980) Potential years of life lost in countries of South-east Asia. *Social Science and Medicine, 14*, 277-81

Ministry of Health (1980) *Bulletin of Health Statistics, 2*, Health Planning Unit, Lusaka, Zambia

Moser, J. (1980) *National and sub-national profiles of alcohol use, alcohol-related problems and preventive measures, policies and programmes.* World Health Organization, Geneva

Nair, V.R., and M.D. Khan (1977) A study of accident victims seen at Kitwe Central Hospital, Zambia, January, 1971– December, 1972. *Medical Journal of Zambia, 11*, 11-15

Neame, P.B., and S.M. Joubert (1961) Post-alcoholic hypoglycaemia and toxic hepatitis. *Lancet, 2* (October 21), 893-7

Noak, J.L. (1967) Urban clinics in Lusaka. *Medical Journal of Zambia, 1*, 113-21

Okada, E.E. (1967) Excessive drinking and crime: a survey of selected court cases from Central Province. Mimeo, Research Unit, Lusaka

Otsyula, W. (1974) Problems caused by excessive drinking in Kenya. Proceedings of a Workshop on Alcohol and Drug Dependence of the Association of Psychiatrists in Africa, ICAA Publication, Nairobi, Kenya, pp. 63-6

Owosina, F.A.O. (1981) The traffic scene in Nigeria—an African example. Document prepared for a conference on Traffic Accidents in Developing Countries, Mexico City, November, 1981

Patel, N.S., and G.P. Bhagwat (1977) Road traffic accidents in Lusaka and blood alcohol. *Medical Journal of Zambia, 11*, 46-9

Rittay, D.A.W., and W.M. Castle (1972) Suicides in Rhodesia. *Central African Journal of Medicine, 18*, 97-100

Sarungi, P.M., and A.J. Kaduri (1980) Epidemiological aspects of trauma in children in Dar-es-Salaam. *Dar-es-Salaam Medical Journal, 8*, 4-8

Shaw, L. (1965) The practical use of projective personality tests as accident predictors. *Traffic Safety Research Review, 9*, 2, 34-72

Southall, A.W. (1960) Homicide and suicide among the Alur. In P. Bohannan (ed), *African homicide and suicide.* Princeton University Press, Princeton, pp. 214-29

Swift, C.R. and T. Asuni (1975) *Mental health and disease in Africa: with special reference to Africa south of the Sahara.* Churchill Livingston, Edinburgh

Tongue, E. (1976) Alcohol-related problems in some African countries. *African Journal of Psychiatry, 3*, 351-63

Willcox, P., and M. Gelfand (1976) Spontaneous hypoglycaemia in Rhodesian Africans. *Central African Journal of Medicine, 22*, 57-60

World Health Organization (1976) *The epidemiology of road traffic accidents*. Regional Office for Europe, European Series No. 2, Copenhagen

— (1978) *Medical monitoring of road traffic accidents*. Report on an Ad Hoc Technical Group, Regional Office for Europe, Copenhagen

— (1979) *Road traffic accident statistics*. Report on an Ad Hoc Technical Group, Regional Office for Europe, Copenhagen

— (1981) Major issues in road traffic safety. Document prepared for a conference on road traffic accidents in developing countries, Mexico City, November, 1981, Geneva

4

Alcohol-Related Casualties in Oceania

Sally Casswell

Oceania is an area of considerable geographical fragmentation. It includes 789 island units (Douglas 1969) which are subdivided into the geo-ethnic regions of Melanesia, Micronesia and Polynesia (Figure 4.1). In the west is Papua New Guinea, second largest island in the world and, with a population of 3 million, one of the largest nations in the region. As one travels eastward into the Pacific, the islands are increasingly smaller and geographically more isolated. The region is tropical apart from the one industrialised country, New Zealand.

The geographical isolation, small populations and lack of natural resources have kept many of the island states of Oceania very poor. Western Samoa, for example, is classified with Bangladesh and other 'drastically poor' countries on the basis of its GNP (Rajotte 1980). Some parts of Melanesia and Polynesia, such as Fiji and Tahiti, have relatively well-developed tourist industries but apart from New Zealand the strongest independent economies in the region are those such as Nauru and Papua New Guinea which have mineral resources. The relative affluence of some Polynesian and Micronesian countries reflects their strategic importance to France and the United States. For example, the Republic of Belau, with a population of about 15,000, received $20 million (US) in aid from the US in 1983/1984.

Oceania is clearly a region of considerable diversity. However, one characteristic shared throughout the region is that nowhere, prior to its introduction by Europeans and Asians, was alcohol used by the indigenous people. The history of alcohol's introduction and the development of a pattern of indigenous use varies, depending in part on the origins of the colonising forces. The French in parts of Polynesia appear to have been more permissive in the access to alcohol allowed indigenous

112

Figure 4.1: *The Pacific*

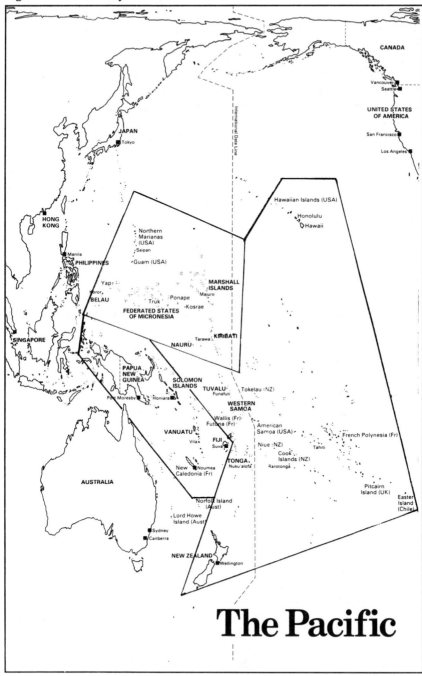

The Pacific

Source: The Middle East Review Co. Ltd. (1984)

people, compared with the approach taken by the Japanese and Americans in Micronesia, and by the Germans, the British and their colonial descendants — Australians, and New Zealanders. In Tahiti (part of French Polynesia) access to alcohol by the indigenous people was legalised in 1920 (Lemert 1964), whereas in areas where the Anglo-Saxon approach prevailed prohibition against alcohol use by indigenous men was commonly not lifted until the early 1960s (Casswell 1985, Hezel 1981). In such countries, access to alcohol became an important political issue tied to the acquisition of independence.

The countries in the region also varied in the extent to which production and use of locally produced 'homebrew' became an integral part of the social and economic scene. In Micronesia a low alcohol content toddy, fermented from coconut milk or yeast, is drunk in some areas. Both here and in parts of Polynesia the widespread production and use of different kinds of homebrew, such as the orange beer of the Cook Islands and *fa'amafu* brewed with imported malt in Western Samoa, can be traced back to European origins. In Melanesia homebrew is apparently less common; in Vanuatu for example, production of 'Jungle Juice' never became widespread, despite encouragement from US servicemen. This may reflect the easier access to commercial alcohol which accompanied the French in the Pacific (the New Hebrides were administered by a joint Anglo-French Condominium) and the traditional use of the indigenous drug, *kava* (piper methysticum).

There is some evidence that an increase in consumption of commercial alcohol in the Polynesian islands of Tokelau (1968-76) was accompanied by an increase in consumption of the local toddy (Stanhope and Prior 1979). However, it appears likely that in most of the countries of the region, including those with developed traditions of non-commercial alcohol use, the association of modernisation and prestige which accompany commercial alcohol currently make it the preferred beverage over homebrew, and in some areas, over the indigenous *kava* (Marshall 1982a, Finau *et al.* 1982).

Alcohol Consumption

Few data are available on the consumption of alcohol in the less developed countries of Oceania. Statistics on the production or importation of commercial alcohol have been obtained for some countries (Figure 4.2). These indicate that, on a per capita basis, estimated consumption of commercially produced absolute alcohol in most of the less developed countries is considerably below that of New Zealand (and of most industrialised countries throughout the world).

Figure 4.2: *Estimated per capita consumption of absolute alcohol in Oceania*

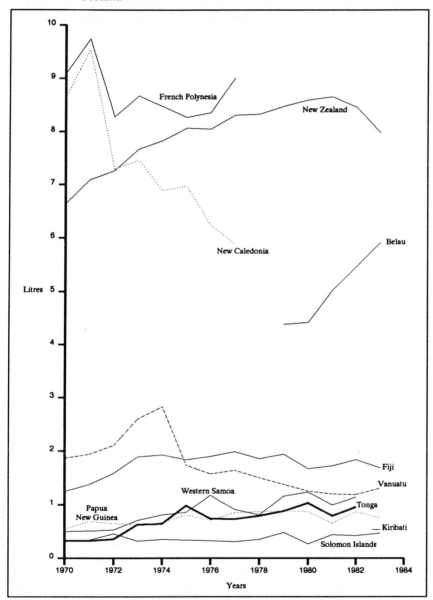

Sources: Various Departments of Statistics, New Zealand, Fiji, Vanuatu,
           Western Samoa, Tonga, Papua New Guinea; *Addiction Research Foundation*
           (1985); and Reports at a regional workshop on national policy and programme
           formulation for the prevention and control of alcohol-related problems (1984).

However, French colonisation has been an obvious influence on *per capita* consumption levels, as the figures for New Caledonia and French Polynesia indicate. Of course these estimates of *per capita* consumption do not exclude the consumption of either tourists or the expatriate population. In French Polynesia, expatriates of European or part-European origin account for 28 per cent of the population and in New Caledonia for 37 per cent. No other countries in the region, apart from New Zealand, had more than 5 per cent European population.

A relationship between affluence and consumption is suggested by the estimated *per capita* consumption levels for the two Micronesian countries for which data are available and also by survey data from Nauru. A nutritional survey of a random sample of Nauruans in the late 1970s revealed an average daily intake of 140 ml of absolute alcohol among males aged 20 to 39 and just over half of this amount for men aged 40 or older (Ringrose and Zimmet 1979). This is higher than the self-reported average daily intake of a random sample of New Zealand males in the same age groups (Casswell 1980).

It is apparent from what little ethnographic and survey data are available that commercial alcohol use is not as widely distributed in the less-developed countries in the region. Its use tends to be more closely confined to adult men, to those living in urban areas and to those involved in the monetary economy (Hezel 1981, Marshall 1982b, Finau *et al.* 1982, Stanhope and Prior 1979, Ringrose and Zimmet 1979, Mahoney 1974).

In many of the less developed countries alcohol is bought mainly for off-premise consumption but drinking is nevertheless primarily a social and public behaviour (in contrast to the family and meal based tradition of the Mediterranean). Drinking occasions tend to be episodic, often linked with pay days and commonly last until all available alcohol has been consumed. The amount drunk varies between individuals and ethnographic data from rural areas of Papua New Guinea show that it depends on a complex set of social, political and economic factors. Drunken comportment has been reported as a frequent outcome of drinking in all areas of the region (Hocking 1970, Lemert 1964, Marshall 1975, Marshall 1982b). Based on ethnographic data, Marshall (1982b) states that, for Papua New Guinea: 'the physical state of inebriation — even to the point of vomiting, losing consciousness and making a public spectacle of oneself — carries no stigma of shame or negative moral evaluation for men in most parts of the country'.

However, in a survey of the perceptions of university students about the effects of drinking, Papua New Guinean students, while agreeing that drinkers drank as fast as possible until there was no more alcohol left, felt that it was a sign of weakness to lose coordination or consciousness (Wilks and Callan, 1984).

One survey of three urban samples in Papua New Guinea has obtained self-reports of the amount of alcohol usually consumed during a drinking session. Among the two employed samples, almost one-fifth reported drinking thirteen or more bottles of beer (170 ml of absolute alcohol) at a session (Marshall 1983). While the samples surveyed were chosen to represent those most likely to be alcohol consumers, these data do indicate that, despite the very low *per capita* consumption levels indicated by production figures, some drinkers in the less developed countries are clearly consuming at levels likely to increase the risk of alcohol-related casualties.

The risk of alcohol-related casualties will, however, be far less widespread in the less developed countries. An illustrative comparison is the distribution of drinking found, from survey data, among the New Zealand population. The proportion who report consuming 100 ml or more of absolute alcohol on a drinking occasion is, similar to the Papua New Guinea sample, one in five, but this is representative of all young male New Zealanders (aged 16 to 24), not of a small selected group. Alcohol-related casualties in this less developed country would therefore, if considered purely in terms of the spread of heavy drinking, be expected to be considerably fewer than in New Zealand.

Cultural Factors Affecting Alcohol-Related Casualties

There are, of course, other factors which are likely to affect the incidence of alcohol-related problems. The exact role alcohol plays in alcohol-related casualties is not well understood or documented (Roizen 1982), but clearly it will be affected by the cultural expectations of alcohol's effect on behaviour (MacAndrew and Edgerton 1969) as well as the less culturally bound physiological effects of the drug.

That drunken comportment is, in part, a matter of learned expectations in the highlands of Papua New Guinea, as elsewhere in Oceania, has been well illustrated by ethnographic observation:

People begin to display drunken comportment almost as soon as they open the first bottle or can of beer. Drinkers talk loudly, sing, laugh and express anger. They make complaints against each other that they may make in everyday life, but they make them more vociferously when drunk. (Sexton 1984)

Similarly, in Micronesia, there is comment on the role of shared expectations influencing drinking and its consequences. One Trukese informant offered an example: 'Suppose I want to take revenge? First I will get drunk. Then I can beat up the man on whom I want revenge. Nobody will say very much because I'm drunk' (Mahoney 1974). In both Papua New

Guinea and Micronesia ethnographers have compared drunken comportment with a dramatic performance (Marshall 1975, Strathern 1982).

Expectations about drunken comportment which are relevant to alcohol-related casualties are certainly not confined to the less developed countries in the region. People's descriptions of the 'effects of a few drinks' reflect their expectations and in New Zealand the cluster of young men most likely to have been suspended from driving and stopped while driving after drinking were twice as likely to describe themselves as feeling aggressive after a few drinks (Perkins 1975).

In most countries alcohol appears to be accepted as 'causing' or allowing disinhibiting changes in behaviour which might, in certain circumstances, increase the risk of casualties. However, it is clear that these changes are always within certain limits (MacAndrew and Edgerton 1969). In a detailed ethnographic study of drinking and its major disruptive effects in Truk, Micronesia, Mac Marshall has demonstrated the shared awareness and acceptance of limits on drunken behaviour:

> Drunks are given *carte blanche* to approach anyone, but they may not attack just anyone. Children and the elderly are absolutely off limits. Although drunks may strike women, they do not actually do so very often. Drunks may chase women, say bad things to them, threaten and frighten them, but they may not beat them up with impunity...Drunks may not physically attack their parents although they may verbally unburden themselves of their aggression and can and do destroy property belonging to their parents...Finally, although drunks may attack adult men, they rarely attack physically. Often they scream out their anger and frustration at an older male. Drunks may attack other young men, of course, and it is among drunken young men that the great majority of physical aggression rises to the surface. (Marshall 1979: p. 122)

Marshall (1979) implies that the individual's own control over his drunken behaviour remains fairly intact. An observer of drunken comportment in Vanuatu, Melanesia, describes customary precautions which are taken prior to intoxication, but which are equally indicative of limits on drunken comportment:

> People expect drunks to fight and their expectations are often realised...Men choose drinking partners carefully. The person they punch should be someone with whom they have no serious dispute...If a previous and serious dispute separates two men they usually are careful not to drink together. If they did, violence could easily get out of hand and become irresolvable by some simple subsequent exchange. (Lindstrom 1982: p. 432)

Despite the existence of limits on drunken comportment, it is obvious from much of the ethnographic data available that drinking in many countries in Oceania is associated with drunkenness and an increase in aggressive behaviour. This is particularly apparent in the behaviour of young men. The exception may be French Polynesia where there appears to be little public drunkenness (Carter 1981, Room 1984).

To the extent that the association between alcohol and aggression is relatively strong in Polynesian, Melanesian and Micronesian cultures, alcohol-related casualties of certain sorts might be greater than would be expected from the estimated *per capita* levels of alcohol consumption.

Alcohol-Related Casualties

Not surprisingly, there are very few data on the role of alcohol in casualties in Oceania, particularly in the less developed countries, and what few data are available describe alcohol use at the time of the serious event, rather than assessing the drinking history of those involved or the experience of casualties among those known to be heavy drinkers (Roizen 1982).

It is obvious that casualties generally make a significant contribution to mortality and morbidity in the less developed countries in Oceania, particularly where the contribution made by infectious disease has been somewhat reduced by socio-economic development (Taylor and Thomas 1985). There is a contrast, for example, between Kiribati and Guam within Micronesia, which differ considerably in their level of modernisation. In Kiribati the prominent causes of mortality in 1980 were infection and respiratory disease, whereas in Guam cardiovascular causes accounted for 30 per cent, neoplasms for 15 per cent and accidents for 11 per cent of mortality.

Similarly, in Nauru accidents and injuries were the most important cause of death and the most significant contributor to years of life lost by adults' premature death—the majority (60 per cent) of accidental deaths involved a motor vehicle (Taylor and Thomas 1985).

In Melanesia, statistics indicate that trauma is an important contributor to morbidity. In both Papua New Guinea (Sinha *et al.* 1981) and Fiji 'accidents, poisoning and violence' featured among the top five causes of admission to hospital and health centres during the late 1970s. However, the contribution is lower than in New Zealand where 14 per cent of hospital admissions in 1982 were so classified. In Fiji (1978-82) and Micronesia (1983) accidents, poisoning and violence accounted for 5 per cent or more of hospital cases.

Traffic Accidents

The roads in the less developed countries in the region are generally narrow and twisting with long flat stretches along the shoreline which invite speed. They have few signs, markings and footpaths and are often in a state of disrepair. The vehicles too tend to be poorly maintained and often overloaded. Not surprisingly, the rate of traffic accidents in the less-developed countries in the region appears to be relatively high. In Papua New Guinea, for example, there was a '400 per cent increase' between 1968 and 1978 and there were thirteen times as many fatal accidents per 10,000 registered vehicles as there were in Britain (Wyatt 1980). The rate in Nauru was similarly relatively high; on the basis of the age-specific mortality from road accidents in Australian males, one would have expected 4.2 deaths in the Nauruan male population (1976-80) — there were, however, 21 (Taylor and Thomas 1985).

Most of the less developed countries in the region do not have the technology in place to allow measurement of the extent of alcohol involvement in traffic accidents, let alone to assess the causal role alcohol plays. (The Republic of Belau in Micronesia is apparently an exception to this, having breath analysis available (Polloi 1984) and Papua New Guinea is probably about to acquire it.)

Papua New Guinea is unique among less developed countries in the region in that some analyses of blood-alcohol levels, obtained at *post mortems*, have been published. Wyatt (1980) examined *post mortem* records, which covered 80 per cent of those dying in road crashes 1975-78. One-third of the dead drivers (N = 19) had BACs of 80 mg/100 ml or greater and the mean level was 212 mg/100 ml. Analysis of an overlapping series of *post mortems* (1976-80) found similar results: half of the dead drivers (N = 29) had a BAC of 80 mg/100 ml or greater and one-third had a BAC below that but which was detectable (Sinha *et al.* 1981). (Both authors comment that the level of alcohol involvement will be underestimated by these analyses because of the time interval between the accident and blood samples being taken.)

These proportions are similar to those found in industrialised countries (Roizen, 1982). A study of fatal accidents in New Zealand in 1977 found an alcohol involvement (in this case defined as a BAC of 50 mg/100 ml) among 39 per cent of all drivers involved and 46 per cent among drivers who were at fault (Bailey 1979).

Between 30 and 40 per cent of the studied traffic accident fatalities in Papua New Guinea were of pedestrians. The shorter time series found that about two-thirds of the male pedestrians killed had BACs of 80 mg/100 ml or over and 62 per cent had a concentration above 120 mg/100 ml (Wyatt 1980) while the 1976-80 series found 90 per cent of pedestrians whose blood-alcohol level was measured were above 80 mg/100 ml and 55 per cent were greater than 150 mg/100 ml (Sinha *et al.* 1981). In the New Zealand analysis, pedestrians aged 15 to 64 had a level of alcohol involvement similar to that of the drivers (54 per cent) (Bailey 1979).

None of the less developed countries in the region, apart from Papua New Guinea, have any estimates of alcohol involvement in fatal traffic accidents. In Nauru the clustering of accidents during weekends and the proportion which involve loss of control or collision with a stationary object, plus anecdotal evidence, suggest significant alcohol involvement in traffic accidents (Taylor and Thomas 1985). In Fiji most accidents similarly occur on Fridays and Saturdays in the afternoon and evenings. The majority of accidents are classified as caused by dangerous driving and only 3 to 4 per cent were classified as caused by the driver being drunk and incapable (Prasad and Mar 1981).

Only in New Zealand is there any information available on alcohol involvement in traffic injury accidents which is based on breath or blood analysis. A survey of injured drivers (N = 461) admitted to the casualty department of a major metropolitan hospital in 1972 (Hart *et al.* 1975) and another of road casualties (N = 1720) admitted to a provincial hospital in 1979 (Bailey 1984) found 25 per cent and 27 per cent respectively of injured drivers had positive blood-alcohol levels and 16 per cent and 19 per cent respectively had BACs of 100 mg/100 ml or more. Both surveys found that drinking drivers were more likely than sober drivers to have been judged responsible for the accident and the larger study found a much higher proportion of single vehicle accidents among injured drinking drivers (Bailey 1984).

Because of difficulties in assigning ethnicity it is impossible to say whether Maoris were disproportionately represented among the injured drivers. It was apparent, however, that the most notable difference between the two ethnic groups was in alcohol involvement. More than double the proportion of injured Maori car drivers had a positive blood-alcohol level compared with the Pakeha (New Zealanders of European origin) (Bailey 1984). It is not known what proportion of the heavy drinking episodes led to drinking-driving behaviour but it is known from survey data that Maori men tend to consume larger quantities during a drinking occasion than do Pakeha men (Casswell 1980).

In several less-developed countries in the region, police estimates (based on smell and speech impairment) of alcohol involvement in traffic accidents are published. These range from 10 per cent of all traffic accidents in Papua New Guinea in 1982, to 45 per cent in the Cook Islands in 1984 (Teariki 1984). In Vanuatu the local epidemiologist estimated that, of the 700 people 15 years and older who were treated at the Vila Central Hospital in 1983, two-thirds had complaints related to alcohol consumption, mainly through auto accidents and fights (Montaville 1984).

Non-Traffic Accidents and Violence

Very little is known about the role of alcohol in either non-traffic accidents or violent behaviour in New Zealand and in the less developed countries in the region. In a study which concentrated on minor head injuries sustained by men in regular employment, Wrightson and Gronwall (1981) found that 18 out of 66 New Zealand men (27 per cent) showed evidence of having previously taken alcohol. However, since none of the 37 who were injured in sporting activities had previously been drinking, the incidence of alcohol involvement in injuries that were caused in other activities was much higher (62 per cent). A recent study of drowning (N = 225) in New Zealand found that, of the accidental drownings, three-quarters of those who died in boating accidents and half of those who drowned after falling in the water had blood-alcohol concentrations above 100 mg/100 ml (Cairns *et al.* 1984).

With regard to accidents generally, a national general population survey revealed that very few respondents (2 per cent) reported drinking prior to work-related accidents and heavier drinkers were not more likely to do so (Casswell, 1980). The survey did not include information concerning accidents at recreation or in the home.

Once again, in less developed countries the only information about alcohol involvement in non-traffic casualties which is based on blood or breath analysis comes from the retrospective analysis of *post mortems* carried out in Papua New Guinea (Sinha *et al.* 1981). The 1976-80 series of *post mortems* discussed earlier included all deaths following trauma (N = 305). Over half of these were road traffic fatalities and the remainder were largely caused by blunt instruments (55 per cent of non-traffic fatalities) and sharp penetrating wounds due to axe or stab wounds (35 per cent). Brawls and domestic fights were the major cause of blunt injuries while sharp penetrating wounds were generally caused during a fight or an attack by unknown assailants. Almost one in five of these trauma fatalities were found to have BACs greater than 80 mg/100 ml (Sinha *et al.* 1981). A study of all presentations to a village clinic in Papua New Guinea also reported that severe lacerations were often alcohol-associated, stemming from fights which arose in drinking groups (Maddocks and Maddocks 1977).

Domestic violence was often cited as an alcohol-related problem in the region and general practitioners in Fiji reported a relatively high level of involvement with this issue (Robinson and Morrisey 1984). In Papua New Guinea a survey of women who were assaulted by their husbands and sought treatment indicated that alcohol had been drunk before the assault in 30 per cent of the cases (Ekeroma 1983).

Perhaps the most useful information in the region, in terms of assessing alcohol's role in casualties, comes from the wealth of ethnographic data available in Papua New Guinea (Marshall 1982b). For example, one study, carried out in the Highlands province of Simbu, reports on the relationship between drinking, disputes including marital disputes and violence. Violence was observed to be more likely during disputes if drinking had taken place: 68 per cent of the disputes when alcohol had been drunk became violent, compared with 28 per cent of the disputes which occurred when no drinking had taken place (Warry, 1982).

In another Highland village, in which one-third of village income from coffee sales is spent on alcohol, the ethnographer reported that fights and accidents were a common part of drinking:

> Unfortunately, a party rarely lasts the night without a fight...Young men have a bad reputation for starting fights when drunk and those older men less prone to fighting sometimes request that members of the younger age group stay away from their parties. All serious intra-village fights resulting in major physical injuries in 1976-1977 occurred during times of drunkenness... Personal injuries increase with drinking. Inebriates are more prone to injure themselves by being badly burned, cutting their feet on open tin cans or on broken bottles or by falling into a drainage ditch. (Grossman 1982: p. 66)

However, it is noted by some writers that violent behaviour is relatively common when drinking is not taking place and some ethnographers are reluctant to claim that aggression, which is at a high level among the sober, is significantly increased during drunkenness. However, even in these cases, the local people believed drunkenness contributed to the violence (Chowning 1982).

In most of the countries, published comments, such as police and other authorities' reports, impute a causal role to alcohol, particularly in relation to violent behaviour. For example, the Tongan Police Report of 1980 commented:

> It is clear from available evidence that intoxicating liquor is a precipitating factor in many criminal offences committed in the Kingdom. Particular offences which are closely associated with the consumption of alcoholic drinks are assault and bodily injury including those causing death, indecent assault and rape. (p. 51)

Further information on the role of alcohol in casualties may be available from analysis of the effects of the prohibitions on alcohol use which have been the response to perceived problems in some areas of the region, particularly those with relatively intact traditional control systems. However, there are few published reports on the results of such prohibitions. Anecdotal information given to the author in Vanuatu suggested that bans on the islands of Ambae and Ambrym have resulted in decreased availability and decreased alcohol-related problems.

However, Piau-Lynch (1982) cautions against acceptance at face value of reports in the local newspaper that during the liquor ban in Simbu province in the Highlands of Papua New Guinea the crime rate dropped to half its usual number. Other data on bans in Micronesia apparently exist (Dale 1978).

In New Zealand casualties were monitored following a reduction in availability caused by a brewery strike (Brown 1978). Information was gathered from two hospitals, police and traffic departments in Auckland during a four week period. There was a significant reduction in the mean weekly numbers of accident and emergency admissions to one hospital (and a non-significant trend at the other hospital), in the number of Friday road traffic accidents and injuries reported by the traffic department and in the weekly number of arrests for drunkenness and other alcohol-related offences made by the police.

Alcohol involvement in crime is clearly a topic of considerable concern in many of the countries of Oceania and police estimates of alcohol involvement in crime are often made. In the Solomons Islands, for example, 'major offences are arising from consumption of liquor' appear to be routinely recorded (offences apparently doubled between 1975 and 1983) (Takonene 1984). The Marshall Islands' public safety record similarly indicates that alcohol-related crimes more than doubled between 1979 and 1982 (Edwards 1984). The Commission of Inquiry into Alcoholic Drink in Papua New Guinea reported that there was a nine-fold increase in total offences in seven years while the population had increased by only one-fifth. There was 'an indication that offences of which drunkenness is an element are becoming a larger proportion...from 13 per cent in 1967/8 to 28.5 per cent in 1970/1' (New Guinea Commission of Inquiry into Alcoholic Drink 1971). More recently a Papua New Guinea Report on Law and Order presented the results of a multiple regression analysis which estimated the relationship between beer consumption and serious assault; 60 per cent of assault cases were attributed to beer consumption and a further 35 per cent of serious assaults were attributed to unemployment (Morgan 1983).

In both Fiji and Kiribati surveys of prison inmates have been carried out. In Fiji (1974-76), over half of all criminals claimed they had been under the influence of alcohol when committing the offence and in Kiribati 90 per cent of offences were reported as alcohol-related (Yeeting 1984).

Suicide

Suicide has received some attention recently in both Micronesia (the Marshall Islands) and in Polynesia (Western Samoa). In both countries, rates of suicide, particularly among young men, have been reported to be relatively very high. While there has been some comment indicating a link with alcohol consumption, this is far from clear (Edwards 1984).

Discussion

There are very few data on alcohol-related casualties in Oceania in either the less developed countries or in the one industrialised country. There is, however, a considerable amount of concern expressed in many of the less developed countries about the role of alcohol and the problems it is perceived to be causing. This public concern appears to be more obvious in Melanesia and Micronesia compared with Polynesia, but it is not known whether that reflects the relative level of alcohol-related problems, the relative level of public concern or merely the relative existence of organs for public discussion accessible to an outsider.

It does appear from the few data available that, as the countries in Oceania have become more modernised and infectious diseases have been brought further under control, mortality and morbidity from accidents and traumatic incidents of various sorts have become more prevalent. It is also apparent that modernisation and relative affluence are linked with the availability of alcohol and the total levels of alcohol consumed. In addition, there is evidence that the accepted pattern of drinking is of high quantities on infrequent occasions and, particularly in Micronesia and Melanesia, that aggression is often associated with drunkenness. This combination of factors makes it likely that alcohol is involved in a significant proportion of casualties in many of the countries. While few data are available, what evidence is available suggests alcohol-related casualties in the Oceanic region, particularly in the less developed countries, would warrant investigation. Such studies would serve the purpose of providing baseline data for future assessment of the effect and changes in *per capita* consumption levels or specific policy changes. In addition, such data are likely to influence policymakers to take alcohol-related casualties into account when policy decisions are made. Given the possibility of considerable increases in alcohol use in the less-developed countries in the region, research in this area could be of considerable value.

References

Addiction Research Foundation (1985) Statistics on alcohol and drug use in Canada and other countries — Volume 1, Statistics on alcohol uses. Addiction Research Foundation, Toronto

Bailey, J.P.M. (1979) *Alcohol involvement in fatal road accidents.* Chemistry Division, Department of Scientific and Industrial Research

— (1984)*The Waikato Hospital road accident survey, Volume 2, analysis and interpretation.* Chemistry Division, Department of Scientific and Industrial Research

Brown, R.A. (1978) Some social consequences of partial prohibition in Auckland, New Zealand. *Drug and Alcohol Dependence, 3,* 377-82

Cairns, F., T. Koelmeyer and I. Smeeton (1984) Deaths from drowning. *New Zealand Medical Journal, 97,* 65-7

Carter, J. (ed) (1981) *Pacific Islands year book.* Pacific Publications, Sydney

Casswell, S. (1980) *Drinking by New Zealanders.* Alcoholic Liquor Advisory Council and Alcohol Research Unit, Wellington

— (1985) Alcohol in Oceania. A study of five countries. Working Paper, Alcohol Research Unit

Chowning, A. (1982) Self-Esteem and drinking in Kove, West New Britain. In M. Marshall (ed), *Through a glass darkly: beer and modernization in Papua New Guinea,* Institute of Applied Social and Economic Research, Papua New Guinea, pp. 365-78

Dale, P.W. (1978) Restriction of alcohol beverage sales in Truk. Effect on hospital emergency room visits. Manuscript distributed by Trust Territories Mental Health Branch, Saipan

Douglas, G. (1969) Check list of Pacific Oceania islands. *Micronesia, 5,* 327-464

Edwards, R.N. (1984) Country profile on Marshall Islands. Presented to the World Health Organization Workshop on Prevention and Control of Alcohol-Related problems, Auckland, New Zealand

Ekeroma, A. (1983) Sorry plight of the beaten wives. *The Times* (Sept 30), p. 11

Finau, S.A., J.M. Stanhope and I.A.M. Prior (1982) Kava, alcohol and tobacco consumption among Tongans with urbanization. *Social Science and Medicine, 16,* 35-41

Grossman, L. (1982) Beer drinking and subsistence production in a highland village. In M. Marshall (ed), *Through a glass darkly: beer and modernization in Papua New Guinea,* Institute of Applied Social and Economic Research, Papua New Guinea, pp. 59-72

Hart, D.N.J., P.W. Cotter and W.A.A.G. Macbeth (1975) Christchurch traffic trauma survey part 1, blood alcohol analysis. *New Zealand Medical Journal, 81,* 505-7

Hezel, F.X. (1981) Youth drinking in Micronesia. A report on the Working Seminar on Alcohol Use and Abuse Among Micronesian Youth held in Kolonia, Ponape (November), 21-2

Hocking, R.B. (1970) Problems arising from alcohol in the New Hebrides. *The Medical Journal of Australia, 14* (November), 908-10

Holmes, M. (1976) This is the world's richest nation — all of it. *National Geographic, 150*, 344-53

Lemert, E.M. (1964) Forms and pathology of drinking in three Polynesian societies. *American Anthropologist, 66*, 361-74

Lindstrom, M. (1982) Grog blong yumi: alcohol and kava on Tama, Vanuatu. In M. Marshall (ed), *Through a glass darkly: beer and modernization in Papua New Guinea*, Institute of Applied Social and Economic Research, Papua New Guinea, pp. 421-32

MacAndrew, C., and R.B. Edgerton (1969) *Drunken comportment, a social explanation*, Aldine Publishing Co., Chicago

Maddocks, D.L. and I. Maddocks (1977) The health of young adults in Pari Village. *Papua New Guinea Medical Journal, 20*, 110-116

Mahoney, F.B. (1974) Social and cultural factors relating to the cause and control of alcohol abuse among Micronesian youth. Prepared for the Government of the Trust Territory under contract with James R. Leonard Assn, Inc., Trust Territory of the Pacific, Saipan

Marshall, M. (1975) The politics of prohibition on Naumoluk Atoll. *Journal of Studies on Alcohol, 36*, 597-610

— (1979) *Weekend warriors, alcohol in Micronesian culture*. Mayfield Publishing Company, California

— (1982a) A macrosociological view of alcohol 1958-1980. In M. Marshall (ed), *Through a glass darkly: beer and modernization in Papua New Guinea*, Institute of Applied and Social and Economic Research, Papua New Guinea, pp. 15-36

— (1982b) Twenty years after deprohibition (Introduction). In M. Marshall (ed.), *Through a glass darkly: beer and modernization in Papua New Guinea*, Institute of Applied Social and Economic Research, Papua New Guinea, pp. 3-13

— (1983) Patterns of alcohol use in Port Moresby, Papua New Guinea: a quantity frequency survey. Paper presented to a symposium on Alcohol Use and Abuse: Meanings and Context, Vancouver

The Middle East Review Co. Ltd. (1984) *The Pacific Business Guide*. World of Information, Essex, England

Montaville, B. (1984) Epidemiologist. Personal correspondence, Port Vila, Vanuatu

Morgan, L.R. (ed) (1983) Report of the Committee to Review Policy and Administration on Land, Law and Order. Department of Provincial Affairs, Port Moresby

Papua New Guinea Commission of Inquiry into Alcoholic Drink (1971) *Report of the Commission.* Pat Moresby, Government Printer

Perkins, W.A. (1975) The 1975 drinking-driving publicity campaign. Traffic Research Report No 24, Traffic Research Section, Road Transport Division, Ministry of Transport, Wellington

Piau-Lynch, A. (1982) The Simbu liquor ban of 1980-81. In M. Marshall (ed), *Through a glass darkly: beer and modernization in Papua New Guinea*, Institute of Applied Social and Economic Research, Papua New Guinea, pp. 119-29

Polloi, A.H. (1984) Country profile on Palau. Presented to the World Health Organization Workshop on Prevention and Control of Alcohol-Related Problems, Auckland, New Zealand

Prasad, J., and S.W. Mar (1981) Road traffic accidents in the Western Division. *Fiji Medical Journal, August/September,* 129-133

Rajotte, F. (1980) Tourism impact in the Pacific. In *Pacific tourism: as islanders see it,* USP

Ringrose, H. and P. Zimmet (1979) Nutrient intakes in an urbanized Micronesian population with a high diabetes prevalence. *American Journal of Clinical Nutrition, 32,* 1334-41

Robinson, D. and M. Morrisey (1984) The management of alcohol-related problems in general practice. A summary of basic data from fourteen centres, Addiction Research Centre, University of Hull, England

Roizen, J. (1982) Estimating alcohol involvement in serious events. *Alcohol Consumption and Related Problems, 82,*179-219

Room, R. (1984) Observations on alcohol in French Polynesia. *Drinking and Drug Practices Surveyor, 19,* 66-9

Sexton, L.D. (1984) Social and economic impact of the colonial introduction of alcohol into Highland Papua New Guinea. Paper presented at the Conference on the Social History of Alcohol, Berkeley, California, January, 1984

Sinha, S.N., S.K. Sengupta and R.C. Purohit (1981) A five year review of deaths following trauma. *Papua New Guinea Medical Journal, 24,* 222-8

Stanhope, J.M. and I.A.M. Prior (1979) The Tokelau Island migrant study: alcohol consumption in two environments. *New Zealand Medical Journal, 90,* 419-21

Strathern, A. (1982) The scraping gift: alcohol consumption in Mount Hagen. In M. Marshall (ed), *Through a glass darkly: beer and modernization in Papua New Guinea*, Institute of Applied Social and Economic Research, Papua New Guinea, pp. 139-53

Takonene, Z. (1984) Country profile on Solomon Islands. Presented to the World Health Organization Workshop on Prevention and Control of Alcohol-Related Problems, Auckland, New Zealand

Taylor, R. and K. Thomas (1985) Mortality patterns in the modernized Pacific island nation of Nauru. *American Journal of Public Health, 75,* 149-55

Teariki, M.M. (1984) Country profile on the Cook Islands. Presented to the World Health Organization Workshop on Prevention and Control of Alcohol-Related Problems, Auckland, New Zealand

Warry, W. (1982) Bia and bisnis: The use of beer in *chuave* ceremonies. In M. Marshall (ed), *Through a glass darkly: beer and modernization in Papua New Guinea,* Institute of Applied Social and Economic Research, Papua New Guinea, pp. 83-103

Wilks, J. and V.J. Callan (1984) Alcohol-related stereotypes and attitudes: teenagers in Australia, Papua New Guinea and the United States. *Journal of Drug Addiction, 14,* 119-32

Wrightson, P. and D. Gronwall (1981) Time off work and symptoms after minor head injury. *Injury, 12,* 445-54

Wyatt, G.B. (1980) The epidemiology of road accidents in Papua New Guinea. *Papua New Guinea Medical Journal, 23,* 60-5

Yeeting, D. (1984) Country profile on Kiribati. Presented to the World Health Organization Workshop on Prevention and Control of Alcohol-Related Problems, Auckland, New Zealand

Section II:

CONCEPTUAL ISSUES AND METHODS

5

Drinking, Alcohol Availability and Injuries: A Systems Model of Complex Relationships

Harold D. Holder

Injuries are the concurrent result of many factors including human behaviour (or misbehaviour) and the environment. Any consideration of injuries must be prepared to deal with complexity, particularly if we seek to prevent injuries or reduce their likelihood of occurrence.

There are many types of injuries; each has its unique configuration of contributing factors which is actually a network of factors linked together in some fashion. Injury reduction and prevention become more problematic when we introduce drinking. The ingestion of alcohol can alter behaviour. In fact the 'high' of alcohol is one of its properties which gives it social value. Alcohol in a social setting can relax people, increase interaction and contribute to positive experiences. However, alcohol also alters motor skills, reaction time and judgement (see Clayton 1980, Allen and Schwartz 1978, Moskowitz and Burns 1971, Sutton 1983). Alcohol can increase our risk of injury to ourselves, to others and from others (Fell 1983, Malin *et al.* 1982, Owens *et al.* 1983, MacArthur and Moore 1975, Haberman and Baden 1978).

Estimates of the level of alcohol involvement in injury ranges from 50 per cent of fatal auto crashes (US Department of Transportation 1984), up to 38 per cent for fatal recreational accidents and 10 to 25 per cent for home accidents (Centers for Disease Control 1983, Lang and Mueller 1976, Levine and Radford 1977, Planek 1982). In other words, we cannot ignore the substantial contribution of drinking to increased risk of injury.

While the potential contribution of alcohol to accidents and injuries, as well as to violent crime, has been noted, we lack a systematic discussion of this relationship. Both the public and scientific community have tended to oversimplify the complex interaction of drinking and injuries.

Often we make unwarranted conclusions from spurious correlation – that is, things are happening together in time but they may be actually unrelated or related in a fashion not immediately obvious.

For example, consider a newspaper article in *The Toronto Sun* (August 12, 1985: 14), which was entitled 'A-G's Beer Outlet Stand Challenged'. The article noted that Provincial Attorney General Mr. Ian Scott had cited a study in Quebec that showed the number of impaired driving cases had decreased since the introduction of wine in the corner grocery stores. Scott was reported as saying, 'There is...a connection between impaired driving and going out to get it. And if you just walk down to the corner, it's different than if you have to drive across town.' Given the amount of alcohol involvement in auto crashes following drinking in public establishments, it is unlikely that increased grocery store purchases of wine for private consumption would alone reduce traffic crashes. Many other factors, including employment and disposable income, could have a greater impact.

Much of our alcohol-related injury research and prevention has tended to deal with drinking and injury primarily as an individual-based problem. While there is no question of the importance of individual differences and personal drinking behaviour, alcoholic beverages and their social and economic roles in modern society are often overlooked.

My objective in this paper is to present the alcohol and injury relationship as a larger systems problem. In this manner, the significant role and contributions of other parts of the total system can become more relevant to research and prevention policy. My intent is to outline a conceptual framework for discussion and to integrate some of what we know about the relationship of injury and drinking and identify areas of research of importance to improved understanding.

Need for a Systems Perspective

Awareness of the complexity of factors surrounding injuries is an essential first step toward better research and better prevention programming; improved understanding of the system which includes alcohol and injuries is equally essential. We are both participants and observers in this system. Our observations, values and perspectives are not independent of our participation. As Pogo (the cartoon character) once said, 'We have met the enemy and he is us.'

Epistemologically, one does not discover 'reality' but rather one develops and adopts a theory or model which provides understanding of or a means to organise one's experience. Too often we use statistical methods and existing data (measurements) as though they are independent of the conceptualisation (model) on which they are based.

Relationship of Drinking and Injuries

Most of our research evidence to date suggests a strong association (correlation) between alcohol consumption and many non-traffic injuries. This supports our basic model of drinking as a contributor to increased risk of injury — not just for alcoholics and other heavy chronic drinkers — but potentially for any drinker.

While drinking and many injuries are largely independent of one another, a significant proportion of injuries are connected to alcohol use. This relationship can simplistically be represented in Figure 5.1.

Figure 5.1: *Injury risk increased by alcohol consumption*

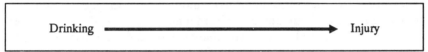

In this figure and in subsequent figures, the lines are used to illustrate contribution or relationship (not single causation). Here the drawing makes the point that drinking contributes to (increases the risk of) injury.

This simple relationship obscures the complex system in which alcohol and injury are a part. Consider the following propositions:

1. Alcohol use, its misuse and resulting injuries are part of a complex system. This system is dynamic (changing over time) and non-linear in nature. Because it is non-linear and dynamic, I suggest that linear descriptive statistics may have limited utility in understanding this system.

2. The system is made up of multiple feedback loops, and as such the identification of purely 'independent' and 'dependent' variables is problematic. For example, if we have variables A, B, C and D in a system such that A can affect B (along with variables C and D) and B in turn can later affect A (i.e. A is in a feedback loop with B), what then are the true 'independent' variables?

3. The 'systemness' of the multiple relationships between alcohol use and injury make it difficult to isolate a single and specific causality. Someone (on the average) who drinks to a BAC level greater than 10 mg/ 100 ml incurs greater incidence of non-traffic accidents (such as falls). These falls are also the resulting interaction of a person's age and gender, the hazard of a person's physical environment, such as stairs or steps at home, and the type of work he or she does, e.g. clerk versus heavy equipment operator. The social acceptance of drinking, both at home and at work, as well as the proximity and/or convenience of alcohol also contributes to the frequency and quantity

per occasion which in turn contributes to the greater risk of accidents. In short, in such a network of variables, one is not able to singularly isolate the amount of individual drinking from other physical and social variables.

If we employ a systems perspective in examining any causal relationships between alcohol and casualties, we place a greater conceptual demand on our research and prevention policy. We are required to make more explicit the postulated (hypothesised) relationships which exist. It also establishes a greater requirement for careful and appropriate use of aggregate measurements.

As systems are complex and time varying, we must make better use of time-series data and of longitudinal studies. Interestingly, a major confounding feature of current statistical techniques for analysing time-series data is auto-correlation or the tendency of single observations to be dependent upon other observations. From a systems perspective, it is exactly this time dependency (as a reflection of the interaction of system variables over time) which reflects the complex network that surrounds and unites drinking to aggregate levels of alcohol-related injuries.

Non-traffic injuries are related to risk activities (in addition to drinking), the conditions of the environment in which the activity occurs and equipment involved such as snowmobiles, power boats or snow and water skis. In like manner, traffic injuries, whether as driver, passenger or pedestrian, are related to driving behaviour, the condition of the vehicle (road worthiness), the use of seat belts and driving conditions including other traffic as well as the weather. Given these factors, drinking can increase the risk of injury. This is illustrated in Figure 5.2.

Alcohol, its use and misuse are not independent of its availability (Figure 5.3). While such a relationship may appear to be self-evident to

Figure 5.2: *Relationship of drinking to casualty outcomes*

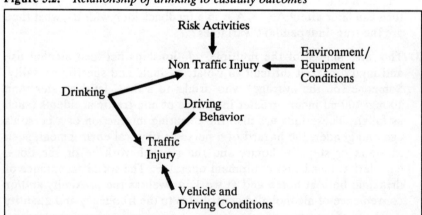

some, the relationship between availability and misuse of alcohol has been a point of some considerable debate in the past 15 or so years (Bruun *et al.* 1975, Parker and Harman 1978 and 1980, Schmidt and Popham 1978 and 1980, Rush *et al.* 1986). Following the repeal of Prohibition in the United States, the regulations on alcohol availability were gradually relaxed. Only individuals who chronically and addictively misused alcohol were targeted for prevention or treatment, not the context in which alcohol was promoted, sold or used. Over the years following the repeal, major prevention emphases in America in addressing alcohol abuse have been to identify and treat alcoholics.

Figure 5.3: *Relationship of drinking to availability*

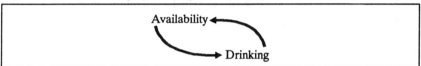

During the past decade, public awareness of alcohol-related problems has gradually increased and a renewed interest in the role of alcohol availability in alcohol misuse and in alcohol-related problems, such as injuries, has occurred. This new perspective includes not only individual addiction but also the destructive use of alcohol by a much greater part of the American population.

This perspective is concerned with alcohol abuse as a problem of public health and welfare. Notable characteristics of this public health perspective include the following views or beliefs.

1. Alcohol abuse is the destructive use of alcoholic beverages in any situation by anyone. Therefore, alcohol abuse includes not only drinking by those unfortunate individuals who, because of their social, emotional or genetic heritage, use alcohol compulsively and without control, i.e. alcoholics, but any use of alcohol by any other drinker that is destructive to or endangers the drinker and others.

2. Destructive misuse of alcohol directly or indirectly affects all citizens, i.e. it is a public health problem.

3. Public health problems are not limited to the individual choices of selected members of society but must be considered as a part of the social system in which we all live and work.

4. Reducing alcohol-related problems requires intervention both in individual lives and in the environment.

5. Prevention must include not only public information and education but also limits on the availability of alcoholic beverages. Limits can be

based on appropriate minimum age of purchase, price of alcoholic beverages relative to the other goods and services, appropriate locations of beverage outlets and their hours of sale, and law enforcement against dangerous alcohol use, such as drinking and driving.

6. Alcoholic beverages are high-risk beverages if used inappropriately. They are not harmless, they are not like soft drinks or juice and they are not just another form of food. As mood altering beverages, they require unique attention on the behalf of the public's well-being and safety.

Regulation and Promotion of Alcoholic Beverages as Commercial Products

The availability of alcoholic beverages is a function of both production and regulation as illustrated in Figure 5.4. In the United States, both federal and state regulations govern production. The specific volume of alcoholic beverages produced is carefully monitored and each ounce is registered and accounted for in production.

Figure 5.4: *Relationship of drinking to regulation and production*

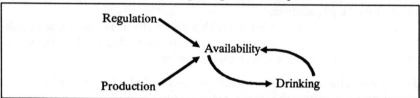

Once alcoholic beverages are shipped for wholesale and retail distribution, they are carefully inventoried, often in government-controlled warehouses for distribution and taxation, before entering the retail market. The retail market is controlled by government restrictions through licensing of two kinds of outlets: those for on-premise drinking and those that sell only for consumption elsewhere (off-premise). In the case of 17 states, the state alcohol beverage commission operates state off-premise stores for bottle sales of distilled spirits. The state controls the number, location and suitability of ownership of privately owned outlets.

A minimum age of purchase for alcoholic beverages exists in all 50 states; most states (and some localities if permitted by state) regulate hours and days of sale as well. Retail prices are affected by state regulation of retail sale and by federal, state and local taxes. Unlike another family of products which are universally used and sometimes also misused — motor vehicles — no special training and certification (licensing) is required to use the product. No special enforcement of alcohol misuse exists except when drinking takes place in conjunction with other behaviour such as driving an automobile, displaying public drunkenness or committing a crime. Absences from work or on-the-job accidents resulting from drinking are not uniformly policed or regulated. Increased costs for medical care resulting from excessive alcohol use are distributed to abstainers and moderate users through medical care charges and health insurance premiums. On the other hand, higher-risk drivers such as those with traffic violations or young drivers are required to pay higher automobile insurance premiums.

No laws govern frequency or quantity of consumption for such high-risk activities as swimming, boating or operating heavy machinery. Few if any public school curricula train students about appropriate and safe consumption. In short, in terms of the potential high-risk use of alcoholic beverages, alcohol may be actually less regulated than other potentially dangerous and misused products.

Often overlooked in discussions about regulating alcoholic beverages is that no commercially available, over-the-counter product has so direct an impact on the biochemistry of the body or the functioning and awareness of individuals. Even at low levels of consumption, ethanol (the intoxicating ingredient in alcoholic beverages) affects functioning (Clayton 1980, McNamee *et al.* 1980, Tong *et al.* 1980). While legal limits of blood-alcohol concentration have been established for arrest and conviction for 'driving under the influence' (DUI) while operating a motor vehicle, impaired or small losses of awareness and reflex occur with much lower levels of alcohol, particularly in young drivers (Fell 1982, Perrine *et al.* 1971).

We do not drink alcohol at levels below the legal DUI limit with no impact on motor skills and then suddenly become seriously impaired at the legal limit. The legal limit is a statutory and judicial compromise at establishing a level of blood-alcohol concentration at which anyone can be considered legally impaired and accountable. A curve which describes impairment for each gender and body weight would be a continuous (but not necessarily linear) line beginning with small amounts of alcohol in the blood and progressing upward as more and more alcohol is absorbed.

Some desirable impairment is actually obtained by drinking. For example, loss of self-consciousness and inhibition often makes a social gathering more enjoyable. But the same, relaxed person operating a power boat can use bad judgement, lack quick enough response in a risky situation and cause a crash and personal injury.

Problems with Regulation for the Alcoholic Beverage Industry

The so-called 'alcoholic beverage industry' is not a unified, monolithic corporate structure but rather a loosely associated collection of private producers, distributors and retail sellers. Three types of alcoholic beverages, i.e. wine, beer and distilled spirits, are competitive products whose makers do not always share common interests and concerns. The term 'alcoholic beverage industry' refers to the total collection of privately owned corporations, companies and small enterprises concerned with producing, distributing and selling alcoholic beverages. While we refer to this collection with an overarching label 'alcoholic beverage industry', we must recognise the diversity and competitiveness of those who make up the industry.

The alcoholic beverage industry, like other private industries, seeks profit. Therefore, maximising profit by increasing sales and lowering production costs is a major objective. The major marketing problem for the beverage industry is that about 50 per cent of alcoholic beverage volume is consumed by 5 per cent of the drinking population (Moore and Gerstein 1981: 29). In the United States, the number of abstainers has remained relatively constant in the 1970s at about 33 to 35 per cent (Johnson *et al.* 1977, Clark and Midanik 1980), yet *per capita* consumption of alcohol has risen. Therefore, increased consumption by existing drinkers and, in particular, increased use by the heaviest consumers would seem to account for most of this increase. Yet these heavy, regular consumers are the population most at risk for alcohol-related problems for themselves, their families, their employers and their communities.

Drinking and Social and Economic Factors

The quantity and frequency of drinking are related to a number of other factors (in addition to availability and promotion), including the price of alcoholic beverages and the disposable income to purchase, as well as cultural values and norms which govern drinking behaviour. This is illustrated in Figure 5.5 which adds these factors to the network of variables previously mentioned.

Since price and income are generally studied together in econometric studies of demand, the research literature on these two factors is essentially the same. While researchers do not have a consensus on the precise level of price sensitivity, they do agree that alcoholic beverage consumption does respond to changes in retail price. The recent research of Ornstein and Hanssens (1983), Cook (1981), Cook and Tauchen (1982), Levy and Sheflin (1983), and Hoadley, Fuchs and Holder (1984) all confirm the inverse relationship between price and consumption. Grossman,

Coate and Arluck (1984) determined the differential price sensitivity of consumption by young people (16 to 21 years old) for all beverages. For beer, the alcoholic beverage of preference for the young, they estimated that a 10 per cent increase in beer price will result in a 14.8 per cent decrease in the number of youthful heavy beer drinkers (three to five drinks per day). Their research indicated that a 30 per cent increase in distilled spirits prices is estimated to lead to a 27.3 per cent decline in the number of youthful heavy liquor drinkers (three to five drinks of liquor per day).

Figure 5.5: *Relationship of drinking to larger social and economic system*

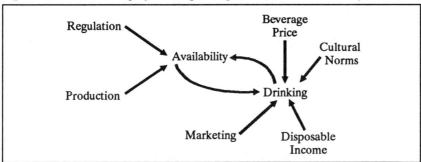

Just as the price of alcoholic beverages relative to other goods is an important factor in demand, so is the availability of income to purchase them. Ornstein and Hanssens (1981) and Cook and Tauchen (1982) documented the impact of disposable income on demand for alcoholic beverages and Cook (1981) concluded that the economic factors of price and income are among the important determinants of demand for alcoholic beverages.

Cultural norms are illustrated in our conceptual model as an aggregate factor which seeks to represent the contribution of changes in regional, religious and other norms inhibiting drinking, as well as the movement toward mass culture and increased cosmopolitanism and thus their impact on drinking behaviour. The importance of social norms concerning drinking have been documented by Pittman and Snyder (1962), Wilkinson (1970), Rabow and Watts (1982) and Parker (1984). Brenner (1975) suggested that social instability can function as an intervening variable to explain the relationship between increased consumption and increased alcohol-related problems.

Tying It All Together: The Prevention of Alcohol-Related Injuries

To this point, I have noted some of the parts and relationships which surround drinking and which link drinking to injuries. In other words, I have sought to illustrate parts of the system. An overall system as the collection of all the elements I have outlined is shown in Figure 5.6. It is important to note that the alcohol availability sub-system is not designed to increase injuries. It is a by-product of the total system. The individual drinker and his or her decision about the amount of and the setting for alcohol consumption are parts of the system but insufficient to understand the totality.

Figure 5.6: *Relationship of drinking, social and economic factors and casualty outcomes*

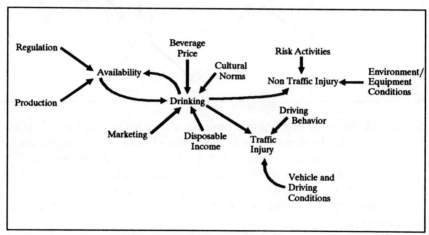

As Ackoff (1974) has observed:

> ...a set of elements that forms a system always has some characteristics, or can display some behaviour, that none of its parts of subgroups can. *A system is more than the sum of its parts.* A human being, for example, can write or run, but none of its parts can. (p. 13)

Many of our efforts to reduce drinking-related injuries and to conduct research have been limited to the individual drinker and his or her behaviour. While this perspective is essential, it is not complete. It fails to take into account the larger system in which alcohol use and misuse are a part. Most previous prevention efforts by the government and by industry have focused on individual decisions to get consumers to moderate their use of alcohol.

These efforts primarily use the mass media; they have heightened public awareness but have not had much success in reducing heavy, high-risk drinking or alcohol-related problems (Wallack and Barrows 1983, Blane and Hewitt 1977, Cameron 1979). However, more optimistic proposals for the potential for well-designed public education as a means to reduce alcohol misuse are provided by Cellucci (1984) and Hochheimer (1981). Nevertheless, the lack of success via mass communications alone is not surprising. Alcohol use is part of a social system in which an individual's actions are influenced by his or her own cultural and physiological heritage as well as by the promotion, availability and price of alcoholic beverages.

For example, it is difficult for a teenage alcohol education program to be effective while beer (the beverage of choice of adolescents and young adults) is frequently and effectively marketed to the young, is cheap (in many areas beer is as inexpensive as carbonated drinks) and is readily and widely available. It is also difficult for education to moderate teenage drinking when drinking is seen as an adult behaviour which the young eagerly seek as a part of growing up. In addition, adult misuse of alcohol sets an inappropriate example for the young. As if to counter teenage alcohol-education programs, adult drinking behaviour can send an indirect message to teenagers from adults, 'Do as I say, not as I do.' In fact, many messages, hidden as well as overt, from our adult-controlled society encourage consumption and characterise drinking as an essential part of routine living.

Preventive approaches to alcohol-related injuries must necessarily broaden the view of injuries and drinking to the community and more general systems. Research and policy objectives should be to sweep in more and more variables, as complexity will increase rather than reduce variables. The field of prevention is clearly moving along these lines. Prevention agendas have moved from the individual to the family and the community and now encompass broader regulatory and legal, as well as social and cultural variables.

Summary

The systems framework enables us to understand how a multi-faceted approach to the prevention of drinking-related injuries can have complementary and interactive effects. With such a systems model we can understand how (and account for) factors like increased disposable income, which is outside the control of prevention efforts, can increase consumption of alcoholic beverages and potentially increase drinking-related injuries both in traffic and in other activities.

If we fail to understand complex systems in which drinking-related injuries are a part, we are most likely to treat symptoms not the causes of problems. Our personal experience with simple stimulus-response relationships may lead us to select the wrong approaches. As Forrester (1969) has pointed out, complex systems, such as the one illustrated here, behave quite differently from simple systems and, therefore, are quite counter-intuitive.

The primary purpose of this paper has been to outline how drinking, alcohol availability and injuries are linked together in a complex system. With this understanding, it is essential that we consider the total system in identifying needed areas of research and potential approaches to prevention.

Beyond our scientific interest, we are concerned about alcohol and injuries as an issue of public health and welfare. We have at least two challenges in attempting to understand the relationship of alcohol to problems such as accidents and injuries, suicides and violent crimes. They are:

1. Documentation: We need to increase scientific and public understanding of the role of alcohol use in injuries in general, as well as specific jurisdictions or cultures. This requires better conceptual models of drinking and alcohol misuse than we currently have and thus better means to measure the relationships between consumption and the risk of casualty.

2. Prevention or problem reduction: We need better models in order to identify appropriate preventive interventions. All preventive efforts, whether educational or environmental, occur in complex systems. As a result of system variables of which we may have no awareness, prevention programs can achieve no significant problem reduction and/or they can be counter-intuitive, i.e. produce unexpected and undesirable results.

Equipment, physical environment and individual skill are important considerations in efforts to reduce injury. However, a comprehensive prevention program to reduce alcohol-related injuries must include a concern about alcohol availability including demand, production and promotion; social and economic factors such as price; cultural values and norms surrounding the use and misuse of alcohol; and the increased risk of injury associated with an individual's drinking.

References

Ackoff, R. (1974) *Redesigning the future*. John Wiley and Sons, New York

Allen, R.W. and S.H. Schwartz (1978) The effects of alcohol on the driver's decision-making behavior. *Proceedings of the Human Factors Society*, 22nd Annual Meeting, NIDA, Rockville, MD

Blane, H.T. and E. Hewitt (1977) *Mass media, public education and alcohol: a state of the art review*. Prepared for the National Institute of Alcohol Abuse and Alcoholism under purchase order NIA-76-12

Brenner, H.M. (1975) Trends in alcohol consumption and associated illnesses: some effects of economic changes. *American Journal of Public Health, 65*, 1279-92

Bruun, K., G. Edwards, M. Lumio, K. Mäkelä, L. Pan, R.E. Popham, R. Room, W. Schmidt, O-J. Skog, P. Sulkunen and E. Österberg (1975) *Alcohol control policies in public health perspective*. Volume 25, Finnish Foundation for Alcohol Studies, Helsinki

Cameron, T. (1979) The impact of drinking-driving countermeasures: a review of the literature. *Contemporary Drug Problems, 8*, 495-565

Cellucci, T. (1984) The prevention of alcohol problems: conceptual and methodological issues. In P.M. Miller and T.D. Nirenberg (eds), *Prevention of alcohol abuse*. Plenum Press, New York, pp. 15-54

Centers for Disease Control (1983) Perspectives in disease prevention and health promotion: alcohol as a risk factor for injuries – U.S. In *US Morbidity and Mortality Weekly Report. Vol. 32, No. 5*. DHHS Publ. No. 83-8017, Superintendent of Documents, U.S. Government Printing Office, Washington, DC

Clark, W.B. and L. Midanik (1980) Results of the 1979 national survey. Social Research Group, University of California at Berkeley, Report to the National Institute on Alcohol Abuse and Alcoholism

Clayton, A.B. (1980) Effects of alcohol on driving skills. In M. Sandler (ed), *Psychopharmacology of alcohol*, Raven Press, New York, pp. 73-8

Cook, P.J. (1981) The effect of liquor taxes on drinking, cirrhosis and auto fatalities. In M. Moore and D. Gerstein (eds), *Alcohol and public policy: beyond the shadow of prohibition*, National Academy of Sciences, Washington, DC, pp. 255-85

Cook, P.J. and G. Tauchen (1982) The effect of liquor taxes on heavy drinking. *Bell Journal of Economics, 13*, 379-90

Fell J.C. (1982) *Alcohol involvement in traffic accidents: recent estimates from the National Center for Statistics and Analyses*. National Highway Traffic Safety Administration, Technical Report No. DOT HS-806 269, Washington, DC

— (1983) *Tracking the alcohol involvement problem in US highway crashes*. DOT National Center for Statistics and Analysis. DOT No.

HS 806-489, Superintendent of Documents, US Government Printing Office, Washington, DC

Forrester, J.W. (1969) *Urban dynamics.* MIT Press, Cambridge, MA

Grossman, M., D. Coate and G. Arluck (1984) Price sensitivity of alcoholic beverages in the United States: youth alcohol consumption. In H.D. Holder (ed), *Control issues in alcohol abuse prevention: Strategies for states and communities.* JAI Press, Greenwich, Conn. pp. 169-98

Haberman, P.W. and M.M. Baden (1978) *Alcohol, other drugs and violent death.* Oxford University Press, New York

Hoadley, J.F., B.C. Fuchs and H.D. Holder (1984) The effect of alcohol beverage restrictions on consumption: a 25-year longitudinal analysis. *American Journal of Drug and Alcohol Abuse, 10,* 375-401

Hochheimer, J.L. (1981) Reducing alcohol abuse: a critical review of educational strategies. In M. Moore and D. Gerstein (eds), *Alcohol and public policy: beyond the shadow of prohibition.* National Academy Press, Washington, DC, pp. 286-335

Johnson, P., D.J. Armor, S. Polich and H. Stambul (1977) *U.S. adult drinking practices: time trends, social correlates and sex roles.* Prepared for NIAAA, US Dept. of Commerce, National Technical Information Service, Pub. #ADM-281-76-0020, Washington, DC

Lang, G.E. and R.G. Mueller (1976) Ethanol levels in burn patients. *Wisconsin Medical Journal, 75,* S5-S6

Levine, M.S. and E.P. Radford (1977) Fire victims: medical outcomes and demographic characteristics. *American Journal of Public Health, 67,* 1077-80

Levy, D. and N. Sheflin (1983) New evidence on controlling alcohol use through price. *Journal of Studies on Alcohol, 44,* 929-37

MacArthur, J.D. and F.D. Moore (1975) Epidemiology of burns: The burn-prone patient. *Journal of the American Medical Association, 231,* 3, 259-63

Malin, H.J., J. Trumble, C.T. Kaelber and B. Lubran (1982) Alcohol-related highway fatalities among young drivers. *US Morbidity and Mortality and Weekly Report, 31,* 641-4

McNamee, J.E., J.E. Tong and D.J. Piggins (1980) Effects of alcohol and velocity perception: stimulus velocity and change in performance over time. *Perceptual and Motor Skills, 51,* 779-85

Mitroff, I. and F. Sagasti (1983) Epistemology as general systems theory: an approach to the design of complex decision-making experiments. *Philosophy of the Social Sciences, 3,* 117-34

Moore, M.H. and D.R. Gerstein (eds) (1981) *Alcohol and public policy: beyond the shadow of prohibition.* National Academy Press, Washington, DC

Moskowitz, H. and M. Burns (1971) Effects of alcohol on response in the psychological refractory period. *Quarterly Journal of Studies on Alcohol, 32,* 782-90

Ornstein, S.I. and D.M. Hanssens (1981) Alcohol control laws, consumer welfare, and the demand for distilled spirits and beer. Working paper series #102, Graduate School of Management, University of California at Los Angeles

— (1983) Alcohol control laws and the consumption of distilled spirits and beer. Working paper, Research Program in Competition and Business Policy, Graduate School of Management, University of California at Los Angeles

Owens, S.M., A.J. McBay and C.E. Cook (1983) Use of marijuana, ethanol and other drugs among drivers killed in single vehicle crashes. *Journal of Forensic Sciences, 28,* 372-79

Parker, D.A. (1984) Alcohol control policy in the United States. In P.M. Miller and T.D. Nirenberg (eds), *Prevention of alcohol abuse,* Plenum Press, New York, pp. 235-44

Parker, D.A. and M.S. Harman (1978) A critique of the distribution of consumption model of prevention. *Journal of Studies on Alcohol, 39,* 377-99

— (1980) A critique of the distribution of consumption model of prevention. In T.C. Harford, D.A. Parker and L. Light (eds), *Normative approaches to the prevention of alcohol abuse and alcoholism.* Report of a conference in San Diego, California, April 26-28, 1977. The National Institute on Alcohol Abuse and Alcoholism, US Dept. of Health, Education and Welfare, Rockville, MD, pp. 67-88

Perrine, M.W., J.A. Waller and L.S. Harris (1971) *Alcohol and highway safety: behavioral and medical aspects.* National Highway Traffic Administration, Report No. DOT HS-800 600, Washington, DC

Pittman, D.J. and C.K. Snyder (eds) (1962) *Society, culture and drinking patterns.* Wiley, New York

Planek, T.W. (1982) Home accidents: a continuing social problem. *Accident Analysis and Prevention, 14,* 107-20

Rabow, J. and R.K. Watts (1982) Alcohol availability, alcoholic beverage sales, and alcohol-related problems. *Journal of Studies on Alcohol, 44,* 767-801

Rush, B.R., L. Gliksman and R. Brook (1986) Alcohol availability, alcohol consumption and alcohol-related damage. I. The distribution of consumption model. *Journal of Studies on Alcohol, 47,* 1-10

Schmidt, W. and R.E. Popham (1978) The single distribution model of alcohol consumption: a rejoinder to the critique of Parker and Harman. *Journal of Studies on Alcohol, 39,* 400-19

— (1980) Discussion of paper by Parker and Harman. In T.C. Harford, D.A. Parker and L. Light (eds), *Normative approaches to the preven-*

tion of alcohol abuse and alcoholism. Report of a conference in San Diego, California, April 26-28, 1977. The National Institute on Alcohol Abuse and Alcoholism, US Dept. of Health, Education and Welfare, Rockville, MD, pp. 89-105

Sutton, L.R. (1983) The effects of alcohol, marijuana, and their combination on driving ability. *Journal of Studies on Alcohol, 44*, 438-45

Tong, J.E., P.R. Henderson and B.G.A. Chipperfield (1980) Effects of ethanol and tobacco on auditory vigilance performance. *Addictive Behaviour, 5*, 153-8

US Department of Transportation (1984) *The 1983 Traffic Fatalities Early Assessment*. E.C. Cerelli (ed), DOT No. HS-806-541, Superintendent of Documents, US Government Printing Office, Washington, DC

Wallack, L. and D. Barrows (1983) Evaluating primary prevention: The California 'Winners' Alcohol Program. *International Quarterly of Community Health Education, 3*, 307-35

Wilkinson, R. (1970) *The prevention of drinking problems: alcohol and cultural influences*. Oxford University Press, New York

6

Alcohol in Connection with Industrial and Recreational Accidents: Conceptual and Methodological Issues

Richard Müller

It has often been stressed that alcohol is a major risk factor in the accidental process. A multitude of studies demonstrate a connection but rarely a causal link between consumption of alcohol and the occurrence of accidental events. It is also generally agreed that an accident is the result of a very complex process. Whenever science fails to explain such a phenomenon, there are two strategies available to cope with the problem. The first consists in 'piece-meal engineering' (Popper 1959), which means that the system's complexity is reduced by subdividing it into subsystems whereas the influence of the surrounding systems on the system to be analysed are simply considered as external factors or disturbances. This strategy leads to the famous 'all else being equal' statements, well known in alcohol and accident research. The second possibility of dealing with the problem is the adoption of the risk-factor concept, meaning, in epistemological terms, that the system is not defined enough. But what does risk mean subjectively? And how should the 'man-machine-environment relationship' be conceptualised to give the role of alcohol an adequate place in the accident process? Finally, what consequences for future research can be derived by answering these questions?

What is an Accident?

There is no lack of attempts in the literature to define the concept of 'accident'. It is generally assumed that an accident is a process during which man, object and immediate environment come into contact with each other so that damage in the systems involved occurs. Further, it has been

149

suggested that the accident process develops in three distinct stages: the pre-accident stage, where states of the three systems for the following phase are predetermined; the intra-accident stage, where system failures provoke an event in the interaction between man, object and environment; and, finally, the post-accident stage, where the event provokes damages in man, object and/or environment. Hence, an accident is not a singular event but a sequence of incidents. Evidently, accidents may be classified according to the emphasis given to the three stages and to the systems involved (Table 6.1).

Table 6.1: *Classification of accidents*

Stage	1 pre-accident stage (conditioning factors)	2 intra-accident stage (system failures)	3 post-accident stage (consequences of the event)
System:			
man	*e.g.* lack of experience/ alcohol intake	*e.g.* error in manipulation	*e.g.* fatal/non fatal, type of injury
object/ machine	*e.g.* lack of protective measures	*e.g.* systems break down	*e.g.* damage of machine
immediate environment	*e.g.* noise/darkness	*e.g.* vigilance absorbing	*e.g.* damage in physical and social environment

Of course there are other possibilities for constructing typologies of accidents. They may, for instance, be classified according to the primary activity they are associated with (driving, sporting, etc.), to the environment where they occur (recreational, industrial, home accidents, etc.), or finally, according to the responsibility attributed to the individual involved in the accident process.

Research on responsibility attribution for accidents supports the theory that the severity of the outcome is an important factor with respect to assignment of responsibility. In general, an individual who perpetrates an accident is more likely to be perceived as responsible for the accident if it has severe negative effects than if the effects are mild (Mitchell and Kalb 1981). Existing data also suggest that the culpability of drinking and driving appear to depend on the consequences produced. As DeJoy and Klippel (1984) have demonstrated, the perceived seriousness of drinking and driving varies according to whether it leads to a secondary unsafe driving act or whether it is associated with serious harm to others. When neither of these occur, drinking and driving is not viewed as being significantly more serious than any safe behaviour. Research on responsibility attribution has almost exclusively been carried out in the drinking and driving field. Such information, however, is crucial in order to develop prevention measures, as well as for other types of casualties.

Many researchers conceptualise accidents as unintended events. Taylor (1976), for instance, suggests an axiomatic intention of every individual to avoid any accident. Referring to Maslow's need hierarchy, he postulates an eternal need for security which guides all actions of man in situations of danger. Taylor's view primarily neglects the fact that in these situations there are often two conflicting motivations present: the need for security and the need for achievement. Particularly in situations of competition, the security motive may be exceeded by the need for achievement. Secondly, he does not take into account the possibility of self-destructive tendencies, meaning that the accident is an intended behaviour of self-mutilation or self-destruction. Thirdly, one has to remember that failures in the man-system may be produced by carelessness. But, obviously,'carelessness' is a normative term and what seems careless to the observer may not be at all imprudent for the actor, simply because observer and actor do not have the same motivations and/or the same information at their disposal. Thus, the attribution of responsibility and culpability to the individual involved in an accident is, at least from a scientific point of view, a tricky question. Ultimately, the problem of conceptualising man as a voluntary or determined entity remains a question of ethics.

The history of psychology of accidents is the history of the search for the accident-prone personality. This type of research produced a plethora of studies, primarily in the 1960s, which tried to correlate personality factors with accident frequencies. The underlying hypothesis was that a man drives as he lives: he is constant in his behaviour in different situations due to his stable dispositions and properties — as if the individual could be isolated from the conditions of his immediate environment and the effects of time. The concept of the accident-prone individual, therefore, proved not to be a very useful conceptual tool. But it served well to define populations at risk and to focus on individual factors responsible for the accident process. Alcohol researchers are immediately aware of an analogy in their own field: the vain search for *the* alcoholic personality produced a myriad of correlational studies focusing on the individual and not on society.

Nevertheless, within a given population exposed to certain risks, there is probably an unequal distribution of an accident risk among individuals even if the environmental settings are controlled. But at the same time, differentials in danger areas also exist within a homogeneous population. This implies different combinations of risk potentials in individuals and in situations (Marek and Sten 1977). Most of the statistical procedures, however, fail to distinguish between environmental and individual risk potentials.

Man as a Risk-Taking Entity

Risk implies danger – if there is no danger, there is no risk – and strangely enough, it seems to an external observer that man has nothing else to do than to engage in dangerous health- or life-threatening activities, despite the fact that he is in general well informed about the possible outcomes of his behaviour. *Vivere pericolosamente* appears to be the device for millions. Among researchers, too, it is a commonly held view that risk acceptance is a major factor in accident causation (Dunn 1972). But let us look somewhat more closely at the meaning of risk for the individual and its consequences for the accident process.

First, we have to remember that, in absolute terms, an accident is not only a frequent but also an unequally distributed event in technologically advanced societies. A large body of descriptive material demonstrates strikingly the significance of accidents for morbidity and mortality. And whenever we want to improve longevity in our societies, we have to cut down the accident and suicide rate. For the statistician as well as for common people, however, an accident is a rare event. The 'Fatal Accident Frequency Rate' (Gibson 1976) for most industrial and non-industrial accidents proves to be fairly low. In addition, there is little doubt that economically advanced countries are now safer societies than they were 60 years ago (Wingard and Room 1977). The exposure to dangers of everyday life has, therefore, decreased and risky life situations are generally mastered by the individual quite well. Only a marginal fraction of drinking events at home, at work and before driving are associated with accidents. This fact is well perceived by individuals and confirms their behaviour as far as drinking is concerned. Consequently, risk is something which is assigned to the behaviours of others. It seems extremely difficult to teach people the personal consequences of risk because the evidence of everyday life 'contradicts' the scientific material presented to them. The tendency to deny the personal consequences of risk is probably supported by the nature of scientific production and the way its results are disseminated: no day goes by without the propagation of a new substance or of an old behavioural pattern that is seemingly hazardous to life. What else can the individual do than to reject this information?

Second, by coping with dangers, man has the possibility of gathering experiences to deal with the risks of life. Thus – as stated by Shaoul (1976) – we are paradoxically saying that even while exposure to risk increases, exposure to risk decreases. Seemingly, alcohol intake fosters risk behaviour (although the drinking-and-risk-behaviour relation is far from being clear); alcohol appears to be a significant contributor to the home, work and traffic accident picture, but we know very little about the effect of having learned to deal with alcohol in situations of task performance and risk exposure.

Third, we have to keep in mind that for a singular individual, an accident is not only a rare event, but people need to believe that serious accidents could never happen to them or if they could, that no one would ever blame them for the consequences. Common experience suggests that people are often inclined to attribute their aberrant behaviour not to themselves but to contingencies, to environmental conditions or to alcohol. Ego-defensive or ego-protective causal attributions are vital in an environment where only minor failures in the man-system may lead to fatal outcomes.

Fourth, risk-taking and accident causation research is largely experimental in character and hence transferable only with caution to real life situations. For instance, no research exists, to our knowledge, on the conflict between the need for security and the need for achievement and the corresponding acceptance of risk in a peer group situation when alcohol is present or not. What is needed is not experimental, but quasi-experimental research.

Alcohol in the Man-Object (Machine)-Environment Relationship

The relationship between alcohol and accidental injuries and deaths has frequently been investigated, but major research has been limited primarily to traffic accident victims admitted to the emergency department of general hospitals. The bulk of all accidents at the workplace, at home or during sporting, however, result in minor injuries which normally are not treated in general hospitals and which are never investigated carefully. Hence, the prevalence of alcohol-related accidents is unknown and our picture of the role of alcohol in casualties is severely biased by clinical research. Moreover, there are neither national nor international standards and practices for recording the results of home and other recreational accidents. 'On-the-scene-investigations' that are sometimes done when traffic and occupational accidents occur are rare and seldom possible in the case of accidents at home or during sporting. And if such investigations are carried out, they rarely tell us under which social conditions alcohol intake occurred, and they never report the social stress or the perceived alienation at work of the victims. As alcohol in the event could also have severe consequences as far as the financial performance of insurance companies is concerned, the fact of workers having drunk is often kept secret by superiors and medical doctors.

To get some ideas of what 'on-the-scene investigations' should focus on, let us consider the man-machine-environment relationship more systematically. The following scheme (Figure 6.1) displays the principal factors in the alcohol-related accident process. The object/machine-system creates, in combination with the immediate environmental system, a situation to be mastered by the individual. The individual has to perceive the situation, to decide upon possibilities of coping with the exposure to danger, to select one possibility and, finally, to act on the situation. The perception and decision/selection process depend, on the one hand, on the general coping capacity, on the specific acquired experiences and skills, and on the personal risk-acceptance level. On the other hand, this process is influenced by need dispositions created by the mediate environment. These dispositions may induce the individual to drink if an opportunity exists.

Cognitive psychology has provided much evidence for possible impairments of perceptual and decisional capacities due to alcohol intake. Accident researchers have investigated the temporal context of drinking as well as the drinking habits of accident victims. Wüthrich (1981), for instance, has pointed out that most victims in occupational accidents drank during work and not before. In addition, 50 per cent of them were chronic heavy drinkers, and the immediate 'cause' of the accident in most alcohol cases was a failure of the man-system, whereas in the non-alcohol cases, the overwhelming identified 'cause' consisted in a failure of the machine-system.

On the other hand, sociologists have focused on the relationship between mediate environment and need disposition for drinking. Weiss (1981) found that monotonous and repetitive activities at work, combined with social isolation and bad extrinsic work conditions, are associated with high alcohol intake in men and depressive symptoms in women. Task performances requiring high vigilance and tenacity inhibit drinking, but only if extrinsic work conditions are favourable. If they are not, alcohol intake proves to be high, even if the availability of alcoholic beverages is reduced. Data indicate that only under good working conditions does availability play a major role as a moderating variable in drinking on the job.

Similar studies on accidents at home and during out-door activities are not available. The publication of alcohol-related home and other recreational accidents has been minimal, although in the United States, for instance, home accidents account for more than one-fifth of the accidental deaths and approximately for one-third of the disabling injuries each year — without accounting for questionable homicides and suicides that are often classified as 'accident' on the death certificate (Planek 1982). Planek points out that:

> the findings about home accident circumstances have been drawn mainly from broad-based studies that focus on salient features of accidental injury quite apart from the location of occurrence, such as age of victim (e.g. children), type of accident (e.g. stairway falls), type of injury (e.g. burns) and product-involved (e.g. clothing). This situation stems from the troublesome nature of home accident data collection and investigation.... As a result, the information that they collect provides few insights into 'causes' of home accidents. (p. 115)

Even more striking, is the general lack of investigation in alcohol-related accident research which tries to combine the psychologist's and the sociologist's view. More careful in-depth investigation is needed, taking into account not only the immediate pre-conditioning factors of accidents at work, at home and during sporting, but also their connection with factors of the mediate environment (Figure 6.1).

Figure 6.1: *Principal factors in the alcohol-related accident process*

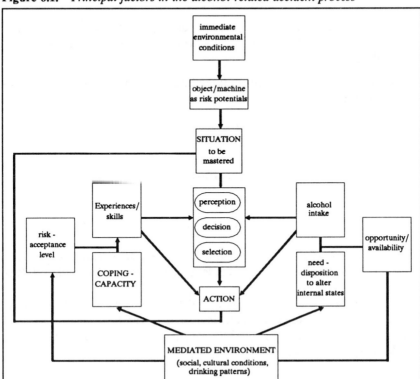

Conclusions

In order to prevent alcohol-related industrial and recreational accidents more effectively, future research should concentrate on the following topics:

- creation of national and international standards for reporting industrial and recreational accidents

- implementation of corresponding meaningful data systems

- study of ego-defensive and -protective causal attribution of alcohol-related accidents at work, at home and during sporting

- enlargement of the almost purely cognitive-oriented approach of information-processing in potentially dangerous situations by introducing affective states of the individual

- development of strategies to teach people the personal consequences of risk

- study of the learning effect of dealing with alcohol in situations of task performance and risk exposure

- investigation by means of quasi-experimental research of the acceptance of risk in different social settings when alcohol intake is controlled

- on-the-scene investigations taking into account not only the immediate but also the mediate environment.

© 1989 Richard Müller

References

DeJoy, D.M., and J.A. Klippel (1984) Attributing responsibility for alcohol-related near-miss accidents. *Journal of Safety Research, 15*, 107-15

Dunn, J.G. (1972) Subjective and objective risk distribution: A comparison and its implication for accident prevention. *Occupational Psychology, 46*, 183-7

Gibson, S.B. (1976) The use of quantitative risk criteria in hazard analysis. *Journal of Occupational Accidents, 1*, 1, 85-94

Marek, J.M., and M. Sten (1977) *Traffic environment and the driver*, Thomas, Springfield

Mitchell, T.R., and L.S. Kalb (1981) Effects of outcome knowledge and outcome valence on supervisor's evaluations. *Journal of Applied Psychology, 66,* 604-12

Planek, T.W. (1982) Home accidents: A continuing social problem. *Accident Analysis and Prevention 14,* 107-20

Popper, K.R. (1959) *The logic of scientific discovery.* Hutchinson, London

Shaoul, J. (1976) Factors which constrain the variability of a group's mileage and other exposure variables, Road Safety Research Unit, University of Stanford

Taylor, D.H. (1976) Accidents, risks and models of explanation. *Human Factors, 18,* 371-80

Weiss, W. (1981) Exzessives trinken: Beruflich bedingte anfälligkeit? *Drogalkohol, 2,* 16-33

Wingard D., and R. Room (1977) Alcohol and home, industrial and recreational accidents. In M. Aarens, T. Cameron, J. Roizen, R. Roizen, R. Room, D. Schneberk, and D. Wingard, *Alcohol, casualties and crime,* Alcohol Research Group, Berkeley

Wüthrich, P. (1981) Alkoholbedingte betriebsunfälle und ihre auswirkungen, leistungskurzungen und schuldfrage. *Drogalkohol, 2,* 3-10

7

Causal Inferences About the Role of Alcohol in Accidents, Poisonings and Violence

Kai Pernanen

In this paper my comments and illustrations range freely between different types of alcohol-related casualties. There will be certain bias in favour of casualties from violence due to a greater familiarity with this type.

What I would have liked to be a systematic treatise is instead a compilation of scattered remarks hopefully relevant to the subject matter of causal inferences regarding the role of alcohol in casualties. There is a definite need for a more systematic treatise. On the other hand, a great deal of naturalistic openness with regard to systematising the analytical problems is a good strategy in such an uncharted research area.

Since only traffic casualties are specifically excluded, I will take the subject matter of this paper to include casualties from intentional physical violence, poisonings, drownings, falls and unintentional fires. (Intentionally set fires, which seem to have a fairly high alcohol involvement in the few scattered studies that exist on the subject, are generally included in statistics on violent crime.) It would probably be unwise not to use some pertinent information from traffic safety research in causal assessments, especially regarding pedestrian casualties. Inevitably, information pertaining strictly to near-casualties or quasi-injuries (such as some outcomes in psychological experimentation) will be relevant to the topic and will be used in this paper in some contexts.

Statistics

'Statistics' in the standard sense, refers mainly to published statistical measures of central tendency, such as *per capita* consumption figures and rates of different types of casualties per 100,000 population, as well as published distributions along certain variables of descriptive interest regarding certain population groups. However, it would perhaps be strategically sound, considering the existing technological possibilities, to focus to some extent on 'statistics' as a user-oriented data base as well as ready-made statistical information. This latter type is unfortunately often the statistical information that individual scientists are limited to, especially in international comparisons. Thus, decisions on what statistics to publish and how to publish them as well as how to facilitate the use of data bases may be as crucial as what data to collect.

It should also be emphasized that the monitoring and policy assessment that statistics enable are in themselves useful and important (although the pitfalls of causal inferences still remain). Consequently, although casualty statistics by themselves provide a rather limited base for causal inferences, other uses well justify the effort of gathering statistical data. As will be discussed below, less finely discriminating 'contributory cause' models are often sufficient as a basis for policy decisions or administrative measures, although statistical data by themselves hardly ever suffice for assessing competing models of 'causal processes'. Often, too, the role of statistics is to provide causal clues to be tested in other ways, such as through more or less controlled studies.

Before discussing the concept of 'cause' a few words may be needed about a couple of preliminary steps to causal accounting, which often are neglected in order to get directly to inferences about causes. These steps in themselves may provide interesting causal clues in explaining alcohol-related casualties.

'Bias' and 'Risk'

In the discussion below I will, for the sake of brevity, assume that the data from one or several jurisdictions, which form the premises of causal generalisations and interpretations, reflect the true state of affairs. Very often, of course, this condition is not met due to at least two major types of bias. There is, first of all, selection bias, exemplified in violent crime statistics by the fact that the police are more likely to apprehend a violent offender if he has been drinking and does not have quite the presence of mind or psychomotor capabilities to remove himself from the scene of the crime or its vicinity, or having a higher than average probability of being known to the police because of a pattern of excessive drinking behaviour, etc. Another type of bias, recording bias, is exemplified by what, according to Crompton (1985), among other criteria, determines the categorisation of a casualty into the accident or the suicide category in England. He states that potential cases of suicide are routinely classified as accidents if the victims had 'consumed so much alcohol that the full significance and consequences of their actions might not have been fully apparent to them at the time'. This, of course, deflates the suicide figures and inflates the accident figures. It also leads to overestimations of the alcohol involvement in accidents and an underestimation for suicides. (If the demarcation is also arbitrary—and especially if it is linked to alcohol involvement—in other jurisdictions (perhaps partly due to consideration of the survivors and their insurance claims), it may be advisable to pool together accidents and suicides, for at least some international comparisons.)

Whether biases directly related to the alcohol involvement shown in statistics are present or not, it is clear that mere recording practices differ greatly between jurisdictions, depending in large part on the institutional structure of control and/or care of casualties, administrative requirements, etc. This, of course, has an impact on the validity of clues for causal models or testings of such.

On the whole, we have to regard the data biases and recording discrepancies as being of a different logical order from the causal questions dealing with the substantive aspects of alcohol's role in casualties. 'Bias' is always bias in relation to the descriptive or explanatory goals of a scientific undertaking. Related to these goals is the question of which of the referents of the term 'alcohol' we are using as the (potential) independent variable. Trying to narrow the focus of the 'alcohol' variable to amounts consumed or BACs we may be playing with a kind of 'uncertainty principle' (by measuring some aspects of 'alcohol' we may be changing the phenomena we measure, for example 'bracketing out' the sociocultural meanings linked to alcohol as a social phenomenon). Policy decisions based on data 'purified' of such bias, may give rise to surprising developments. This possibility bears some analysis but these questions of data biases will not be discussed further, as important as they are in the total process of judging the validity of causal inferences based on statistical data.

Once we have cleared our data of the suspicion of bias, or have been able to adjust or control for biasing factors in some way, we should, on our way toward a causal accounting of a relationship, establish a level of the null hypothesis against which we want to test the strength of the relationship. Thus, one would, on one level of analysis, assume the alcohol involvement in any type of casualty to be higher in a country (or other type of jurisdiction) which has a higher level of consumption. By chance alone, one would expect Finland or Canada to have a lower level of alcohol involvement than France in any type of casualty—at least if we start from a rough working hypothesis implying that distribution and temporal and ecological spacing of alcohol consumption (and a host of potentially conditional cultural factors) do not substantially change the size of this type of null hypothesis. This simple, but central and often substantively interesting, step is often overlooked in discussions of alcohol's causal role in various social problems, although the necessary statistical information seems to be generally available. Deviations from the expected patterns will lead us further toward a true causal accounting of alcohol's role in casualties.

One way of carrying out this step is by relating casualty rates directly to alcohol consumption figures. For example, by relating the annual rate of accidents from falls treated in hospitals to the total alcohol consumption in the jurisdiction, we get a rate of hospital-treated falls per 100,000 litres of alcohol consumed in the country. At least this far we can get with ready-made statistics.

Now, if we have information on the proportion of falls in which the victim had been drinking (or had a BAC above a certain level) and relate these aggregated estimates to *per capita* consumption in the population (or any of its demographic subgroups), we can control for a host of potential causally relevant factors and be closer to a true causal accounting of alcohol-related casualty rates, or differences or changes in these rates. In this way it was calculated in the ISACE study (Mäkelä *et al.* 1981) that official figures on detentions, arrests, prosecutions and convictions for public drunkenness differed greatly between countries, and that these differences remained even when controlling for total consumption. Some differences became even more pronounced while others became smaller than in the simple rates per population unit. These 'purified' rates deserve to be shown for illustrative purposes (Table 7.1).

Table 7.1: *Rates of public drunkenness per a) 100,000 inhabitants aged 15 and over, and b) per 10,000 litres of absolute alcohol for 1975 (for Ontario 1973 figure).*

Jurisdiction	Per 100,000 15 and over	Per 10,000 litres
California	1,325	10
Finland	7,485	94
Ireland	220	2
Netherlands	21	2
Ontario	615	6
Poland	1,646	18

Source: Mäkelä *et al.* 1981

With regard to casualties from violence, I made a similar 'purified' comparison of homicides between Finland and Canada in preparation for a cross-national study on the relationship between alcohol use and aggression (Pernanen 1979). (Unfortunately, no data existed for Canada on the alcohol involvement in non-fatal types of violent crimes.) The results of the comparison are shown in Table 7.2.

Table 7.2: *Rates of alcohol-involved and other homicides per 100,000 persons aged 15 and older, Canada and Finland, 1974*

Country	Alcohol involved	No alcohol	Total rate
Canada	1.1	1.3	2.4
Finland	1.5	0.8	2.3

Source: Pernanen 1979

If we now relate the rates of alcohol-related homicides to the level of alcohol consumption in the two countries, we find that in Finland the risk of a certain amount of alcohol being linked to a homicide is almost twice as large as in Canada, although the risks are still very small: there was one alcohol-involved homicide per 750,000 litres of absolute alcohol consumed in Canada as compared to one per 410,000 litres in Finland.

Calculation of risk figures or other types of quantifications of null hypotheses based on alcohol consumption is only the second step on the road to causal accounting of the role of alcohol in casualties, but it is still an area where pertinent statistical bases can accomplish a great deal. (In addition to comparisons between jurisdictions, this type of risk figure could, of course, also be used in time series analyses with some potentially interesting results. The same goal is accomplished through a host of multi-variate procedures, but with a loss in descriptive impact.)

'Cause' and 'Alcohol'

Two key concepts in the context of this paper are 'cause' and 'alcohol'. The latter is certainly not as determinate and unproblematic in its reference as it may seem, especially as dealt with on the epidemiological level.

'Cause' also has different meanings. This leads to some confusion regarding the causality of alcohol-related phenomena, and distinctions and clarifications are in order so that the nature of causal inferences can be illuminated. Among its epidemiological referents, alcohol has the following: amounts consumed per occasion, BAC, congener content, length of drinking occasion, rising or falling BAC, intoxication, prevalence of withdrawal symptoms, social meaning of different types of beverage, relative incidence of consumption with meals, and beliefs and attitudes with regard to drunkenness (e.g. ideas of responsibility, accountability, 'sacred state' versus degradation, beliefs about stages of drunkenness, etc.). When we speak of the effects of alcohol or increases in alcohol consumption we actually speak in an indeterminate way about all these referents and the causal processes in which they are implicated. Some of these referents we may be able to 'control for' in analyses even of aggregated statistical data, but others have to be taken care of in hypothesising interpretations and/or referred to testing in more controlled settings. In other analyses, the whole conglomerate of 'alcohol', with all the different types of causal processes which take place, will do perfectly well for our analyses. This will be the case if we want to assess, for example, what the total absence of alcohol in society will lead to with regard to casualty rates. (This is possible, within a short-time perspective, in some 'natural experiments' — see below.)

The concept of 'cause' and 'causality' have, of course, been the subject of analysis and speculation over many centuries. The pervasiveness of the concept of cause for the ordering of human experience (individually and collectively) is central in understanding some problems associated with it. This pervasiveness can be exemplified by the fact that the influential philosopher Immanuel Kant gave the concept an *a priori* status as one of the ways that humans by their nature order their experiences. The notion of causality in our outlook on the world is seen as inescapable. There is a certain obvious truth to this notion of inescapability of causal structurings of our world and of acting in it. We do tend to try to ascribe causality even in the most obtuse connections and within the possibilities that we have at our disposal; cognitively we try to build causal models. The resistance to the idea of 'acausal' explanations is well illustrated by the difficulties that physicists have had with the theoretical notions of quantum physics.

Imputations and applications of causality are very closely allied with another principle of human thought which was formalised and elevated to a status as a principle of scientific inference by William of Ockham in the fourteenth century: the principle of parsimony. The combinations of these ordering principles of human thought into causal ascriptions by the most parsimonious available model sometimes lead to unfortunate blockings of progress. We can find this tendency in ascriptions of causal roles to alcohol. Most clearly it is encountered in the ascription of conveniently labeled causal properties to alcohol. Widely accepted is the 'disinhibiting' property of alcohol which is used to explain a wide variety of behaviours in connection with drinking (Pernanen 1976, Room and Collins 1983). The tendency towards somewhat premature parsimonious causal ascription will be illustrated with an example from the possible role(s) of drinking in the explanation of one type of casualty: victimisation by violent crime. This will also be an illustration of the use of rather simple analytical possibilities (which are too often overlooked), which may move us a considerable distance toward revealing causal processes. It is provided by considering two fairly recent Scandinavian contributions to the field of alcohol-related casualties. Considering these in juxtaposition also shows what may hide under the concept of 'alcohol' and the concept of 'cause'.

Despite the generally accepted idea in the public's mind (certainly true of the Scandinavian public) that alcohol is causally implicated in a great deal of violent events occurring in society, only two types of epidemiological/quantitative analyses based on aggregated statistics have been carried out to test this preconception.

By far the most common procedure of assessing (or setting the stage for assessing) alcohol's causal contribution to casualties is by way of the measure of 'alcohol involvement', for example, the extent to which the victim and, in violent events, the offender or both, had been drinking in fairly close temporal proximity to the casualty event. Surprisingly enough, another type of analysis for which aggregated data would be more commonly available has not been used at all to the same extent. However, Lenke (1976) has carried out this second type of analysis with some very interesting results. In a convincingly executed series of analyses, he brought data from several Scandinavian jurisdictions (mainly national data) to bear on the problem of the correlative connection between alcohol consumption and crimes of violence. The findings seemed to have strong causal implications. He found that rates of violent crime over several years and in several different Scandinavian samples closely followed rates in *per capita* consumption.

Even rather abrupt changes in *per capita* consumption (some of these in the nature of natural experiments which increased or decreased the availability of alcoholic beverages) coincided closely with changes in the rate of crimes of violence. Through this type of correspondence in the time series it was rather convincingly established that there was no common cause variable on the aggregate level which could causally account for both the increase or decrease in aggregated consumption and the corresponding changes in violent crime rates.

Up to this point in the history of alcohol-casualty research, alcohol involvement data, in a rather common display of investigative inertia and lack of adequate data, had been focussed on one point in time in a jurisdiction. To the extent that systematic data existed of alcohol involvement in violent crimes, they had been used mainly descriptively or as unqualified (and unproblematic) indicators of the alcohol problems which required policy decisions. Aho (1976), however, cleverly combined alcohol involvement figures in violent crime in a time series analysis pertaining to Finland, with rates of violent crime (which had increased during the period) and *per capita* alcohol consumption figures during this period, which also had increased (i.e. Lenke's findings). Aho deduced, from the general reasoning around the fact that the increase in alcohol consumption was seen as causally responsible for the concurrently increasing rates of violent crime, that the alcohol involvement in violent crime would also show an increase. (One would also assume that the statistical null hypothesis related to the causal importance of alcohol would be elevated with increasing consumption and thus on the basis of chance alone, a higher alcohol involvement would be expected. This, however, was not part of Aho's reasoning and is slightly peripheral also for our illustrative purposes.)

The empirical results as tested on Finnish statistics, however, proved to be different. Despite a steady increase in aggregate consumption and rates of violent crime, there was no systematic increase in the proportion of violent crimes prior to which the offender or the victim or both had been drinking. Thus it was clear that the causal processes related to alcohol-use events or increased amounts consumed could not account for all the increase despite the next to perfect correlation in these measures of central tendency, and in the findings from natural experiments affecting the availability of alcohol which occurred during the study period. The most likely remaining causal explanation, vague and general as it may be, seems to be that increasing the availability of alcohol or increasing the number of alcohol-use events also affects social processes which, independently of alcohol use, increase the risk of violent encounters.

Aho achieved a specification of sorts of a statistical (correlative) relationship which must modify our view of the type of causal relationship that exists between changes in *per capita* consumption and rates of violent crime (at least in this jurisdiction). Thus, even on this still rather superficial level, the causal implications of innovative statistical analyses can be profound indeed.

Aho's example above indicates the power that knowing the causal processes which implicate alcohol in casualties could lend to explanation and prediction. For other purposes, a 'yes-no' answer often suffices: does alcohol use (in all its referents and all the processes in which these are active) contribute to the risk of casualties? To answer this type of question, there exist standard statistical techniques (assuming that the statistical material is available and with their own specific assumptions), but the most dramatic and, by its immediacy, convincing method is that of natural experiments. These are from time to time provided through strikes by liquor or beer store employees, lowering of the drinking age, the opening of new liquor stores (especially appealing if done in previously 'dry' areas), etc. The problem from a researcher's point of view is that the most dramatic changes in alcohol availability tend to be rather short-lived and this limits the possibilities of generalising the results.

When the availability of alcohol approaches zero or is cut drastically very interesting analyses can be made. Takala (1973) showed clear decreases in violent crimes during a six-week strike by liquor store employees, using available statistical material, and Karaharju and Stjernvall (1974) used the opportunity to gather data on patients in the casualty department of a large hospital. Significant decreases in patient loads were observed during the period of the strike, especially on weekends.

Systematic and continuous collection of statistical data with easily achieved temporal cutoff points allow the relatively easy use of natural experiments for causally relevant analytical purposes. If for example a strike of liquor store employees starts on May 12 and ends on June 19 in any given year, it is important to be able to at least approximate the consumption figures from on-premise sales (as a control) and the casualty rates for this idiosyncratic period. This should ideally be taken into account in planning statistical recording systems.

Causal Process

On the statistical/epidemiological level we are mostly dealing with 'contributory causes': how much of the variation in casualty rates do alcohol use variations account for (typically using bivariate or multivariate analyses over time periods and/or jurisdictions); or how much in absolute figures or proportions in casualty rates does alcohol use or changes in the availability of alcohol contribute (typically by using the opportunities afforded by natural experiments).

The relative contributions of different causal processes naturally differ between different types of alcohol-related casualties. In casualties connected with interpersonal violence, we are more directly tied to social processes and intra- and interpersonal dynamics in our explanations, and the 'effects of alcohol' are obviously not as clearcut as with other types of casualties. In falls, poisonings, fires and drownings, the psychomotor effects of alcohol are of greater relative significance than in inter-personal violence. The psychomotor effects are probably less affected by characteristics of the surrounding environment and variations in intrapersonal (i.e. especially psychological) factors, than the factors which determine whether a drinking person will display aggressive behaviour. (A simple 'thought experiment' may clarify matters somewhat: in a situation where subjects under experimental conditions are given increasing doses of alcohol, we can rather safely predict that practically all will at some level of consumption start staggering and falling. However, we do not know if any specific individual will start behaving aggressively towards other persons in the situation and cannot make any general predictions to the effect that at some level of intoxication all subjects will behave aggressively. We do not even have any idea of the proportion of subjects who will become aggressive.)

Still, even preceding falls and drownings, more or less conscious assessments of the situation and its 'task demands' and decisions based on these are taken by the drinking individual. In addition to the psychomotor, attentional and other processes linked to alcohol use, the whole range of social definitions and interpersonal processes is at work in determining the probability of actions that will increase or decrease the risk of an accidental fall or a drowning incident. There is no question but that social attributions of causality to alcohol play a role in these risk-affecting processes. They interact with the attributions that are placed on the type of behaviour to be 'expected from' a drinking or intoxicated person.

More often than not it seems that one of the reasons for drinking is to occasion a redefinition of the acute situation and with it, to some extent, one's own identity, and status. Considering the situational redefinition of identity and status, we may better understand the attempts to change surroundings and context of drink by changing the decor and type of drinking establishment. These have proliferated in the last couple of decades even in previously puritan drinking cultures (Mäkelä *et al.* 1981). We also can understand better, in my view, identity definitions that take the form of bragging in many drinking cultures. 'Risk-taking' behaviour is also one aspect of bragging and of identity redefinition in the situation. It seems that, at least in some cultures, behaviour in drinking contexts is often based on challenges: challenges to drink, to hold one's liquor, to compete in games, etc. These challenges are effected through direct peer group exhortations, for example, or the type of challenge which comes about through perceived or real negative attitudes towards the drinker. In some cultures this seems to be more prevalent than in others. In the midst of other causal processes, these processes would have an impact on the risk of alcohol-related casualties of the most varying types. Statistical material easily leads us into reasoning based on single variables, linear correlations and, at a more sophisticated level, analyses of interactions between variables which can be fitted into a linear model. Despite any level of sophistication much of the causal processes will still be missed and important clues for policy decisions disregarded if the social interactional meaning of drinking, of the different beverages, of the amounts consumed, etc., are not considered and put into the context of cultural/institutional clusters. Were one to only look at the type of beverage that was consumed in, for example, the violent events which took place in the community in North-western Ontario where I carried out a study a few years ago (Pernanen 1979), one would find that beer drinking carried the highest risk of violence compared to liquor and wine, despite the fact that the onset of intoxication is slower and the BACs reached not as high as with the other beverages. Beer, however, is a (young) man's drink in this culture, and much of the consumption of beer occurs in public drinking places. Both of these facts tend to increase the risk of alcohol-related casualties from violence and would show up in statistics as beer-related phenomena.

More generally it can be said that although alcohol consumption—*per capita* or per event—and the resulting BACs are definitely continuous ratio scale variables, 'drunkenness' seen as a cluster of objective and measurable physical signs, and also phenomenologically from the drinking person's point of view, is not. And definitely the social perception of drunkenness is a cluster of nominal scale variables since the individuals whom the drinking person interacts with categorise him and attribute behaviour, motives and moral qualities to him. These categorisations are culturally bound and in this they are dependent on the situational context in which the drinking person is perceived (see studies on permissible drinking situations). They also change over time. Their contribution is potentially as great and, under given circumstances, greater than the purely physiologically determined effects of alcohol use. With regard to different types of alcohol-related casualties, these cultural transformations of the alcohol consumption variable need to be taken into account.

Statistical data will not suffice for the accounting of casualty phenomena by causal processes because of the complexities involved, but they will give important leads, which can be assessed by carrying out special studies collecting primary data or by using other sources of statistics (demographic, economical, political, etc.).

In the frame of causal accounting, when using theories as inference rules in our explanations (and not merely assessing the contributory role of the unspecific conglomerate of 'alcohol') we should not forget that drunken comportment also consists of more or less harmless revelry, of unselfish, affectionate and perhaps emotionally cathartic behaviour, etc. These behaviours should ideally also fit in the same theoretical frame as the behaviours which potentially could and actually do end up as statistical casualties. The alcohol-induced obliviousness to objective risks and to individuals present in the situation is unsystematically documented in, for example, newspaper reports and private recollections of ordinary citizens. Some of these end up in official statistics as casualties or under labels other than casualties, but most (as is true with most falls, violent incidents, etc.) are nowhere recorded. All of these can perhaps be characterised as 'excessive behaviour' —whether that categorisation will help us theoretically (and causally) is another matter.

There is, of course, a great deal of theoretical and causal relatedness with many psychological alcohol studies. I shall here only mention the experiments which during recent years have been carried out on the expectancy effects of alcohol, where a theoretical junction seems to exist to attitudinal studies within epidemiological methodology. This type of study, as well as psychosocial small group observational studies could, if replicated in several cultures, provide fertile insights into differences which might help us explain some characteristics of casualty statistics. More than that, findings based on statistics should help formulate questions for more systematic and controlled testing. The door to other disciplines within alcohol research should be left demonstratively open.

Concluding Remarks

We should take care not to commit the same standard single-focus mistake that was committed over a long period in traffic safety research, when statistics on drinking and driving were considered almost exclusively as atomistic incidents and the contribution to these rates of the same individuals (lopsidedly represented by 'problem drinkers') was not considered systematically. Scandinavian data at least (e.g. Kühlhorn 1984) show that there is a great deal of clustering to the same individuals also in violent crime (often well known to the police from other types of crime incidents). The same 'problem families' also contribute a sizeable part of the alcohol-related violence that shows up in the current Swedish statistics. With regard to other casualties, Waller (1976) has indicated that 'there is some evidence that the individuals who are excessively involved in alcohol-related unintentional injury events often are the same ones involved in deliberate injury' specifically 'drivers in alcohol-related crashes frequently [who] have previous histories of assaultive behaviour while under the influence of alcohol'. It should be possible to build a collection of information on clustering to individuals into at least a subsample of regularly collected statistics.

This is also a reminder in more directly causally motivated research to look into determinants of differing individual risks of aggression and violence in connection with alcohol use. Nothing much is really known about differences between individuals or social categories in the tendency to behave aggressively or in a risk-taking manner after drinking, for example, and even less about variations in the same individual from one alcohol-use occasion to the next in this tendency. Several drinking cultures have shorthand expressions for these individual differences, such as 'happy drunk' versus 'mean drunk', or speaking of a person as having 'a bad beer sense' (Swedish: *daligt olsinne*), or the Finnish references to 'bad liquor head' (*viinapaa*). These individual differences are almost as solidly ensconced in the cultural images of drinking as the picture of the staggering drunk. The distribution curves of alcohol consumption have taught us to look differently at the phenomena of alcoholism, the determinants of alcohol consumption, health risks connected with drinking, etc. In a similar fashion, a frequency distribution curve of alcohol-related violence and other casualty producing behaviour, and changes in this distribution (to the extent that it is possible to systematically collect such data over the fairly long period of time that is needed) might lead us to both descriptive epidemiological and theoretical insights.

Acknowledgement

This work was supported by a grant from the Swedish Ministry of Health and Social Affairs, Delegation for Social Research (Project No. D84/211:1).

References

Aho, T. (1976) *Alkoholi jä vakivalta (Alcohol and violence)*. Selvite Oikeusministeriö, (Report from Ministry of Justice), Publication 7: D Series, Helsinki

Crompton, M.R. (1985) Alcohol and violent accidental and suicidal death. *Medical Science and the Law, 25,* 59-62

Honkanen, R., L. Ertama, P. Kuosmanen, M. Linnoila, A. Alha and T. Visuri (1983) The role of alcohol in accidental falls. *Journal of Alcohol Studies, 44,* 231-45

Karaharju, E.O., and L. Stjernvall (1974) The alcohol factor in accidents. *Injury, 6,* 67-9

Kühlhorn, E. (ed) (1984) *Den Svenska våldsbrottsligheten (Swedish criminal violence)*. Brottsforebyggande rådet, Report 1984: 1, Stockholm

Lenke, L. (1976) Alkohol och våldsbrottslighet (Alcohol and criminal violence). *Alkohol och Narkotika, 17,* 1, 8-17

Mäkelä, K., R. Room, E. Single, P. Sulkunen, B. Walsh *et al.* (1981) *Alcohol, society and the state, volume 1: a comparative study of alcohol control.* Addiction Research Foundation, Toronto

Pernanen, K. (1976) Alcohol and crimes of violence. In B. Kissin and H. Begleiter (eds), *The biology of alcoholism, volume 4: social aspects of alcoholism,* Plenum Press, New York, pp. 351-444

— (1979) *Alcohol and aggressive behavior. A community study with a cross-cultural perspective, volume I, introduction: rationale, methodology and fieldwork.* Addiction Research Foundation Substudy No. 1050, Toronto

Room, R. and G. Collins (eds) (1983) *Alcohol and disinhibition: nature and meaning of the link,* US Department of Health and Human Services, Research Monograph No. 12, Rockville, Maryland

Takala, H. (1973) Alkoholstrejkens inverkan pa uppdagad brottslighet (The effect of the alcohol strike on reported crime). *Alkoholpolitik,* *36,* 14-6

Waller, J. A. (1976) Alcohol and unintentional injury. In B. Kissin and H. Begleiter (eds), *The biology of alcoholism, volume 4: social aspects of alcoholism,* Plenum Press, New York, pp. 307-49

8

Alcohol: Pharmacology, Methods of Analysis and its Presence in the Casualty Room

Bhushan M. Kapur

Pharmacology

Pure ethanol (CH_3CH_2OH, m.w = 46.06) is a clear, colourless liquid with a characteristic but weak odour and a strong, burning taste. At a concentration of 95.6 per cent by weight, alcohol and water form an azeotropic mixture with a minimum boiling point of 78.15°C. Density of ethanol at 20°C is 0.78934 and melting point of absolute ethanol is -114°C.

As a rule, people drink alcoholic beverages which contain mostly ethanol and water. Beverages differ according to the sugar source: from grapes, wine; from grain and hops, beer; from grain and corn, whiskey; from sugar cane, rum and from potato, vodka.

The drug ethyl alcohol is naturally of interest to pharmacologists because of its pervasive clinical and social presence in our society. It also presents an intellectual challenge, in that the simplicity of its chemical structure suggests an unusual mechanism of action. Alcohol is taken in tens of grams (or by the ounce), in contrast to other familiar drugs where the usual dose may be a thousand times lower. Its inertness at low concentrations allows its presence to be raised to very high levels.

The main facts of alcohol metabolism are well established. Human metabolism does not deviate essentially from that of experimental animals. However, species differences as shown by enzymological and metabolic findings are well known and must be taken into consideration when extrapolating from results obtained *in vitro* and/or on experimental animals to the situation prevailing in the human organism (Von Wartburg 1971). In contrast to food, ethanol need not be digested and is readily absorbed in the gastro-intestinal tract. Over 90 per cent of ingested alcohol is oxidised enzymatically to carbon dioxide and water. Only a small percentage of the unmetabolised ethanol is excreted in urine, expired air, perspiration and in milk during lactation. Ethanol is oxidised mainly by alcohol dehydrogenase to acetaldehyde, which is further oxidised to carbon dioxide and water (Kalant 1971).

Absorption

Ethanol is absorbed from the stomach by simple diffusion. Gastric absorption is fastest when strong drinks, distilled spirits containing 40 to 50 per cent ethanol by volume, are consumed. Diluted beverages, such as beer (4 to 5 per cent ethanol) or wine (11 to 12 per cent ethanol) are absorbed slowly. Alcohol is absorbed very rapidly from the small intestines. The essential action of food is to delay gastric emptying and thus slow the absorption process (Lin *et al.* 1976). The type of food seems to make little difference, since the effect has been demonstrated with proteins, carbohydrates and fats. The greater the interval between alcohol ingestion and the meal, however, the less the effect on alcohol absorption. In the fasting state, ethanol is absorbed within an hour.

Distribution

Ethanol rapidly diffuses throughout the aqueous compartments of the body, going wherever water goes. It is not very lipid soluble. Since alcohols diffuse readily across capillary walls, the physical principles governing their distribution from blood to various tissues and body fluids are exactly the same as those governing their absorption through blood. Ethanol is found in all tissues in a concentration that depends on the water content of the tissue.

Miles (1922) examined the time-course of a single oral dose of ethanol in man and showed that the concentration in urine was lower than that in blood during the period of most active absorption, but higher after the peak blood level had passed. The question of alcohol diffusion across the mucosa of the bladder has been of interest primarily for medico-legal reasons. In humans, Haggard *et al.*(1940) found that urine retained in the bladder for various times after consumption of ethanol did not show appreciable changes in ethanol concentration, except for the expected effects of dilution by newly-formed urine of lower alcohol content. This finding simply reflects the time-lag between the formation of urine and its collection in the bladder.

One of the body fluids of special interest is blood. Different investigators have, for various reasons, measured blood-alcohol concentrations in whole blood, plasma, or serum, and found the relationship between these not to be constant. The lower concentration of alcohol in whole blood reflects the lower water content of this fluid. Other body fluids and secretions have been examined less extensively but the general conclusions are similar. The higher the water content, the higher the alcohol concentration in relation to whole blood.

Saliva has also received much attention for medico-legal reasons. In an excellent early study, Linde (1932) collected parotid saliva and found that the time curves of alcohol concentration in blood and parotid saliva were parallel with no appreciable lag in the saliva. The parotid saliva-blood ratio closely approximated the plasma/blood ratio, and confirming again the relationship between alcohol and water content. Recently Jones (1979) in a study based on 336 determinations, confirmed these findings and also showed the mixed saliva-blood ratio to be 1.08:1, as predicted by Linde in the 1932 study. He also confirmed that both the saliva and blood-alcohol concentration curves are parallel and both reach zero simultaneously, with no appreciable time-lag in the saliva.

The passage of ingested alcohol into the milk of lactating women showed the same time-lag with respect to blood-alcohol curve as the other secretions do (Goldstein 1983). There was thus a higher alcohol concentration in the milk than in the blood during the post-equilibration phase. These findings have been confirmed and show that alcohol concentration in the milk bears no relation to the rate of milk excretion; this is in keeping with the process of simple diffusion of alcohol from blood into milk. Qualitatively, similar relationships have been found between alcohol concentrations in the blood and sweat, aqueous humours, vitreous humours, bile, ascitic fluid, amniotic fluid and human fetal blood.

Elimination

The rate of removal of ethanol from the body is the sum of the rates of excretion in urine, breath and sweat, plus the rate of metabolism in the liver and other tissues. In most mammals, metabolism follows zero order kinetics and is largely independent of alcohol concentration in the blood, since the principal enzyme involved reaches its maximum rate of activity at quite low concentrations. In contrast, excretion follows first order kinetics, since all the excretory processes are essentially based on diffusion, and the rate of excretion at any time is proportional to the concentration of alcohol in the blood. Therefore, the larger the dose of alcohol given, and the longer the duration of the measurable blood-alcohol curve, the larger the proportion of the dose excreted when very high blood-alcohol levels are maintained or when diuresis, hyperventilation, or profuse sweating occurs. Alcohol elimination rates have been reported for various ethnic groups by different authors. There seems to be a wide range between them. The range for Caucasians reported to be between 12 mg/100 ml to 22 mg/100 ml; American Indians, between 16 mg/100 ml to 26 mg/100 ml; Eskimos, 16 mg/100 ml and Chinese, 13 mg/100 ml (Goldstein 1983).

Ethanol pharmacokinetics have been reported to be similar in females throughout the menstrual cycle (Marshall *et al.* 1983). No variations were seen in mean peak blood levels or elimination rates in mid-follicular (8-10 days) and mid-luteal (22-24 days) phases. No significant sex differences between males and females in mean ethanol elimination rates have been reported. The apparent volume of distribution of ethanol in females (0.59 $\pm$ 0.02 l/kg) was less than in males (0.73 $\pm$ 0.02 l/kg) ($p < .001$). Both apparent volume of distribution of ethanol and area under curve have been found to be significantly correlated with total body water, suggesting that the differences are due to body water content differences in the two sexes (Marshall *et al.* 1983).

The effects of alcohol depend on how quickly it is absorbed. In general, the faster the rate of absorption, the more striking the effect. Chronic use of alcohol results in an increased capacity to metabolise alcohol, which declines after several weeks of abstinence. Chronic use of alcohol produces pharmacodynamic tolerance, so that a higher blood concentration is necessary to produce intoxication in the tolerant than in the normal individual (Goodmann and Gilman 1980). Chronic maintenance of high concentrations of alcohol in blood produces a state of physical dependence. Individuals tolerant to alcohol usually show cross-tolerance to anesthetics and various sedative-hypnotics, including benzodiazepines (Goodmann and Gilman 198). Chronic exposure to ethanol causes a variety of liver abnormalities, both functional and morphological. Liver cirrhosis is an important cause of death in alcoholics (Goldstein 1983). Peripheral neuropathy, Wernicke-Korsakoff encephalopathy and cerebellar degeneration are among the commonly reported damages to the nervous system (Goodwin 1980).

Alcohol Analysis

There are various reasons why alcohol measurement is done. It is the most commonly observed drug in patients presenting themselves to emergency rooms of hospitals (Peppiatt *et al.* 1978). The presence or absence of alcohol can have major prognostic and diagnostic implications. In a clinically compromised patient, a low blood-alcohol level would indicate to the attending physician that further investigations are necessary. An underlying concurrent disease, a head injury or the potential presence of another drug may be the cause of the compromised clinical condition. If the blood alcohol level is high, alcohol alone may be the potential cause of the clinical condition. In either case, the presence and the approximate blood-alcohol level is an important clue in the management of the patient.

Alcohol analysis is also performed to follow up patients who are in treatment programmes. This is a relatively new application. Alcohol analysis is particularly important when the patient is being treated with alcohol-sensitising drugs such as calcium carbamide or disulfiram (Peachey and Kapur 1986).

Two factors which should be considered before analysis are, body fluid to be analysed and the method of analysis. Breath, blood and saliva levels reflect the current blood-alcohol level whereas urine reflects the average blood-alcohol level between voidings (Kalant 1971). In programs requiring monitoring of alcohol use, urine is probably the better specimen (Peachey and Kapur 1986).

Body Fluids

Body fluids such as sweat, saliva, blood, urine and breath have been used for alcohol analysis. Each of these have advantages and disadvantages. Table 8.1 summarises these data. Breath is commonly used by law enforcement authorities. Although both blood and saliva levels reflect current blood alcohol level, blood specimen are used in hospitals to generally assess patients in the casualty wards. In programs requiring monitoring of alcohol use, urine is probably the specimen of choice. Urine-alcohol level, which represents the average blood alcohol level between voidings, has the potential of testing 'positive' while the blood may test 'negative'. Appropriate selection of urine collection times, i.e. a specimen taken before going to bed or first thing in the morning, can be effectively used in monitoring alcohol use in treatment programs (Peachey and Kapur 1986).

Method

Since the introduction of the micro-method (Peppiatt *et al.* 1978) for alcohol analysis in blood by Widmark (1922), many new methods and modifications have been introduced (Kapur and Israel 1983). The distillation-oxidation methods are generally non-specific for ethanol, whereas the enzymatic (Lindblad 1976; Redetzki and Dees 1976) and gas chromatographic (Jain 1971; Berild and Hasselbalch 1981) methods currently used are specific for ethanol. The most recent introduction is the alcohol dipstick method (Kapur and Israel 1983). This method is not

only sensitive, it also does not require instrumentation. The alcohol dipstick can be used for the detection of alcohol in all body fluids. It provides results in ranges of pharmacological and toxicological interest.
Thus it can be used in casualty rooms of hospitals as well in monitoring
patients' alcohol use in treatment programs. Studies in the 'non-labora-
tory' clinical environment have shown this to be a viable method (Peachey
and Kapur 1986). Table 8.2 summarises and compares the various
methods of alcohol analysis.

Alcohol and Drugs in the Casualty Room

The Toxicology Laboratory of the Addiction Research Foundation is the
central resource for emergency toxicology for most of Metropolitan

Table 8.1: *Assessment of body fluids; biological samples available for analysis*

Breath	Blood	Saliva	Sweat	Urine
Collection - ease of collection				
easy	easy	can be difficult	difficult	easy
non-invasive	invasive	non-invasive	non-invasive	non-invasive
Need for supervision				
yes	yes	yes	no	no
Compliance				
no problem	no problem	no problem	yes, difficult to check compliance	accuracy depends on the authenticity of the patients' sample
Interpretation ratio to blood levels reflect				
current BAL *	current BAL	current BAL	results are reported to reflect the amount of alcohol taken over the duration of the collection	average BAL between voiding
Clinical utility				
potential for accurately reflecting clinical status at the time of sample collection			levels are difficult to interpret	levels are lower during absorption phase and higher during the elimination phase

* BAL = Blood alcohol level

Table 8.2: *Various methods of analysis*

	Breathalyzer		Gas chromatography	Spectro-photometry[c]	Alcohol Dipstick
	Non-portable[a]	Portable[b]			
Analytical Methods					
Technology requirements					
Instruments	Less complex	Simple	Complex	Complex	None
Automation	No	No	Yes	Yes	No
Ease of Operation	Simple	Simple	Complex	Complex	Simple
Portability			No	No	Yes
Sample requirements					
Source	Breath	Breath	All body fluids and breath	All body fluids	All body fluids
Pretest Preparation	Minimal	Minimal	Extensive	Extensive	None
Sample Throughput	Slow	Slow	Medium (with automation)	High (with automation)	High
Economics — cost per test					
- Disposables	$2 - 5.00	$1 - 2.00	$1.00	$3 - 5.00	$1.00
- Labour	Low	Low	High	High	Minimal
Capital expense	1 to 5 K[d]	1 K	10 to 40 K	2 to 50 K	none

[a] e.g. Borkenstein
[b] e.g. A.L.E.R.T.
[c] Includes immunoassay reagent systems
[d] K = $1,000

Toronto's hospital casualty wards. This service, which is available on a 24-hour basis, is used by about 60 different hospitals. General drug screening on serum and urine specimens is done unless specified otherwise by the requesting emergency room physician. Gas chromatography and thin layer chromatography (Kapur 1984) are the main technologies used in the analysis of patients' serum and urine-gastric washing specimens, respectively. All patient demographic data, including the results, are stored in a computer data base using ATLAS (the Automated Toxicology Laboratory Administrative System) software system, which was developed at the Addiction Research Foundation. Although age and sex of the patient are usually requested from the hospital, they are not always supplied. Hence, numbers used in data analysis, based on sex and age reported here, do not add up to 100 per cent.

Recently the emergency room data from January 1984 to July 1985 were reviewed and some of the findings are presented below. Most of the analysis reported below was done on the first six months of 1984 (total samples = 7,940). We found that the patterns and number of specimens were very similar in the following twelve-month period, June 1984 to May 1985 (total samples = 16,043). Detailed alcohol statistics were done on the June 1984 to May 1985 data set.

Between January 1984 and June 1984, 4,566 blood-serum and 3,374 urine-gastric samples were analysed (9,150 and 6,893 for serum and urine respectively between June 1984 and May 1985). Figure 8.1 shows the pattern of positive results and number of drugs per specimen. Table 8.3 shows the data of positive blood specimens. Since some of the patients' specimens were repeated, the actual number of patients is also presented. Alcohol was the most common finding in the emergency room, followed by benzodiazepines and barbiturates. There has been a change in the pattern of barbiturate use in the Toronto region. In the mid-1970s amobarbital and secobarbital were the most common barbiturates. Butalbital has recently replaced these short-acting barbiturates. Table 8.4 lists the most common positive findings in urine specimens; benzodiazepines lead this list, followed by codeine and tricyclic antidepressants.

Table 8.3: *Positive blood drug screen (January - June 1984)*

Drug	Number of samples	Number of patients
Butabarbital	2	2
Barbital	2	2
Butalbital	140	80
Amobarbital	46	38
Pentobarbital	39	16
Secobarbital	79	64
Phenobarbital	316	204
Methyprylon	35	22
Meprobamate	11	9
Methaqualone	34	21
Acetaminophen	302	271
Salicylates	136	87
Methanol	20	3
Benzodiazepine	601	512
Ethanol	1515*	1287
Isopropanol	13	13
Ethylene Glycol	42	3
Aceton	40	78

Total number of samples — 4566 (*3,784 samples screened for ethanol)
Number with ≥1 drug — 2456 (53.7%)

Our data suggest that the number of specimens received is not significantly different on different days of the week. We did not find any significant difference between weekdays and weekends. The peak level of activity appears to be around the early hours of the morning. In our laboratory, results on 90 per cent of blood and urine specimens were reported within three hours to the hospital/physician requesting the tests.

Alcohol in the Casualty Room

Between the period of June 1984 and May 1985, 7,483 serum samples were analysed for ethanol. Of these 3,213 (42 per cent) were found to test positive for ethanol. A very wide distribution pattern of alcohol levels was observed (Figure 8.2). Mean blood level in our emergency room population was 211 mg/100 ml with a range going up to 868 mg/100 ml found in a male comatose patient. Fifty per cent of this population was above 220 mg/100 ml. Among those with positive blood alcohol levels, 23 per cent also had another drug in them (Figure 8.2). As has been reported by others (Ewing and Fox 1961; Boulton and Triger 1981), we also found that there were more males (63 per cent) than

Table 8.4: *Positive urine drug screen (January - June 1984)*

Drug	Frequency
Codine	309
Morphine	41
Amphetamines	11
Methamphetamine	9
Pentazocine	7
Benzodiazepine	365
Amitriptyline, Nortriptyline, Imipramine, Desimipramine, Doxepine	253
Chlorpromazine ⎤	
Perphenazine ⎬	64
Thioridazine ⎦	
Cimitidine	104
Pheniramine	92
Ephedrine	52
Phenylpropanolamine	136
Lidocaine	65
Cocaine	14
PCP - MDA - TMA	7
Unidentified	370

Total number of samples   - 3374
Number with 1 drug   - 1652 (49%)

Figure 8.1: *Frequency distribution of number of drugs detected by serum and urine drug screening*

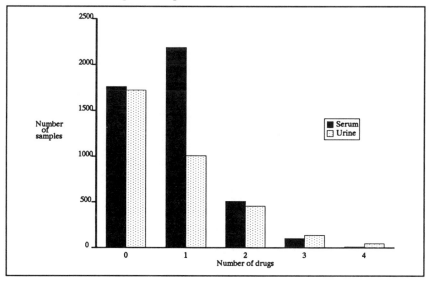

Figure 8.2: *Blood ethanol levels for alcohol only and with multiple drugs[a]*

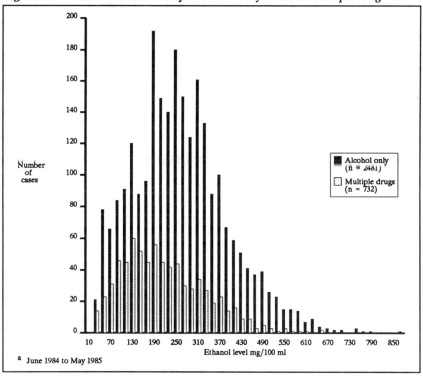

a   June 1984 to May 1985

Figure 8.3: *Blood ethanol levels by sex*[a]

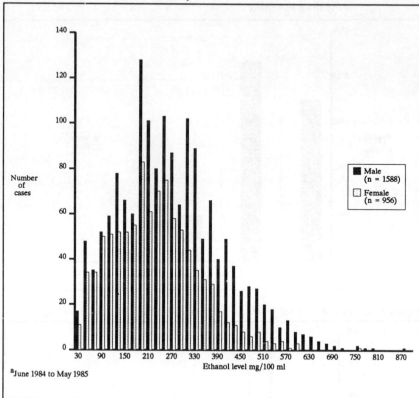

ᵃJune 1984 to May 1985

females (37 per cent) (Figure 8.3) in our population. Levels of consciousness were reported to us in some patients and Figure 8.4 shows the blood levels in 'alert' and 'comatose' patients at the time of admission to the emergency room. Of the 328 comatose patients, 77 (23.5 per cent) also had another drug present (Figure 8.5). These patients generally had lower blood-alcohol levels. There was a linear decline in number of patients with increase in age, although the mean blood-alcohol level is the highest in the 50-60 age bracket (Figure 8.6). Most of the patients were between 20 to 40 years old.

Alcohol is among the most commonly observed drugs in patients presenting themselves to the emergency rooms of hospitals. A study in *The Lancet* (Boulton and Triger 1981) reported that of the 107 admissions in the 6 month period, during 1980, they found alcohol was detectable in the blood of 48 per cent of the patients on admission. More often they were males (69 per cent) rather than females (34 per cent). Earlier studies in the 1960s by Ewing and Fox (1961) had also shown that 25 per cent of

Figure 8.4: *Blood alcohol levels in alert and comatose patients*

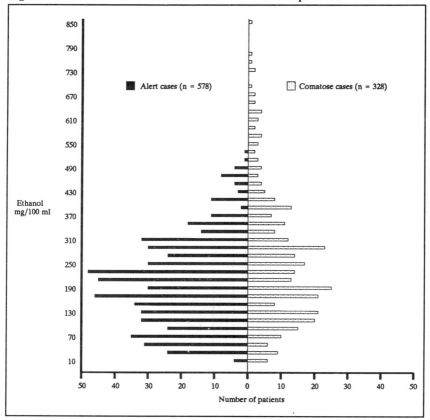

their patients had alcohol present in them. Our studies also show a similar pattern.

A large proportion of patients' specimens analysed in our laboratory showed the presence of drugs including alcohol. Our data suggest that on the basis of a given blood-alcohol level it is not possible to reliably predict the clinical level of consciousness of a patient. Tolerance to alcohol, presence of underlying clinical disorders or the presence of other drugs can complicate the interpretation of blood alcohol levels. In our population, although the highest level observed in a comatose patient was 868 mg/100 ml, some other comatose patients exhibited levels below 80 mg/100 ml, which is the upper limit for legally operating a motor vehicle in many countries. It is not unusual to observe patients who are 'alert' and have a BAL of greater than 400 mg/100 ml. Given our finding and the literature of a high incidence of alcohol in casualty room patients, at least semi-quantitative blood-alcohol measurements should be available in the casualty room of every hospital.

Figure 8.5: *Blood ethanol levels in comatose cases with alcohol only and with multiple drugs[a]*

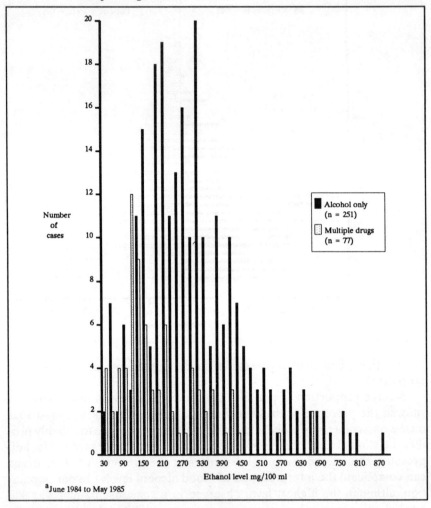

[a]June 1984 to May 1985

Figure 8.6: *Mean age distribution and mean BAL for each age group*

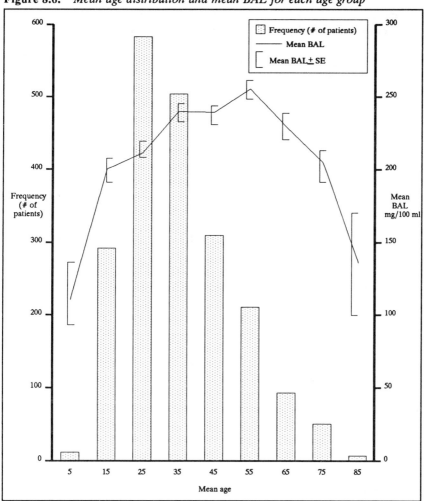

© 1989 Bhushan M. Kapur

185

References

Berild, D. and H. Hasselbalch (1981) Survival after a blood alcohol of 1127 mg/dl. *Lancet,* August 15, 1981, 363

Boulton, A.J.M. and D.R. Triger (1981) Self-poisoning patterns. *Lancet,* December 19, 1981, 1426

Ewing, M.R. and A.R. Fox (1961) Blood-alcohol levels in adult patients admitted to hospital after road traffic accidents. *Medical Journal of Australia, 42,* 2, 976

Goldstein, D.B. (1983) *Pharmacology of alcohol.* Oxford University Press, New York

Goodmann, L.S. and A. Gilman (eds.) (1980) *The pharmacological basis of therapeutics, Sixth edition.* Macmillan Publishing Co., Inc. New York, pp. 552-3

Goodwin, D.W. (1980) The pharmacology of alcohol: Some clinical aspects. In W.E. Fann, I. Karacan, A.D. Pokorny and R.L. Williams (eds), *Phenomenology and treatment of alcoholism.* Spectrum Publications, Inc, New York, pp. 21-31

Haggard, H.W., L.A. Greenberg, R.P. Carroll, and D.P. Miller (1940) The use of urine in the chemical test for intoxication; possible errors and their avoidance. *Journal of the American Medical Association, 115,* 1680

Jain N.C. (1971) Direct blood injection method for gas chromatographic determination of alcohols and other volatile compounds. *Clinical Chemistry, 17,* 82-5

Jones, A.H. (1979) Distribution of ethanol between saliva and blood in man. *Clinical and Experimental Pharmacology and Physiology, 6,* 53-9

Kalant, H. (1971) Absorption, diffusion, distribution and elimination of ethanol. In B. Kissin and H. Begleiter (eds), *Effects of biological membranes: the biology of alcoholism, volume 1, biochemistry,* Plenum Press, New York, pp. 1-62

Kapur, B.M. (1984) Strategies in a drug analysis laboratory: Therapeutic Drug Monitoring and Toxicology Continuing Education and Quality Control Program. *American Association for Clinical Chemistry, 5,* 12, 1-6

Kapur, B.M. and Y. Israel (1983) Alcohol dipstick — a rapid method for analysis of ethanol in body fluids. In N.C. Chang and H.M. Chao (eds), *Early identfication of alcohol abuse,* research monograph no. 17, National Institute of Alcohol Abuse and Alcoholism, 5600 Fishers Lane, Rockville, Maryland, pp. 310-320

Lin, Y., D.J. Weidler, D.C. Garg *et a.* (1976) Effects of solid food on blood levels of alcohol in man. *Research Communications in Chemical Pathology & Pharmacology, 13,* 4, 713-22

Lindblad, B (1976). Unusually high levels of blood alcohol? *Journal of the American Medical Association, 236*, 1600-2

Linde, P. (1932) Der Ubergang des Aethylalkohols in den Parotisspeichel beim Menschen. *Archiv für Experimentelle Pathologie und Pharmakologie, 167*, 285-91

Marshall, A.W., D. Kingstone, M. Boss and M.Y. Morgan (1983) Ethanol elimination in males and females: relationship to menstrual cycle and body composition. *Hepatology, 3*, 701-6

Miles, W.R. (1922) The comparative concentrations of alcohol in human blood and urine at intervals after ingestion. *Journal of Pharmacology and Experimental Therapy, 20*, 265

Peachey, J. and B.M. Kapur (1986) Monitoring drinking behaviour with the alcohol dipstick during treatment. *Alcoholism: Clinical and Experimental Research, 10*, 663-6

Peppiatt, R., R. Evans, and P. Jordan (1978) Blood alcohol concentrations of patients attending an accident emergency department, *Resuscitation, 6*, pp. 37-43

Redetzki H.M. and M.L. Dees (1976) Comparison of four kits for enzymatic determination of ethanol in blood. *Clinical Chemistry, 22*, 83-6

Von Wartburg, J.P. (1971) The metabolism of alcohol in normals and alcoholics. In B. Kissin and H. Begleiter (eds), *Enzymes in the biology of alcoholism, volume 1, biochemistry*, Plenum Press, New York, pp. 63-102

Widmark, M.P. (1922) Eine Mikromethode zür Bestimmung von Athylalkohol im Blut. *Biochemische Zeitschrift, 131*, 474-84

9

Research into and Registration of Alcohol-Related Non-Fatal Casualties in Finland: The Need for Improved Classification

Kari Poikolainen

This paper briefly reviews existing research on non-fatal alcohol-related casualties in Finland, excluding traffic accidents. The principles of alcohol detection in clinical settings and the National Hospital Discharge Register are described. Suggestions for improvements to facilitate research are presented.

Detection of Alcohol in Clinical Settings

In Finland, a minority of hospitals have systematic detection and registration practices concerning alcohol in casualty cases. At the Emergency Station of the Department of Orthopaedics and Traumatology, University Central Hospital of Helsinki, patients are evaluated for the ethyl sign and blood ethanol is either estimated from the breath or measured from the blood when alcohol is suspected to have been related to the injury.

The ethyl sign is a semi-quantitative summary of the clinical evaluation of the degree of alcohol intoxication. The following classifications are being used:

-      no evidence of alcohol use

+   smell of alcohol on the breath and slight behavioural changes

+ +   moderate intoxication: distinct behavioural changes and decreased ability to co-operate

+ + +   heavy intoxication: total loss of ability to co-operate

In 1973, positive ethyl signs were recorded in 13.5 per cent of the patients in the emergency station. Of patients with alcohol in the blood, 50 per cent had a positive ethyl sign while less than 0.5 per cent of patients with no alcohol in the blood had a positive ethyl sign (Honkanen 1976).

Alcohol-Related Casualties at Emergency Stations

Honkanen (1976) studied the role of alcohol in accidents treated at emergency stations. Of the seriously injured patients at the above-mentioned emergency station, 37 per cent had alcohol in the blood. The highest percentage was found among patients injured in fights or assaults (71 per cent). Head injuries predominated among alcohol-related injuries. In an analysis of 182 consecutive adult injury victims at the emergency station of the Jyväskylä Central Hospital in 1974, 30 per cent of patients were found to have alcohol in their blood.

In a case-control study on pedestrian accidents due to falls and hits by motor vehicles, the relative risk was found to be approximately exponentially related to the blood-alcohol level. Compared with pedestrians with no alcohol in the blood, the relative risk associated with a blood-alcohol level of over 200 mg/100 ml was 29. In the 1970s, an estimated 18 per cent of all injury cases were due to alcohol.

Evaluation of Casualty Prevalence

Salaspuro (1978) evaluated the number of hospital days, out-patient visits and primary care contacts related to alcohol in Finland in 1972. Two complicated sets of criteria were used to identify alcohol-related cases, one more and another less stringent. Briefly, the more stringent criteria were fulfilled if the patient had been intoxicated during the injury, presented with an alcohol-related disease, was observed to be intoxicated at the start of the treatment contact, used alcohol during the treatment or if evidence of heavy alcohol use was obtained either from the patient, from medical records or from relatives. The proportion of alcohol-related hospital days was estimated at 4.6 to 5.3 per cent of all hospital days. Alcohol-related casualties (injuries and poisonings) were found to comprise 10 per cent of all alcohol-related hospital days. This was around 0.5 per cent of all hospital days. Among males, 42 per cent of all alcohol-related out-patient visits were due to casualties.

Non-Fatal Alcohol Poisonings

Between 1980 and 1982, the Finnish Poison Information Center was asked for advice concerning 837 cases involving treatment for alcohol or glycol poisoning. The Monthly peaks in incidence were observed in April for preschool children and in December for adults (Eskola and Poikolainen 1985). In 1981, one-half of the poisonings among children aged under 16 years were life-threatening (Eskola 1983).

Casualty Hospitalisations

The Finnish National Hospital Discharge Register is run by the National Board of Health. All terminating hospitalisations and out-patient visits lasting at least 15 hours should be reported to this register. From 1967 onward, data have been derived from all general hospitals, mental hospitals, tuberculosis hospitals and from the hospitals of special institutions (e.g. prison hospitals, alcoholism treatment institutions). The annual number of registered hospitalisations in recent years has been around one million.

The basic tabulations are based on the principal diagnosis, i.e. the diagnostic category demanding most treatment and examination resources. In 1982, the number of hospitalisations in general hospitals due to casualties was around 70,000 (7.7 per cent of the total number of admissions). The percentage of hospitalisations due to casualties was 11 per cent among males and 5 per cent among females. The respective hospitalisation rates were 1.8 and 1.1 per 1,000 of population.

In addition to the principal diagnosis, three other diagnostic codes could be recorded. In casualty cases, one of these should be the code for the external cause of injury (E-code) corresponding to the principal diagnosis which indicates the nature of injury codes. Judging from the number of the nature of the injury codes about 70 per cent of the E-codes are missing (National Board of Health of Finland 1984). The available data suggest that accidental falls, transport accidents and the sub-group 'other accidents' (including drownings) predominate among both sexes (Table 9.1). This is also somewhat true for the sub-group that probably includes the highest proportion of alcohol-related casualties, males aged 25 to 44 years. In this group, the leading casualties are accidental falls (33 per cent), other accidents (28 per cent), transport accidents (16 per cent) and suicide and self-inflicted injury (7 per cent).

The coverage of stroke and myocardial infarction hospitalizations was found to be 78 per cent in the early 1970s (Heliövaara *et al.* 1984). Since then, the coverage has improved and is at present considered to be close to 100 per cent for all hospitalisations (National Board of Health of

Finland 1984). The percentage of agreement between medical records and discharge register data for alcohol-related hospitalisations between 1974 and 1975 has been found to be 98 per cent for date of birth, 96 per cent for date of admission, 91 per cent for the principal diagnosis, 84 per cent for marital status and 76 per cent for the second diagnosis (Poikolainen 1983).

A 1.9-fold increase in hospital admission rates due to alcohol poisoning for females between the years 1969 and 1975 has been described (Poikolainen, 1980). No other studies of hospitalisations due to alcohol-related casualties have been done so far, although some could easily be carried out. Among casualty patients, cross-tabulations of the principal casualty diagnosis with alcohol-related second, third and fourth diagnoses would reveal associations between types of alcohol problems and

Table 9.1: *Casualty discharges from Finnish hospitals in 1982 by external cause of injury and sex, percent*[a]

External cause of injury	Percent		ICD-8 codes
	Males	**Females**	
Transport accidents	17	15	807-846
Accidental poisonings	2	3	859-877
Accidental falls	33	57	880-887
Fire accidents	1	0	890-899
Accidents due to natural and environmental factors	1	1	900-909
Other accidents[b]	22	13	910-939
Late effects of accidental injury	3	4	940-949
Suicide and self-inflicted injury	3	4	950-959
Homicide and injury purposely inflicted by other person	3	2	960-969
Legal intervention	0	0	970-978
Injury undetermined whether accidentally or purposely inflicted	1	1	980-989
Injuries resulting from operations of war	13	0	990-999
Total	99	100	
Number of hospital admissions	34,487	22,113	

[a] Excluding mental and tuberculosis hospitals and the hospitals of special institutions
[b] Includes drowning

Source: Unpublished data sheets of the Finnish hospital discharge register

types of casualties. Since the presence of a unique personal identification number makes record-linkage feasible, follow-up studies of patients with alcohol problems could be carried out to yield estimates of casualty risks in these patient groups.

Comments and Recommendations

Having reasonable coverage and satisfactory reliability, the National Hospital Discharge Register in Finland would, in principle, be a good source of data for studies on alcohol-related casualties. These advantages are undermined, however, by the lack of information about alcohol and by problems with classifications of diseases and injuries currently available.

To have a simple and fairly reliable indicator of the relationship of alcohol to the injury, the concentration of alcohol in the blood (or its estimate from breath) should be measured early during every patient visit to out-patient departments, either in selected age-groups or for all patients during a certain period of time, say, for one month at selected intervals. This information should then be registered in the hospital discharge register. Clinical evaluation of the degree of intoxication (the ethyl sign) might be a useful piece of additional information but should not yet be included in the register because its reliability remains unknown and probably varies considerably between investigators. A clinically applicable method for evaluating the degree of intoxication would be useful, since, together with information on blood-alcohol levels it could be used to evaluate the degree of tolerance to alcohol. The development and testing of such methods should be given high priority.

The ninth revision of the International Classification of Diseases, Injuries, and Causes of Death (ICD-9) (World Health Organization 1977) is tautological and almost useless for research into alcohol-related casualties. Two improvements are needed. First, the coding of alcohol-related conditions needs revision. To facilitate comparisons between countries and years, the following simplifications should be considered:

1. Since criteria of dependence vary considerably and are difficult to measure, the categories 'alcohol dependence syndrome' (303) and 'non-dependent abuse of alcohol' (305.0) should be combined and all kinds of abuse coded into the category 303. The category 303 should exclude 'alcohol withdrawal syndrome' (291.8) and 'toxic effect of alcohol'(980) as well as 'alcohol inebriation'. Category 305.0 should not be used.

2. 'Alcohol inebriation' should be given a code of its own. One possibility would be the code 305.0. This would help make a distinction be-

tween the behavioural symptoms of alcohol intoxication (inebriation) and the toxic state itself (alcohol intoxication). This is important because individuals with high tolerance may exhibit no behavioural symptoms, yet have their bodies poisoned by alcohol. The word 'intoxication' comes from the words 'intensive' and 'toxon', the latter a Greek word for poison, and should not be used as a synonym for drunkenness.

3. To increase consistency, the category 'toxic effect of alcohol' (980), a synonym for alcohol intoxication, should be used as the principal diagnosis in hospital cases only if the main cause of treatment is respiratory failure due to alcohol intoxication, and in death certificates as the underlying cause of death only if the death is due to alcohol-induced aspiration, respiratory paralysis or toxic shock. The category 'excessive blood level of alcohol' (790.3) should not be used since there is no sense in dividing blood-alcohol levels into excessive and non-excessive.

The fact that around 70 per cent of the E-codes for injuries are missing in the Finnish hospital discharge register is not only an indication of a lack of interest on the part of the certifying physicians and surgeons but also a symptom of the impractical structure of the E-code. As a matter of urgency, a simple and more informative E-code should be developed along proposed lines (Baker 1982). A multi-axial system based on four dimensions (injury mechanism, site of occurrence, activity, and intent), developed by NOMESCO (1985), is worth considering. Users of this classification need to remember only 41 distinct options instead of the 192 categories in the E-codes of ICD-9. Yet these options combine to yield a theoretical maximum of 32,400 categories.

A good hospital discharge register would benefit research in many ways. Casualty hospitalisation trends could be monitored to describe seasonal variation and to find out effects of changes in alcohol availability, price and drinking habits. Cross-regional comparisons could examine the effects of the aforementioned and other factors on casualty admission rates and help in resource allocation. Moreover, the length and the cost of treatment could be compared between various regions and various types of patients. Among casualty patients, cross-tabulations of the principal casualty diagnosis with both possible alcohol-related additional diagnoses and with information on blood-alcohol concentration, and the degree of inebriation would reveal associations between types of alcohol problems and types of casualties. From such a register, patients for epidemiologic case-control studies could easily be found. And finally, when unique personal identification numbers make record-linkage feasible, follow-up studies of patients with alcohol problems could cost-efficiently be carried out to yield estimates of casualty risks in these patient groups.

© 1989 Kari Poikolainen

References

Baker, S.P. (1982) Injury classification and the International Classification of Diseases codes. *Accident Analysis and Prevention, 14*, 199-201

Eskola, J. (1983) *Lasten myrkytykset Suomessa: myrkytystietokes kuksen aineiston analyysi (Childhood poisoning in Finland: analysis of the data from the Finnish Poison Information Center)*. Health services research No. 26, National Board of Health of Finland, Helsinki

Eskola, J., and K. Poikolainen (1985) Seasonal variation and recurring peaks of reported poisonings during a three-year period. *Human Toxicology, 4*, 609-15

Heliövaara, M., A. Reunanen, A. Aromaa *et al.* (1984) Validity of hospital discharge data in a prospective epidemiological study on stroke and myocardial infarction. *Acta Medica Scandinavica, 216*, 309-15

Honkanen, R. (1976) Alcohol involvement in accidents: the role of alcohol in injuries treated at emergency stations. Department of Public Health Science, University of Helsinki, Helsinki

National Board of Health of Finland (1984) *Poistoilmoitusjärjestelmän kehittäminen (Developing the hospital discharge register)*. Lääkintöhallituksen työryhmien mietintöjä No. 7 Helsinki

Nordic Medico-Statistical Committee [NOMESCO] (1985) *Nordic classification for accident monitoring*, Copenhagen

Poikolainen, K. (1983) Accuracy of hospital discharge data: five alcohol-related diseases. *Drug and Alcohol Dependence, 12*, 315-22

— (1980) Increase in alcohol-related hospitalisations in Finland 1969-1975. *British Journal of Addiction, 75*, 281-91

Salaspuro, A. (1978) *Alkoholiin liittynyt terveyspalvelukäyttö Suomessa vuonna 1972 (Alcohol-related use of health services in Finland in 1972)* Volume 29, Finnish Foundation for Alcohol Studies, Helsinki

World Health Organization (1977) *Manual of the International Statistical Classification of Diseases, Injuries, and Causes of Death, Ninth Revision, Volume 1*, Geneva

Section III:

STUDIES OF NATIONAL SYSTEMS

10

Alcohol-Related Casualty Statistics in Australia

Robyn Norton

Statistical information on alcohol use and abuse has been collected in Australia since 1800. As the number and diversity of services has increased, the amount of available information has increased correspondingly.

Within the last few years, consideration has been given to the establishment of a national drug-related statistical collection. It is envisaged that a national statistical collection would co-ordinate drug-related data from a range of sources, including health, welfare and law enforcement departments and agencies. As an initial step, a concerted effort has been made to identify existing national, state and territory data collection systems relating to drugs, including both alcohol and tobacco. Currently, a range of data collection systems has been identified and details have been collected on the information available from each system.

The majority of collection systems are not specifically 'alcohol-related', but information on alcohol-related behaviours can be drawn from them. In some collections, the role of alcohol can only be ascertained by referring back to the original data sources. In other collections, it is necessary to employ 'indices' of alcohol's involvement from studies that have previously investigated the role of alcohol in behaviour.

Alcohol-related casualties, excluding motor vehicle accident casualties, have not been a particular focus of interest or concern in Australia. However, statistics on alcohol-related casualties are available from the existing data collection systems. In almost all of the collection systems, the role of alcohol in casualties is not defined, and reference must be made to the original data sources or to studies undertaken previously.

For the purpose of this paper casualties are defined as accidents, poisonings and violence involving injury or death to a person or persons. Motor vehicle accidents have not been included, given the large body of research already devoted to this topic. Casualties are also defined as persons attending hospital casualty/emergency departments. Persons attending casualty/emergency departments following a motor vehicle accident have not been included in the discussion.

The aim of this paper is to provide information on alcohol-related casualties and alcohol-related casualty statistics in Australia. Initial consideration is given to existing systems of recording and analysis of alcohol-related casualties. The causal role of alcohol in casualties is then discussed, followed by an assessment of the prevalence of alcohol-related casualties in Australia. The use of casualty statistics for curtailing and managing casualties is considered and, finally, proposals for new initiatives in this area are discussed.

Existing Systems of Recording and Analysis

The National Mortality Data System

Data on alcohol-related deaths in Australia are available through the annual collection of mortality data undertaken by the Australian Bureau of Statistics. Basic data on all deaths have been published annually since the early 1900s and further data are available on microfiche and computer tapes.

The registrars of births, deaths and marriages in each state and territory are responsible for routinely forwarding copies of all death certificates to the Bureau of Statistics for tabulation and coding according to the International Classification of Diseases. An examination of this procedure has shown that information recorded from the death certificate is reliably classified and coded (Drew 1982a). Cause of death, age, sex, marital status and country of birth are recorded on each death certificate. Alcohol-related deaths are not necessarily reported as such in this collection, which uses the ICD-9 categories of diseases and external causes of death. Although the number of categories identified as alcohol-related has increased in recent years, few deaths from specifically alcohol-related casualties are identified.

Since 1978, data concerning selected alcohol-related mortality have been brought together in three publications, providing a summary of alcohol-related statistics in Australia (Commonwealth Dept. of Health 1978, 1979, 1984). The analysis and publication of the data have been undertaken by the Central Statistical Unit of the Commonwealth Department of Health, employing data provided by the Bureau of Statistics. For a range of deaths, a conservative estimate or 'index' of the proportion of deaths in which it can be assumed that alcohol has played a significant role, has been calculated. In determining the indices for specific causes of death, reviews of studies reported in the world literature, in addition to Australian studies, have been considered.

State/Territory Hospital Morbidity Data Systems

Unlike the mortality data systems, statistics on hospital discharges are not collected on a national basis in Australia. Each state or territory has responsibility for the collection of data on hospital morbidity within its own region. However, both the period of time over which data have been collected and the quality of the data available from each state or territory vary considerably. Published data with almost 100 per cent coverage of public and private hospitals are available from three states: Queensland, New South Wales and Western Australia. Data are available from both Queensland and Western Australia since 1973, and from New South Wales since 1977. Of the remaining states and territories, the coverage and the quality of data in two states are incomplete; in the third state, publication of data has recently been discontinued; and in the two territories, although collected, no published data are available.

As with the mortality data, even where published morbidity data are available, alcohol-related hospital admissions are not necessarily reported as such. In only a few instances does the International Classification of Diseases allow for the identification of an alcohol-related illness. To date, no attempt has been made to develop any 'indices' of alcohol's involvement in selected hospital admissions. As a consequence, although some state morbidity data systems exist, and, potentially, hospital morbidity alcohol-related casualty statistics are available, no systematic collation of such statistics has yet been undertaken.

Casualty-Specific Data Systems

In addition to the National Mortality Data System and the hospital morbidity data systems, a number of additional data systems exist which provide information on specific casualties.

Accidents

Industrial accidents. Data on industrial accidents are collected nationally by the Australian Bureau of Statistics, but the collection is deficient in specifically identifying those accidents which are alcohol-related. In addition to this collection, each of the states and territories maintains a collection system on work-related accidents through the framework of the

Worker's Compensation Commission. Again, however, information identifying alcohol-related accidents is deficient. The primary reason for the
difficulty in identifying alcohol-related accidents relates to the nature of
the compensation system. As the system is not a 'no-fault' system, the in-
centive exists to minimize the possible involvement of alcohol in the accident (Frommer 1985).

Aviation accidents. The Federal Department of Aviation maintains a
data system on all aviation accidents, involving air transport where a li-
cence is required. The system has been maintained since 1969, and although record of alcohol is not mandatory in the reports, its presence is
generally noted.

Water accidents. During the summer months in Australia, many of the
more populous beaches are patrolled by members of the Surf Life Saving
Association of Australia. Resuscitation report forms are completed for
each person requiring any form of resuscitation by a member of the Association (Mackie 1978).

Although the recording of alcohol is not mandatory, its presence or
absence is generally noted. The proportion of both near-drownings and
drownings that involve members of the SLSAA has not been calculated.
A unique and very comprehensive collection system exists on all fatal
drownings occurring in and around the Victorian town of Geelong. The
director of pathology at Geelong Hospital has maintained an interest
over the last 25 years in the role played by alcohol in drownings. As a
consequence, all fatal drownings in the area over the last 25 years have
been autopsied, and the presence or absence of alcohol has been recorded (Plueckhahn 1984).

Poisonings

A National Poisons Case Reporting System was established by the Commonwealth Department of Health in 1966 (Newman-Martin 1985) and
detailed statistics from the system are available from 1982 (Drew 1982b).
Two sources of information are used in the reporting system: data from
each state and territory Poisons Information Centres, and data from
hospital casualty departments. The Centres provide telephone information on poisonings and data are recorded on all notified poisonings. The
use of alcohol, alone or in association with other substances, is noted on
the report form. The proportion of all poisonings that are notified is unknown, and it is possible that some poisonings may also be included in the
hospital casualty statistics. At present, only 15 per cent of all hospitals
report poisonings seen in their casualty departments in full detail. As
reporting of poisonings is undertaken on a voluntary basis, not all hospi-

tal staff within a hospital participate in the scheme, nor do all hospitals participate. In addition, the extent to which alcohol overdose is uniformly recorded as 'poisoning' has not been determined.

Violence

Although the Federal Police Department maintains a collection system on drug-related crime, the emphasis is on illicit drugs and, as such, the system is deficient in identifying crimes that are specifically alcohol-related (McLauglan 1985).

Within each state and territory, incident reports are filed by investigating police and data from these reports are published annually. Although information indicating the presence or absence of alcohol in a particular incident may be noted in the police report, this information is not uniformly collated and published in the annual reports. Detailed analyses of the police reports has been undertaken in some states, and the results of these analyses published (New South Wales Bureau of Crime Statistics and Research 1973, 1974, 1975a, 1975b, Office of Crime Statistics 1981).

Court reports of cases where an alleged offender has been charged are collated in all states and territories. As with the police reports, although alcohol involvement may be noted in the reports, the collated statistics do not include detailed information on the presence or absence of alcohol.

In addition to the above systems, a data collection system is maintained in each state or territory through the coroner's courts. In cases of 'unnatural' death, an autopsy is often required by the court, involving among other procedures, the measurement of blood alcohol. In many of the states, although reports on all investigations have been kept, annual collection and analysis of the reports have not been undertaken.

Within New South Wales, the Bureau of Crime Statistics and Research has established a 'firearms casualty reporting system'. Records are maintained on all gun-related accidents, suicides and attempted suicides, and criminally influenced deaths or injuries. Information is obtained on both shooters and victims, including, where possible, data on the presence or absence of alcohol.

Data Systems Within Hospital Casualty Emergency Departments

Data collection systems specifically recording details on all persons attending casualty/emergency departments do not currently exist. Statistics of all admissions can be obtained through the hospital morbidity collections, and information detailing alcohol use at the time of the admission can be obtained by reading through individual case files. Blood-alcohol readings are taken routinely on all motor vehicle casualty admissions. However, no legal requirement exists for taking of such measurements in other admissions. Although in many hospitals staff routinely record information on 'usual' alcohol consumption, in addition to recording information on the presence or absence of alcohol at the time of admission, it is not undertaken by all staff in all hospitals.

The Causal Role of Alcohol in Casualties

Indices used in the Assessment of National Data on Casualty Mortality

The first attempt to investigate the role of alcohol in mortality in Australia was made by Derrick in 1967. He derived a comprehensive list of indices for alcohol-related deaths, employing both Australian and overseas studies. Based on an Australian study by Adams in 1966, he suggested that 13 per cent of all drownings and 20 per cent of those occurring in persons over 15 years of age were alcohol-related. On the basis of an Australian study by Birrel in 1965, he suggested that 50 per cent of homicides were alcohol-related. From a series of reports on suicide, he concluded that at least 20 per cent could be attributed to alcohol.

The list was revised by Drew in 1976 and 1982. Drew's indices, which were developed as conservative indices, based on studies reported in the world literature, have been adopted by the Central Statistical Unit in preparing their published estimates on the extent of alcohol-related mortality in Australia. Despite the problems inherent in using information from studies conducted in other countries, where quantities and patterns of consumption may be different, the Central Statistical Unit has adopted Drew's approach given the paucity of Australian studies.

On the basis of two overseas studies, Drew concluded that, conservatively, 10 per cent of falls were alcohol-related. The lack of Australian reports on the relationship between alcohol and burns, combined with the small numbers of deaths involved, led Drew to disregard this in his assessment of alcohol-related mortality. By comparison, comprehensive reviews of the literature on drowning by Mackie (1978) and Plueckhahn (1984), pointed to the fact that alcohol was involved in 30 per cent of all drownings in persons 15 years and older. Drew's review of the suicide literature led him to suggest conservatively that alcohol was involved in 20 per cent of all suicides. Finally, after consideration of the literature on homicide, Drew suggested an alcohol index of 33.3 per cent.

Australian Studies Investigating the Causal Role of Alcohol in Casualties

Both Derrick and Drew, in preparing their mortality indices, reviewed many of the Australian studies that had been undertaken to investigate the causal role of alcohol in both mortality and morbidity. However, a comprehensive review of studies in this area was published in 1983 by Smith. Although his review includes overseas studies, prominence is given to Australian studies. Almost all the studies undertaken in Australia provide little more than data on the presence or absence of alcohol in the person's body at the time of the event. Little attempt has been made to assess the presence or absence of alcohol in persons at risk, who were not involved in the event. As a consequence, minimal data are available on the risks associated with the consumption of alcohol, in relation to the occurrence of a particular casualty.

In addition to the above limitations, many of the studies suffer from the fact that only a proportion of the cases under consideration have information recorded on alcohol. Few of the studies have attempted to determine or even discuss the biases that may result as a consequence.

Accidents

Industrial Accidents. Although many reports, particularly those advocating the introduction of Employee Assistance Programmes in industry, suggest that alcohol contributes significantly to industrial accidents, no studies of this sort have been undertaken in Australia. Two surveys of management personnel, reported in a recent review, found that the majority of personnel staff perceived a relationship between drinking and accidents in their companies (Schlosser and McBride 1984). However, neither study was able to provide comprehensive evidence of the fact.

Aviation Accidents. An assessment by the Federal Department of Aviation of all aviation accidents occurring in Australia from 1969 suggests that alcohol is involved in 0.6 per cent of such accidents. However, information on alcohol was not available in all cases.

Water Accidents. A study of accidental drownings reported by Adams in 1966 found that of 163 accidental drownings, 22 persons (13.5 per cent) were intoxicated at the time of death. Mackie refers to the Water Safety Council of New South Wales's 1976-7 report, suggesting that raised blood-alcohol levels were found in 30 per cent of all adult drownings occurring in New South Wales in that year. In the same review, Mackie references an analysis of the Life Saving Association of Australia's resuscitation report forms, in which 26 per cent of adults who had drowned and 30 per cent of adults who had nearly drowned, had imbibed alcohol.

Over the 25 years of Pleuckhahn's research, 265 persons have died as a result of either accidental or purposeful immersion in fresh or salt water. Except in those cases where the bodies had disintegrated, 100 per cent of persons drowned were autopsied. Of the 135 'accidental' drownings occurring in persons 15 years and older, 45 per cent had consumed alcohol prior to their deaths, and 29 per cent had BACs greater than 80 mg/100 ml. Only one of the thirteen women had consumed alcohol, but 60 of the 122 men (49 per cent) had imbibed. Thirty-two per cent of the men had BACs greater than 80 mg/100 ml, with the highest proportion being men in the 30 to 64-year age group. Of those who had been swimming or surfing at the time of their deaths, 20 per cent had BACs greater than 80 mg/100 ml; of those who had fallen and slipped immediately before death, 62 per cent had BACs greater than 80 mg/100 ml; and of those drowning following a water transport accident, 17 per cent had BACs greater than 80 mg/100 ml.

Poisonings

The role of alcohol in persons presenting to hospital casualty departments following 'overdose' has been investigated in three studies. Freeman *et al.* in 1968-9 found that 42 per cent of males and 12 per cent of females arriving at the Royal Hobart Hospital in Tasmania had consumed large quantities of alcohol before overdosing. A study undertaken at Box Hill District Hospital in Victoria found that 53 per cent of males and 31 per cent of females had consumed alcohol before overdosing (Brentnall 1985). Over a three-month period, Reilly *et al.* (1983) investigated all acute and chronic drug problems, excluding alcohol, presenting to the accident and emergency department at St. Vincent's Hospital in Sydney, New South Wales. Alcohol was present in 44 per cent of the 158 overdose cases that were assayed. (Forty-one overdose cases either refused to be assayed or discharged themselves before an assay could be done.)

Analysis of the Poison Information Centre reports for 1983 indicated that alcohol, either alone or in combination with other drugs, was involved in 1.8 per cent of poisonings. Alcohol alone represented only 0.95 per cent of all poisonings notified through this reporting system. Analysis of the hospital reports for 1982 suggested that alcohol, either alone or in combination, was involved in 20.5 per cent of poisonings, with only 4.3 per cent involving alcohol alone. In 1983, 16.2 per cent of the reports involved alcohol alone or in combination, and 4.2 per cent involved alcohol alone. A breakdown of these statistics indicates that alcohol alone was involved in a higher proportion of poisonings due to misuse than those due to suicide. Alcohol was minimally involved in poisonings due to accidents (Newman-Martin 1985).

Table 10.1: *The causal role of alcohol in attempted suicides*

Authors	Year	Alcohol involvement
James *et al.*	1961-62	62% had BAC of 0.05% and over – 69% M & 59% F. 50% M & 20% F had BAC > 0.015%. 27% M & 6% F were alcoholics
Buckle *et al.*	1963-64	19% were under the influence – 17% M & 23% F. 52% M & 12% F were alcoholics (c.f. 19% M & 4.7% F controls)
Krupinski *et al.*	1963	13.2% M & 2.6% F were alcoholics
Edwards *et al.*	1965-66	48% M & 16.5% F had consumed alcohol before attempt. 38% M & 9% F were alcoholics
Krupinski *et al.*	1967	> 25% M & almost 12.5% F were under the influence
N.S.W. Bureau of Crime Stats.	1973-74	34.3% of gun suicides had been drinking prior to shooting
Goldney	1975-80	in F high lethality group reported less use of alcohol c.f. lower lethality groups

Table 10.2: *The causal role of alcohol in completed suicides*

Authors	Year	Alcohol involvement
James *et al.*	1961-62	37.5% had BAC > 0.04% – 47.8% M & 38.5% F. 6.7% had a history of alcoholism
Krupinski *et al.*	1963	32.8% M & 21.9% F were alcoholics
Gay *et al.*	1965-66	20% M & 6.5% F had taken alcohol
Burvill	1967	14% M & 7% F had evidence of heavy drinking. 6% M & 2% F were alcoholics
Chynoweth *et al.*	1973-74	34% M & 33% F had been heavy drinkers
Goldney	1975-80	28% F had alcohol in blood
Renwick *et al.*	1976-78	almost 50% had alcohol in blood. (20% of total of whom 50% had no BAC)

Violence

Suicides. A substantial body of research has been undertaken in Australia on both attempted and completed suicides. Summaries of these studies are presented in Tables 10.1 and 10.2, respectively.

In studies of attempted suicide, alcohol involvement ranges from 19 to 62 per cent for males and females combined (Table 10.1). With one exception, all the studies suggest that alcohol is involved in a higher proportion of male attempts. In studies of completed suicides, alcohol involvement ranges from 28 to 50 per cent, for males and females combined, with alcohol being involved in a higher percentage of male suicides (Table 10.2).

Of those studies comparing attempted suicides with completed suicides, it was found that a higher percentage of attempted suicides, compared with completed suicides, had consumed alcohol prior to the event (James *et al.* 1963, Krupinski *et al.* 1965).

Homicides and assaults (other than domestic and sexual assaults). The first study reporting on the role of alcohol in homicides was that by Birrel in 1965. He found that alcohol was present in 76 per cent of the homicide victims that he studied. More extensive research in this area has been undertaken and reported by the New South Wales Bureau of Crime Statistics and Research (1973). An assessment of gun and knife attacks occurring in 1972 suggested that 62 per cent of the attackers in serious assaults and 69 per cent of those responsible for homicides were at least partially affected by alcohol. Information on alcohol was recorded in only half of these cases. An assessment by the Bureau of all criminal firearm offences occurring between 1973 and 1974 found that in cases where information on alcohol was available, 40 per cent of the victims and 44 per cent of the shooters had been drinking. Information on drinking was available in two-thirds of the reported cases. It was noted that information on drinking was recorded less often when the victim had died.

A study of homicides and serious assaults occurring in 1978, 1979 and 1980 was undertaken by the Office of Criminal Statistics in South Australia. Of the 38 per cent of the cases for whom information was available, the victims only, had consumed alcohol in 22 per cent of the cases; the offenders only, in 25 per cent of the cases; both the victim and the offender had consumed alcohol in 35 per cent of the cases; neither had consumed alcohol in the remaining 18 per cent of the cases.

A personal assessment of 100 persons accused of murder and who underwent a psychiatric assessment was reported recently (Parker 1979). A third of the cases had been drinking prior to the offence. However, the extent to which this group differed in their behaviour to those who had not undergone a psychiatric assessment was not discussed by the author.

Further support for the role of alcohol in violent offences is available from a study of prison inmates (Drew 1967). Among males imprisoned for violent offences for a period of more than three months, 47.2 per cent indicated that they were under the influence of alcohol at the time of the offence.

Domestic Assaults. The New South Wales Bureau of Crime Statistics and Research undertook a comprehensive assessment of all cases of domestic assault that were handled by chamber magistrates at 22 courthouses throughout the state between mid-April and the end of June, 1975. In the victims' statements, nearly 60 per cent of the attackers had been drinking before the assault. In 14.5 per cent of the cases, the complainant had also consumed a quantity of alcohol, either separately or in the company of the alleged attacker.

The results of two surveys of individuals reporting, by telephone, their experiences of domestic violence have provided further evidence of alcohol's involvement in domestic violence (Stewart 1982, Scutt 1983).

Sexual Assault. A 1968 study of imprisoned sexual offenders found that 30.1 per cent were under the influence of alcohol at the time of the offence (Bartholomew). Research on sexual assault was reported by the New South Wales Bureau of Crime Statistics and Research in 1973. Of 169 reported 'genuine' rapes, information on alcohol was available in 102 cases. In 34.3 per cent of the cases, both the victim and the offender had been drinking together before the offence; in 30.4 per cent of the cases, offenders only had been drinking, and in 19 per cent, the victims only had been drinking.

A comprehensive study of rapists in Victoria was reported by Cordner *et al.* in 1979. Of 103 alleged rapes occurring between January and October, 1976, information on alcohol abuse was available in 84 cases. Of these, 17.5 per cent of the victims of single offenders and 14.8 per cent of the victims of multiple offenders had been drinking. Information on offenders was available in 66 of the cases and of these, 48 per cent had been drinking. By comparison, Hodgens, in an earlier study, found that 12 per cent of the victims of single offenders and 57 per cent of victims of multiple offenders had been drinking. Sixty-eight of the 69 offenders in this study had been drinking.

The Causal Role of Alcohol in Casualty/Emergency Departments in Australia

To date, the causal role of alcohol in casualty/emergency departments in Australia has not been extensively investigated. In 1970, Gay *et al.* published a study in which, over a seven-day period, BACs were determined in all persons attending a casualty/emergency department in a large hospital in Melbourne, Victoria. Two hundred and forty-six persons, between 18 and 65 years of age were studied, with a further 31 persons refusing to have BACs taken. Of those studied, 30.7 per cent gave BACs greater than 10 mg/100 ml (32 per cent of males and 38 per cent of females). BACs greater than 50 mg/100 ml were found in 26 per cent of males and 13 per cent of females. After excluding persons attending the casualty department following a motor vehicle accident, 24 per cent of persons were found to have BACs greater than 10 mg/100 ml, 19 per cent were found to have BACs greater than 50 mg/100 ml and 8 per cent were found to have BACs greater than 150 mg/100 ml.

Since the publication of that paper, there have been no further published studies. However, the situation is likely to change within the next few years. As part of the World Health Organization's collaborative study on the identification and treatment of persons with harmful alcohol consumption, a study is currently being conducted to address the question of alcohol's role within casualty departments at Royal Prince Alfred Hospital in Sydney, New South Wales (Saunders 1985).

The Prevalence of Alcohol-Related Casualties

Given the minimal attention focused on alcohol-related casualties in Australia, few systematic attempts have been made to document their prevalence.

Alcohol-Related Casualty Mortality

Data on alcohol-related mortality in Australia in 1965 is provided in Derrick's 1967 paper. Alcohol-related mortality from poisonings, drownings, homicides and suicides accounted for 0.5 per cent of all deaths.

Data are available from the Central Statistical Unit on alcohol-related mortality for 1981. The indices calculated by Drew in 1982 have been applied to the total mortality for each specific cause of death.

In 1981 there were 591 deaths from alcohol-related poisonings, falls, drownings, homicides and suicides. These deaths represented 17 per cent of the total deaths that were attributed to alcohol. Deaths from alcohol-related motor vehicle accidents accounted for 57 per cent of the total deaths that were attributed to alcohol. The 591 alcohol-related 'casualty' deaths accounted for 0.5 per cent of the total deaths for that year and represented a rate of 3.96 alcohol-related casualty deaths per 100,000 population. Of these 591 deaths, suicides comprised the largest proportion (56.7 per cent), followed by homicide (15.9 per cent), accidental falls

(15 per cent), accidental drownings (11.2 per cent) and accidental poisonings (1.35 per cent).

Comparison of these 1981 data with previous years suggests that alcohol-related casualty mortality as a percentage of total alcohol-related mortality has changed little over time. Similarly there has been little change in the percentage of alcohol-related casualty mortality as a percentage of total mortality, in the rate of deaths per 100,000 population or in the percentage contribution of each casualty to the total casualty mortality.

Alcohol-Related Casualty/Emergency Department Admissions

As discussed above, data from Gay *et al.'s* 1970 study suggest that 24 per cent of persons being admitted to the casualty/emergency department, excluding admissions from motor vehicle accidents, had been drinking prior to admission. Nineteen per cent had a BAC greater than 50 mg/100 ml and 8 per cent had BACs greater than 150 mg/100 ml. The age group with the highest percentage of positive BACs was the 35 to 59-year olds, with the 26 to 35-year olds having the lower percentage.

The Use of Casualty Statistics in Developing Policies and Programs

The Development of National Policies and Programs

The development of a national policy on alcohol use and abuse in Australia is seen as a priority within the Commonwealth Department of Health (Grigson 1985). Recent discussions have focused on the particular direction that the policy should take. The general consensus has been to emphasize the reduction of drinking behaviours that lead to problems, rather than an overall reduction in consumption *per se*. The development of 'responsible' drinking behaviour and the identification of 'high risk' individuals have also been expressed as particular foci of a national policy. Casualty statistics have contributed to the development of this policy as they form part of the general body of statistical knowledge about alcohol use and abuse. While programs aimed at curtailing or managing specific casualties may be initiated as a consequence of a national policy, these are likely to be developed within the context of a range of strategies aimed at achieving the broad goal of a reduction of harmful drinking behaviour.

The Development of State and Territory Policies and Programs

Concern about alcohol misuse and its associated problems has led some states and territories to consider the development of specific policies on alcohol and other drugs. In New South Wales, a draft policy has been prepared by the Department of Health (1984) and has recently undergone discussion and comment. As a preamble to the specific policy statement, the role of alcohol in specific casualties has been discussed. As with the proposed national policy, the New South Wales policy statement is concerned with the broader issues of the prevention and minimisation of adverse consequences of use. However, within the stated specific policy objectives, a reduction in the incidence and prevalence of drug and alcohol-related accidents and trauma, in addition to an overall reduction in the incidence and prevalence of drug and alcohol-related illness and death, has been stated as a specific policy objective.

Programmes and strategies aimed at achieving the stated objectives are likely to be emphasized if the policy document is accepted. Persons interested in undertaking research and other activities aimed at curtailing or managing casualties, would presumably have a strong mandate for support.

The Development of Casualty-Specific Policies and Programs

Employee assistance programmes have gained considerable support in Australia through the activities of a number of organisations and industries. However, their implementation has occurred in the absence of statistical data on the role of alcohol or the numbers of alcohol-related accidents in the Australian workplace.

The work of Plueckhahn has contributed significantly to concern about alcohol's role in water-related accidents. As a consequence, educational programs aimed at reducing the numbers of alcohol-related water accidents have been developed in many state and territory government departments concerned with water safety, sport and tourism.

Future Proposals

As was discussed in the opening paragraphs, the establishment of a national drug-related statistical collection has recently been considered. This proposal was given considerable impetus as a consequence of a special premiers' conference on drugs, held in Canberra on April 2, 1985 (Office of the Prime Minister). At that meeting, the establishment of national and state drug data collections were endorsed and resources made available. The potential now exists for improvements in the existing systems, for the establishment of new systems and for detailed analyses of all available data. In addition, co-ordination of drug-related data from a variety of sources will enable comprehensive analyses not only of the causal role of alcohol in casualties, but also of the prevalence of alcohol-related casualties within Australia.

The establishment of a national morbidity data system on drugs has been proposed (Drew 1985). Comparable data on drug-related morbidity is perceived as essential for obtaining accurate information about the importance of drugs in health services, health costs and the priorities required in professional training. In addition, the monitoring and modifying of policies and programs in accordance with assessed trends is being stated as a justifiable reason for the establishment of such a system. Detailed discussion of the proposal is currently being undertaken.

Support for ongoing and future proposals aimed at identifying and recording alcohol-related casualties and investigating the causal role of alcohol in casualty/emergency departments in Australia is increasing. In particular, there is growing support from the recently formed Australasian College of Emergency Medicine (Fulde 1985). Members of the College have expressed a great deal of concern about the number of casualty/emergency department admissions which appear to be alcohol-related. Despite their own limited resources, they see the need for alcohol-related work as a priority, and are willing to co-operate and collaborate with others interested in this area.

Summary and Conclusions

Although statistics on alcohol-related use and abuse have been collected in Australia for many years, alcohol-related casualty statistics have not generally been identified as a sub-category. Alcohol-related casualty mortality statistics have been obtained through the application of alcohol 'indices' that have been developed following reviews of both Australian and overseas literature. Use of these indices suggests that alcohol-related casualties have contributed to 0.5 per cent of all deaths in the last 20 years, and approximately 17 per cent of all alcohol-related deaths. Suicides comprise the largest proportion of alcohol-related casualty mortality. Theoretically, alcohol-related casualty morbidity statistics can also be obtained in this way. However, to date, appropriate 'indices' have not been developed.

Casualty-specific data collection systems currently exist for a number of casualties. Many of the systems and the research undertaken using the statistics collected in the systems suffer in that the collection of information on alcohol is voluntary. As a consequence, the role of alcohol in casualties is difficult to ascertain. The outstanding exception is the collection system on drownings, maintained by Plueckhahn. Data from this system suggest that alcohol is a factor in approximately 30 per cent of accidental drownings in persons 15 years and older.

Information on the role of alcohol in casualty/emergency department admissions in Australia is limited. Research undertaken in 1969 suggests that alcohol was present in 24 per cent of admissions excluding motor vehicle accident admissions. Studies currently being undertaken in a number of hospitals may provide an updated assessment of this figure within the next year.

Although alcohol-related casualty statistics have contributed in part to the development of proposed national and state policies on alcohol, their contribution has been within the context of a broad assessment of the total available alcohol-related statistics.

Acknowledgements

I would like to acknowledge the many people who gave both time and information in the collection and preparation of data for this paper. In particular, the assistance of Col Parrett, Social Health Branch, Commonwealth Department of Health, was invaluable in establishing many of the initial contacts. The paper was prepared, in part, with the support of a grant from the Utah Foundation.

References

Adams, A. (1966) The descriptive epidemiology of drowning accidents. *Medical Journal of Australia, 2*, 914-99

Australian Bureau of Statistics [no date] *Causes of Death, Australia*, Catalogue No. 3303

— [no date] *Hospital morbidity, Queensland*, Catalogue No. 4303.3

— [no date] *Hospital inpatient statistics, New South Wales*, Catalogue No. 4306.1

— [no date] *Hospital inpatient statistics, Western Australia*, Catalogue No. 4301.5

Bartholomew, A. (1968) Alcoholism and crime. *Australian and New Zealand Journal of Criminology, 1*, 76-99

Birrel, J.H.W. (1965) Blood alcohol levels in drunk drivers, drunk and disorderly subjects and moderate social drinkers. *Medical Journal of Australia, 2*, 949-53

Brentnall, E. (1985) Personal communication

Buckle, R.C., J. Linane and N. McConachy (1965) Attempted suicide presenting at the Alfred Hospital, Melbourne. *Medical Journal of Australia, 1*, 754-8

Burvill, P.W. (1971) Suicide in Western Australia, 1967: an analysis of coroner's records. *Australia and New Zealand Journal of Psychiatry, 5*, 37-44

Chynoweth, R., J.I. Tonge and J. Armstrong (1980) Suicide in Brisbane. A retrospective psychosocial study. *Australian and New Zealand Journal of Psychiatry, 14*, 37-45

Commonwealth Department of Health (1978, 1979, 1984) *Alcohol in Australia. A summary of related statistics*, AGPS, Canberra

Cordner, S.M., C.G. Ainley and M.A. Schneider (1979) Rape and rapists in Victoria. *Australia and New Zealand Journal of Criminology, 12*, 41-50

Department of Health, New South Wales (1984) Alcohol and other drug use problems. Draft policy statement

Derrick, E.H. (1967) A survey of mortality caused by alcohol. *Medical Journal of Australia, 2*, 914-99

Drew, L.R.H. (1967) Alcohol offenders in a Victorian prison. *Medical Journal of Australia, 1*, 575-8

— (1982a) Death and drug use in Australia, 1969 to 1980. *Technical Information Bulletin, 69*, 1-44

— (1982b) Monitoring drug use in Australia: National Poisons Case Reporting System. In preparation

— (1985) Personal communication

Edwards, J.E. and F.A. Whitlock (1968) Suicide and attempted suicide in Brisbane I. *Medical Journal of Australia, 1*, 932-8

Freeman, J.W., C.A. Ryan and R.R. Beattie (1970) Epidemiology and drug overdose in Southern Tasmania. *Medical Journal of Australia, 2*, 1168-72

Frommer, M. (1985) Personal communication

Fulde, G. (1985) Personal communication

Gay, T.J., R.L. Coates, G.L. Coggins, R.D. Alexander and J. Nayman (1970) Blood alcohol concentrations upon admission to a hospital based casualty department. *Medical Journal of Australia, 2*, 778-81

Gibson, M. (1985) Personal communication

Goldney, R.D. (1981) Alcohol in association with suicide and attempted suicide in young women. *Medical Journal of Australia, 2*, 195-7

Grigson, B. (1985) Personal communication

Hodgens, E.J., I.H. McFadyen, R.J. Failla and F.M. Daly (1972) The offence of rape in Victoria. *Australia and New Zealand Journal of Criminology, 5*, 225-40

James, I.P., S.P. Derham and D.N. Scott-Orr (1963) Attempted suicide: a study of 100 patients referred to a general hospital. *Medical Journal of Australia, 1,* 754-8

Krupinski, J., P. Polke and A. Stoller (1965) Psychiatric disturbances in attempted and completed suicides in Victoria during 1963. *Medical Journal of Australia, 2,* 773-8

Krupinski, J., A. Steller and P. Polke (1967) Attempted suicides admitted to the Mental Health Department, Victoria, Australia: A socio-epidemiological study. *International Journal of Social Psychiatry, 13,* 5-13

Lee, R. (1985) Personal communication

Mackie, I. (1978) Alcohol and aquatic disasters. *Medical Journal of Australia, 1,* 652-3

McLauglan, B. (1985) Personal communication

New South Wales Bureau of Crime Statistics and Research (1973) Gun and knife attacks. *Statistical Report 9, Series 1*

— (1974) Rape offences. *Statistical Report 21, Series 1*

— (1975a) Intentional shootings. *Statistical Report 2, Series 2*

— (1975b) Domestic assaults. *Statistical Report 5, Series 2*

Newman-Martin, G. (1985) Personal communication

Office of Crime Statistics (1981) *Homicide and serious assault in South Australia, Series 11, No. 9*

Office of the Prime Minister (1985) 'Special Premiers' Conference on Drugs: Canberra — 2 April, 1985, Communique

Parker, N. (1979) Murderers: a personal series. *Medical Journal of Australia, 1,* 36-9

Plueckhahn, V.D. (1984) Alcohol and accidental drowning. A 25 year study. *Medical Journal of Australia, 1,* 22-5

Reilly, D.K., J.E. Ray and R.O. Day (1983) Emergency room drug problems: A preliminary report. In J. Santamaria (ed), *Proceedings of the 1983 Autumn School of Studies on Drugs and Alcohol,* pp. 59-72

Renwick, M.Y., G.G. Olsen and M.S. Tyrrel (1982) Suicide in rural NSW. *Medical Journal of Australia, 1,* 377-80

Saunders, J. (1985) Personal communication

Schlosser, D. and J.W. McBride (1984) *Estimating the prevalence of alcohol and other drug-related problems in industry,* NSW Drug and Alcohol Authority, Sydney

Scutt, J. (1983) *Even in the best of homes. Violence in the family,* Penguin, Australia

Smith, D.I. (1983) *Indices for the use and abuse of alcohol: a literature review,* Western Australia Drug and Alcohol Authority, Perth

Stewart, D.E. (1982) Violence and the family, Discussion Paper No. 7, Institute of Family Studies, Melbourne

11

Finnish Statistics on Alcohol-Related Accidents

Esa Österberg

There is no country in the world where accidents do not have a major bearing on public health. At a crude estimate, one million or so of Finland's roughly five million inhabitants fall victim to one kind of accident or another each year. The fact that younger people are especially accident-prone makes the accident rate even more important to public health. An added difference between accidents and many other public health problems is that many accidents can be prevented by policy measures.

There are a variety of reasons for collecting data on the prevalence of accidents and their distribution among different segments of the population. The information is, for instance, necessary to help plan ambulance services, medical care and rehabilitation. Similarly, there is a call for knowledge of the preventable causes which underlie accidents and the efficacy of treatment and rehabilitation. The data may be gathered by conducting specific studies, by means of registers or by employing both simultaneously.

In Finland accidents are registered by numerous bodies. Each organisation records accidents mainly for its own purposes; in consequence, the items recorded and the coverage of the registers vary considerably. The different registers also overlap to some extent.

There are a host of other considerations which affect recording procedures. The various classification categories involve different causal and disability profiles and it follows that it is impossible to use the same data collection procedures for different purposes. For example, one important factor is the severity of the injury which is usually classified in two different ways. Accidents are classified as fatal, occasioning permanent disability or resulting in temporary disability; or they are classified as fatalities, accidents resulting in hospital admissions, or accidents calling for medical attention. A further factor which governs recording practices is the type of accident. Traffic and industrial accidents are generally recorded as separate categories; the third category used, 'other accidents', mainly covers unintentional injuries which befall people when they are at home or off work.

This paper concentrates on three chief issues. It first looks at how accidents are registered and recorded in Finland and examines how the role which alcohol plays in accidents is taken into account. Second, it examines the Finnish accident rate in the light of current data and research findings. It concludes by looking at alcohol-related accidents and discussing the problems of current recording methods from an alcohol research point of view.

Permanent Finnish Registers on Accidents

Register of Causes of Death

The Finnish register of causes of death takes comprehensive account of fatal accidents. Indeed, Finland has recorded causes of death for more than 200 years. Since 1936, the system in operation has been based on certificates of death issued by physicians. The WHO classification of causes of death (the seventh ICD revision) was put into use in 1951 and E-codes have been employed since 1961. Beginning in 1969 Finnish records of causes of death have been kept in accordance with the eighth ICD revision. The Central Statistical Office publishes these data in its statistics of Causes of Death.

In about 85 per cent of fatalities where injury constitutes the cause of death, death certificates are issued as a result of forensic medical autopsies. In the remaining 15 per cent, the deceased is either examined by a hospital physician prior to death or the death certificate is based on a forensic medical examination of the corpse, or medical autopsy (Honkanen 1983).

The register of causes of death provides information specified according to sex and age on the principal and external cause of death. From the point of view of research into accidents, however, the register fails to shed light on several important points. For instance, it gives no indication of whether the accident occurred at work or at home and says nothing about the blood-alcohol level of the deceased and what time he or she died.

In fatalities where the deceased was a victim of accident, the physician issuing the death certificate is asked to answer three questions: When?

Where? and How? In practice, however, where alcohol-related fatal accidents are concerned, the register of causes of death only provides information in cases where alcohol constitutes a direct agent under the terms of the ICD classification – say, alcohol poisoning – or when alcohol is otherwise known to have played an important role – drowning, for instance.

National Hospital Discharge Register

Finnish hospital records have a history which stretches back more than one hundred years. A computerised register of discharges from hospital covering all hospitals controlled by the National Board of Health has been in operation since 1967. The data in it are gathered from forms completed by patients upon discharge from hospital.

The information which the discharge records provide includes the duration of the treatment, diagnoses, E-codes and supplementary treatment. From the viewpoint of studies of accidents, the discharge records fail to provide information about what patients were doing when the accident occurred – whether they were at work or taking part in sports, for instance. Nor do the records say anything about when and where the accident happened or how serious the resulting injury was. In recent years, furthermore, nearly one-third of all discharge certificates have been completed without indicating an E-code (Honkanen 1983).

In principle, the National Hospital Discharge Register makes it possible to assess the prevalence of accidents and injuries which necessitate hospital treatment. Unfortunately, the usefulness of the register is limited. The fact that an E-code is not always indicated, for instance, means that no distinction can be made between accidents, deliberately inflicted injuries, after-effects of injuries and complications which arise during treatment. These shortcomings where the E-code is concerned also make it impossible to distinguish between traffic accidents and accidents which take place at home or at work.

Registers of Out-Patient Treatment

The sole Finnish agency which maintains a continuous computerised register of the treatment given to ambulatory patients is the emergency unit of the Department of Orthopaedics and Traumatology of the Helsinki University Central Hospital. The register was set up in 1972 and has, from the outset, included codes for external causes (nature of accident), location and state of intoxication and blood-alcohol content (*see* Chapter 9). The location code distinguishes between domestic and industrial accidents and accidents which occur during leisure.

The Social Insurance Institution's Register

Finland's Social Insurance Institution is responsible for numerous wide-reaching sectors of social insurance. The Institute's work obliges it to keep diverse data registers; these are chiefly used in the Institute's administrative duties but they are also available for research and statistical purposes. There are three registers which contain diagnostic data: the work disability pension register; the sample register on per diem disability benefits and maternity leave allowances; and the rehabilitation register.

The work disability pensions register includes all the work disability pensions of Finns aged 16 to 64 years. The register has not included the E-code or any other accidents code since 1980.

The register on per diem disability benefits provides a good picture of how many persons of working age are incapacitated for work for periods of more than seven working days. Where accidents in particular are concerned, however, the per diem allowance register furnishes a less complete picture. Under Finnish law, the Accident Indemnity Act and the Traffic Insurance Act have priority. In other words, the Social Insurance Institution's records do not include persons injured in traffic or industrial accidents. It is estimated that the Institution's statistics only cover some 50 per cent of accidents (Honkanen 1983). Neither do rehabilitation schemes run by the Social Insurance Institution cover a major part of accident victims since there are other organisations and programmes concerned with the rehabilitation of injuries (Gustafsson 1982).

Registers of Industrial Accidents

The National Board of Labour Protection has registered industrial accidents since 1976. The records are based on notices of accidents given by employers which are also sent to insurance companies, together with medical certificates, and constitute insurance claims. The Board uses this information to publish details of industrial accidents which result in victims being incapacitated for work for at least three days and come under the terms of the Accident Indemnity Act. Its register contains, for instance, information on types of accidents, their causes, the varieties of injuries suffered and how long the victims were absent from work.

The notices sent to insurance companies specify whether alcohol was involved in the accident. It should be noted that if alcohol is seen as a cause of the accident, victims lose their compensation. It is, therefore, in the victims' interests that intoxication should not be reported as a cause.

The National Board of Labour Protection keeps a special accident report register for serious industrial accidents. When an especially serious accident occurs, local labour protection inspectors visit the scene of the event and report on how the accident took place, what caused it and how it might have been prevented.

Registers of Traffic Accidents

The Central Statistical Office of Finland keeps a register of all traffic accidents involving human injury that come to the attention of the police force. The register gives details of the time of day the accident occurred, the conditions which prevailed, the type of accident, the number of persons injured and the blood-alcohol levels of the parties involved.

The insurance companies also keep records of traffic accidents. Their register is based on claims for compensation made by policy-holders; the notices sent to insurance companies also include information on alcohol's role in the accident. Once again, however, mentioning alcohol is against the interests of the policy holder, especially if he or she is held to be the guilty party.

More traffic accidents come to the attention of the insurance companies than to official bodies or other record-keeping organisations. In 1979, for example, the statistics issued by the insurance companies cited some 74,000 traffic accidents. Some 14,300 of them involved human injury. The corresponding numbers for the records kept by the Central Statistical Office were, respectively, 28,700 and 9,400 (Hantula 1982).

The insurance companies' committees for examining traffic accidents also keep records that include a large number of detailed data. The number of accidents investigated is some 500 a year.

Register of Privately Insured Accidents

The Statistical Centre of the Finnish Federation of Insurance Companies receives information on about 80 per cent of all accidents covered by private insurance policies. The Central Statistical Office of Finland publishes general information on the number of accidents and policy-holders. The register of privately insured accidents includes the following variables: the conditions which pertained when the accident took place, the accident's cause, the nature of the injury incurred, the number of days the victim was off work and the severity of any possible permanent disability (Honkanen 1983).

Register of Poison Information Centre

The Finnish Poison Information Centre was founded in the early 1960s mainly in response to a relatively large number of deaths among young children as a result of poisoning. In the late 1950s, for instance, between 20 and 30 children died each year. The figure fell steadily in the 1960s and, since the early 1970s, the annual number of juvenile fatalities has been zero and three. The number of telephone inquiries made to the Poison Information Centre has increased at an even rate. It is estimated that the Centre received some 12,000 calls in 1981 (Vilska 1982).

Accidents in Finland

Fatal Accidents

In 1980, some 11 per cent of all deaths among Finnish men were due to casualties, if the term 'casualty' is understood to refer to both unintentional accidents and intentional or self-inflicted injuries. The corresponding proportion for Finnish women was 5 per cent. These figures are not very different from the 1955 data; they are, however, somewhat lower than the figures for the early 1970s. Approximately 80 out of 100,000 Finns died through accident in 1980.

One aspect of the accidental death rate fell markedly between 1969 and 1980 when fatal traffic accidents decreased dramatically (see Table 11.1). This decline is a good example of how accidents can be prevented

Table 11.1: *Violent deaths in Finland by external cause of injury, 1969 - 1980*

External cause of injury	1969	1970	1973	1975	1977	1980
Motor vehicle	1,068	1,191	1,112	916	703	569
Water traffic	156	201	170	168	154	125
Other traffic	80	97	88	81	55	49
Accidental poisoning	271	294	258	289	420	314 [a]
Falls and drops	486	529	446	445	490	548
Suicide	1,096	1,003	1,097	1,178	1,222	1,226
Homicide, manslaughter	120	126	125	171	135	158
Unclear	112	90	117	121	159	172
Other accidents	678	674	716	682	603	526 [b]
Total	4,067	4,205	4,129	4,051	3,941	3,687

[a] Includes 238 alcohol poisoning cases
[b] Includes 149 deaths due to drowing

Source: Causes of death in Finland 1969-1980, Central Statistical office of Finland

(Mäki 1984). Also, over the last 20 or 30 years, the number of accidental child fatalities has fallen notably.

Approximately 550 fatalities a year are the result of falls — roughly the same number of people die on the roads annually. The majority of persons who die through falls are more than 64 years old. The importance of falls as a cause of death has been about the same during the last years.

The number of deaths due to poisoning, on the other hand, went up sharply between 1969 and 1980. There was an especially large increase in the number of deaths due to alcohol poisoning. Whereas some 60 per cent of all Finnish deaths due to poisoning were the result of alcohol intoxication in 1965, in 1980 the corresponding figure was 76 per cent.

The Finnish suicide rate has also increased. Currently, about twice as many people take their own lives as die in traffic accidents and it is evident that some unclear deaths are actually due to suicide. The greatest increase in suicide has occurred among men between the ages of 15 and 24 years and it is interesting to note that there has been no drop in the traffic accident death rate in this group either. The number of homicides and cases of manslaughter also rose in the 1970s.

Finland has the highest Nordic accidental death rate. The likelihood of Finnish men dying because of violence, for instance, is 1.5 times greater than their Swedish counterparts (Korhonen and Honkanen 1983). In 1980, Finnish men were 2.9 times more likely to die through accident than Finnish women.

Non-Fatal Accidents

According to the National Hospital Discharge Register, about 7.5 per cent of all treatment given in Finnish hospitals in 1978 was occasioned by accidents and injuries. This represents some 61,000 courses of treatment, equivalent to some 1,280 hospitalisations per 100,000 inhabitants. Injuries sustained as the result of falls and the like accounted for about half of all the therapy given to accident victims (*see* Chapter 9). In real terms, the number of traffic accident victims who needed hospital treatment fell during the 1970s.

As we noted earlier, there is no nationwide record of outpatient care. The emergency unit of the Department of Orthopaedics and Traumatology of the Helsinki University Central Hospital is the largest Finnish clinic for accidents and treats some 30,000 patients each year. In 1980, the breakdown of its patients by type of accident was as follows: traffic accidents, 10 per cent; industrial accidents, 19 per cent; domestic accidents, 21 per cent; other accidents occurring out of working hours, 41 per cent; and intentional or self-inflicted injuries, 9 per cent (Honkanen 1982).

A special study was conducted in 1968 to ascertain the nationwide incidence of accidents which called for medical attention. It was found that 9.5 per cent of all visits to medical practitioners were caused by accidents—some 7,500 visits for every 100,000 inhabitants.

Using available statistics and the findings of specialized research, Honkanen estimated that about 700,000 accidents requiring medical attention occurred annually during the early 1980s. Some 70,000 were traffic accidents, 180,000 were industrial accidents, 150,000 were domestic accidents, while other accidents occurring outside working hours totalled about 300,000 (Honkanen 1982). Compared to the late 1960s, industrial and traffic accidents had fallen and domestic accidents had remained more or less stable. Other forms of accidents that took place during people's leisure hours had, however, increased.

Disabilities

In the early 1980s, approximately 10,000 accident victims were in receipt of occupational disability pensions as laid down in the National Pension Act. This figure is equivalent to 310 pensioners per 100,000 inhabitants and represents some 3.9 per cent of all Finnish pensions. In 1979, 819 new disability pensions stemming from accidents were granted; this figure works out to 26 pensions per 100,000 inhabitants (Järvikoski 1982).

According to the register kept by the National Pensions Institution, injuries caused by accidents account for some 50,000 periods of per diem disability benefits payment. The figure is equivalent to 12 per cent of all benefit payment periods.

Handicapped persons whose injuries stem from accidents account for only a small proportion of the National Pension Institution's overall rehabilitation budget. In 1979, for example, the Institution financed rehabilitation therapy for some 16,000 persons, no more than 300 to 400 of whom were accident victims. The exact proportion of Finland's overall rehabilitation figures accounted for by the National Pension Institution has yet to be estimated.

The Central Statistical Office's Study of Victims

In 1980, the Central Statistical Office of Finland conducted a study where 15- to 74- year-olds were interviewed. The size of the sample was 10,533 and the interviews were either conducted by telephone (78.5 per cent) or took place in the respondents' homes (21.5 per cent). The inquiries had to do with any accidents which might have occurred during the past twelve months. Accidents which caused the victim to lose at least one day's work or necessitated medical attention were classified as serious. On average, it was found that 15,400 accidents took place per 100,000 inhabitants. This total was made up of 1,200 traffic accidents, 5,800 industrial accidents, 2,700 domestic accidents, 3,900 sports accidents and 1,800 other forms of mishap. For every 100,000 inhabitants, furthermore, an annual average of 800 violent assaults which resulted in injury took place.

Alcohol and Accidents

In recent years, approximately 30 per cent of adults receiving treatment for injuries resulting from accidents at out-patient clinics have been under the influence of alcohol. Two-thirds of the patients, moreover, have been found to have blood-alcohol levels of over one part in 1,000 (approximately 100 mg/100 ml), the average being two parts in 1,000. About one-half of all the accidents which adults suffer in Finland during the night or on Saturday occur to people who have been drinking (Honkanen 1976).

Not surprisingly, industrial accidents involve alcohol less often than other types of accident (see Table 11.2). When industrial accidents occur, moreover, blood-alcohol levels are generally lower than is the case with mishaps occurring outside working hours.

The role which alcohol plays in traffic accidents in Finland varies considerably with the type of incident in question. Over the last few years, about 50 per cent of the drivers and adult pedestrians involved in single-vehicle or single-party accidents have been intoxicated. The corresponding proportion for drivers involved in collisions with other vehicles, however, is no higher than about 15 per cent (Honkanen 1979).

Domestic accidents involving alcohol appear to be rare. Nevertheless, young adults who suffer accidental injury when not at work are often found to have been drinking, the most common cause of injury being a fall.

In Finland, three out of every four cases of accidental fatal poisoning are due to excessive drinking. And even when the immediate fatal agent involved is not alcohol but a medicinal drug or carbon monoxide, for example, nearly one-half of the corpses are later found to have high blood-alcohol levels (Alha and Korte 1976).

More than half of all persons who drown in Finland perish while under the influence of alcohol. Hirvonen and Ojanen (1973) found that 74 per cent of all drowned adults had blood-alcohol levels in excess of 80 mg/100 ml [0.8 parts per 1,000]. The majority of adults who freeze or burn to death are also intoxicated.

Yet it is less usual for alcohol to play a part in accidents that are due to an external factor beyond the victim's control and not attributable to negligence on his or her part. The 1973 records for the emergency unit of

Table 11.2: *Percentages of accident victims found to be intoxicated in certain studies*

Author, country or area, date	Subjects/ sample	Blood-alcohol (0/00)	Work	Traffic	Domestic or other leisure accident	Violence	Suicide	Overall data
Lahelma, E., Finland, 1973[a]	337/959	0.1-	6-16					
Alha, A. *et al.*, Province of Uusimaa 1974[a]	417/417	0.1-	9	22	26	57	32	32
Traffic Insurance Association, Finland, excluding Helsinki, 1987[a]	2735/ (over 90%)	0.1-		26				
Honkanen, R. and T. Visuri, Emergency station of the Department of Orthopaedics and Traumatology of the Helsinki University Central Hospital, 1976	1012/1313	0.1 (0.1-)[b]	19 (9)[b]	38 (25)[b]	36 and 45 (25 and 28)[b]	71 (54)[b]	64 (45)[b]	37 (24)[b]
Honkanen, R. and J. Ottelin, Central Hospital of Central Finland, 1976	182/187	0.1- (1.0-)[b]	9 (4)[b]	17 (17)[b]	40 and 29 (27 and 17)[b]	86 (71)[b]		30 (20)[b]
Honkanen, R. *et al.*, Helsinki Out-Patient Clinics, 1978	203/ (90%)	0.1-		15				
Järvinen, P. and O. Kari-Koskinen, Kemi Central Hospital 1978	83/83	0.1-	?	54	?	?		31

[a] Forensic medicine data; other data refer to hospitals
[b] The proportion of victims with blood-alcohol levels over 1.0 per mille are given in parenthesis

Source: Honkanen, 1979, p.431

the Department of Orthopaedics and Traumatology of the Helsinki University Central Hospital, for instance, show that no more than 1 per cent of the persons who were injured during their leisure by accidents involving machinery had been drinking — the corresponding figure for patients treated as the result of a fall was 19 per cent (Honkanen 1976).

On average, two out of three persons wounded in violent assaults are inebriated when the incidents occur; most of the injuries sustained affect the skull.

In Conclusion

Whether one is trying to plan the prevention of accidents or implement existing schemes, one needs to know all one can about the prevalence of accidents. Information about the causes and consequences of accidents is at a special premium — especially when the mishaps might have been prevented. In general, the priority of prevention depends on the prevalence of the health problem in question, its severity and how easily it might be forestalled. The prevention of injuries caused by accidents constitutes a priority area.

In Finland, domestic accidents and other mishaps which occur during leisure time are highly significant. First, they accounted for 36 per cent of the overall loss of working years due to accidents in 1972. Second, between the mid-1960s and 1980, the proportion of all accidental injuries incurred in domestic or leisure situations and requiring medical attention grew from less than half to approximately two-thirds. Third, domestic and other leisure accidents account for an average of 60 per cent of all injuries leading to hospitalisation. In all age groups, this figure is greater than the corresponding ratio obtained when traffic and industrial accidents are combined (Honkanen 1983).

From the point of view of research into alcohol-related accidents, there are two chief reasons why domestic accidents and other mishaps which take place during hours of leisure deserve special attention. The first is that alcohol is not an important factor in industrial accidents. The other is that Finland has scrutinised the role which alcohol plays in traffic accidents very closely and this has resulted in fewer traffic accidents and lower blood-alcohol levels when accidents do occur. The fall in traffic accidents emphasizes the importance of domestic and other leisure mishaps and indicates that efficacious prevention would yield valuable results.

Present statistical and registering practices do not focus on alcohol to any marked extent. One of the tasks for the future is, therefore, the development of procedures which would elucidate alcohol's role in accidents. Regarding permanent registers, a first step would be to have procedures which differentiate between domestic and leisure accidents and other types of accidents. In general — and this applies to most countries — it is during leisure and the time people spend at home that drinking takes place. Yet while few people drink at work or use the roads when intoxicated, it remains true that alcohol use at work or in traffic can cause far greater havoc than drinking at home. Second, classification procedures which indirectly furnish information on alcohol should be encouraged. Besides concentrating on domestic and leisure activities in general, investigations should pay attention to the time of day when accidents occur since alcohol-related mishaps tend to take place at certain hours. Third, it would also be desirable to measure blood-alcohol levels when accidents take place because the victim's state of intoxication indicates how great a role alcohol played in a given accident. In addition to measuring blood-alcohol levels, we should also differentiate between the time when the accident took place and the hour at which the patient came to be medically treated. The registration should also take into account the fact that alcohol affects different people in different ways according to how old they are and how experienced they are in using alcohol.

The Finnish example shows that there seem to be special problems when incorporating alcohol-related behaviour in permanent registers. For this reason, future studies of alcohol and accidents might also focus on three other issues. First, more surveys about the prevalence of accidents and alcohol-related accidents should be carried out. Second, special investigations of all severe accidents should be carried out in the same manner as is the case with severe industrial and traffic accidents. Third, special studies should be carried out in order to pinpoint how much hospital and medical treatment alcohol is responsible for.

© 1989 Esa Österberg

References

Alha, A. and T. Korte (1976) Alkoholi väkivaltaisissa kuolemissa (Alcohol in violent deaths). *Alkoholikysymys, 44,* 3-8

Gustafsson, F. (1982) Tapaturmia koskevat tiedot Kelan rekisterissä (Accidents in the Registers of the Social Insurance Institution). In R. Honkanen and A-S. Pilli-Sihvola (eds.), *Tapaturmatutkimus ja tapaturmien rekisteröinti Suomessa (Accident Research and Accident Registration in Finland)*, Suomen Akatemia, Helsinki

Hantula, L. (1982) Liikennetapaturmien rekisteröinti (Registration of traffic accidents). In R. Honkanen and A-S. Pilli-Sihvola (eds.), *Tapaturmatutkimus ja tapaturmien rekisteröinti Suomessa (Accident Research and Accidents Registration in Finland)*, Suomen Akatemia, Helsinki

Hirvonen, J. and K. Ojanen (1973) Analysis över drunkningsolyckor i Uleåborgs län 1969-72 (Analysis of drownings in the Oulu province in 1969-72). *Nordisk Rättmedicinsk Förenings Förhandlingar*, No. 253, Nordisk Rättmedicinsk Förening, Lund

Honkanen, R. (1976) *Alcohol involvement in accidents. The role of alcohol in injuries treated at emergency stations*, Department of Public Health Science, University of Helsinki, Helsinki
— (1979) Alkoholi ja tapaturmat (Alcohol and accidents). *Duodecim, 95*, 429-35
— (1982) Näköhtia tapaturmien epidemiologiasta ja sen tutkimisesta (Some views of the epidemiology and research of accidents). In R. Honkanen and A-S. Pilli-Sihvola (eds.), *Tapaturmatutkimus ja tapaturmien rekisteröinti Suomessa (Accident research and accident registration in Finland)*, Suomen Akatemia, Helsinki
— (1983) Tapaturmien rekisteröinti. Katsaus, arviointi ja rekisteröintimallien kehittäminen terveydenhuoltoon (Accident registration. Review, evaluation and developments of registration methods). *Lääkintöhallituksen julkaisuja*, No. 41, Lääkintöhallitus, Helsinki (Same in an abridged version: R. Honkanen (1984) Finnish Accident Registration Project (FARP). *Publications of the National Board of Health in Finland*, No 50, National Board of Health, Helsinki
Järvikoski, A. (1982) Tapaturmapotilaiden kuntoutuksen tutkimus (Research of the rehabilitation of the victims of accidents). In R. Honkanen and A-S. Pilli-Sihvola (eds), *Tapaturmatutkimus ja tapaturmien rekisteröinti Suomessa (Accident research and accident registration in Finland)*, Suomen Akatemia, Helsinki
Korhonen, K. and R. Honkanen (1983) Väkivaltainen kuolleisuus Suomessa ja Ruotsissa vuosina 1955, 1965 ja 1975 (Mortality for violent causes of death in Finland and Sweden in 1955, 1965 and 1975). *Sosiaalitieteellinen aikakauslehti, 20*, 21-7
Mäki, M. (1984) Suomen liikenneturvallisuustilanteesta ja maailman terveysjärjestön onnettomuuksien ehkäisyprojektista (Traffic and traffic safety). In R. Honkanen and A-S. Pilli-Sihvola (eds), *Tapaturmatutkimuksen 2. kansallinen tutkijakokous, 10*, 261-67 (The Second National Multidisciplinary Meeting on Accident Research in Finland, 1983)
Poikolainen, K. (1989) Research into and registration of alcohol-related non-fatal casualties in Finland: The need for improved classification. In N. Giesbrecht, R. González, M. Grant, E. Österberg, R. Room, I. Rootman and L. Towle (eds), *Drinking and casualties: Accidents, poisonings and violence in an international perspective*, Routledge, London, pp. 188-94
Vilska, J. (1982) Myrkytystietokeskuksen toiminta (The activities of the Poison Information Centre). In R. Honkanen and A-S. Pilli-Sihvola (eds), *Tapaturmatutkimus ja tapaturmien rekisteröinti Suomessa (Accident research and accident registration in Finland)*, Suomen Akatemia, Helsinki

12

Alcohol-Related Casualty Statistics in Canada

Manuella Adrian

An alcohol casualty is one where injury or death occurs directly as a result of alcohol use by the injured or deceased, or by other persons involved in the circumstances leading to injury or death. It is also something which is likely to be treated in a casualty or emergency department.

While some jurisdictions have developed systems for reporting on emergency room episodes (Department of Health and Human Services 1983), Canada, unfortunately, has no current statistical system which measures the number of alcohol-related casualties. However, there are several well-established national or provincial statistical systems which can provide us with an indirect indication of the level of alcohol-related casualties.

This paper briefly reviews what some of these systems are and discusses how, by statistical manipulation, it is possible to get an indication of the total burden placed on hospital emergency departments by alcohol-related casualties.

Canada is a relatively small country in terms of population (25 million inhabitants) with a long-standing statistical tradition that began in the seventeenth century, during the French colonial era when the first superintendent general ordered our first official census.

Alcohol and drug problem statistics have been compiled for over a century (Government of Canada 1883), with historical series going as far back as 1871 (Popham and Schmidt 1958). Data for the latest year available have been published in *Statistics on alcohol and drug use in Canada and other countries - Volume I: statistics on alcohol use, data available by September 1984* (Adrian 1985). This is a compilation of national, provincial, regional and international data on alcohol with several sections devoted, indirectly, to alcohol casualties. These indirect alcohol casualty statistics are concerned with traffic crashes, hospital treatment and deaths. These statistics are based on administrative reporting systems intended to monitor enforcement or compliance with various government regulations; their coverage is universal for their jurisdiction.

In order to obtain an estimate of the burden imposed by drinking-related casualties, one would need to have a count of all events (accidents) where one of the parties was alcohol-involved and a count of all sober and inebriated persons involved, injured, or killed. In traffic accidents, for example, this would include drivers, passengers, pedestrians and bystanders. Similar data would be needed for other casualties, for example, for casualties on the job, at home, in the event of fires, etc. We will consider to what extent available data meet these criteria of full coverage.

The first section presents data from published sources with the information organised by type of casualty. A short section indicates what data are available from unpublished sources. Several related topics are addressed in the third section: the number of casualties treated in hospitals, health problems of alcohol patients, kinds of injuries diagnosed, external circumstances leading to injuries and the estimated total alcohol-related casualties.

Casualties as Indicated in Published Statistics

Traffic Accidents

In Ontario in 1982, alcohol-related non-fatal injuries in traffic accidents occurred in 554 accidents where the pedestrian was impaired by drink or had been drinking; they involved 12,384 drivers who were impaired by drink or who had been drinking and 86 impaired drivers of snowmobiles. Fatalities occurred in 56 accidents involving impaired pedestrians; traffic fatalities involved 491 impaired drivers and 9 impaired snowmobile drivers (Adrian 1985: Tables 26-28).

Statistics are collected in such a way that, although there is a count of events when death or injury occurs, it is not always clear who was injured or killed in these traffic accidents, i.e. the pedestrian, the driver, the passenger(s) or the bystander(s). Indeed, as traffic accidents are categorised in terms of the most serious outcome, a 'fatal accident' may involve not only one or several deaths, but also one or several injured persons. The figures given above represent a minimum count of traffic alcohol-related casualties.

Data collected from the coroner's offices by the Traffic Injuries Research Foundation of Canada (TIRF) for seven provinces including Ontario do relate to persons, specifically to driver fatalities. However, due to the technical aspects of blood collection and laboratory testing, it is not possible to test the blood of all drivers dying as a result of a car crash. Of the 75.3 per cent traffic deaths TIRF did test in 1982, 59.7 per cent had a positive blood-alcohol concentration (BAC). This figure has held steady at about 60 per cent for the past ten years (Adrian 1985: Table 25). In order to have a notion of total alcohol traffic fatalities, TIRF figures would have to take into account the BAC of passengers or of pedestrians killed in traffic accidents.

Fires

Statistics on injuries and deaths occurring in fires due to impairment by alcohol, drugs and medicaments relate to events (183 fires in 1982 in Canada) and to persons who are injured (36) or deceased (23). However, as published, they do not distinguish between impairment due to alcohol or other drugs (Adrian 1985: Table 62). They also do not indicate how many fire victims were themselves impaired or how many impaired persons provoked fires.

Murders

In the period between 1961 and 1974, there were 1,498 solved murder incidents; or 41.4 per cent of all solved murders, in which the suspect, the victim or both had ingested alcohol prior to the murder incident. Another 113 or 3.1 per cent of all solved murder incidents occurred when alcohol and/or other drugs had been ingested prior to the murder. Most solved murders occurred when there was a known relationship between the suspect and the victim, especially a family relationship. The highest percentage of murders (62.4 per cent in the period 1961 to 1974 involving alcohol occurred in common law families.

Murders in bar brawls accounted for a certain number where there was no known relationship between victim and suspect. Of victim-precipitated murder incidents in the period 1961 to 1974, 29.3 per cent occurred in bar brawls instigated by the victim and, of non-victim precipitated murder incidents, 7.8 per cent occurred in bar brawls not instigated by the victim.

In murders committed during sexual assaults on children, 15.6 per cent occurred when the suspect had been drinking or was drunk. In murders involving sexual assault on adults, 40.7 per cent occurred when the suspect had been drinking or was drunk and 23.7 per cent when the victim had been drinking or was drunk.

In robbery-murder incidents, 11.1 per cent occurred when the victim was drunk or had been drinking, 17.9 per cent when the suspect was drunk or had been drinking, 2.1 per cent when the suspect had been drinking and using drugs, 23.7 per cent when the suspect had been using alcohol or drugs and 3.7 per cent when the suspect was on drugs or an addict (Adrian 1979: Table 31).

Morbidity and Mortality

National published morbidity and mortality statistics are somewhat less helpful in identifying alcohol-related casualties. Published tabulations include only the most responsible diagnosis or the primary cause of death.

The alcohol diagnoses are easy to identify in the statistics. They consist of alcoholic psychoses (diagnostic category 291 in the ninth edition of the International Classification of Diseases (World Health Organization 1978)), alcohol dependence syndrome (303), non-dependent abuse of alcohol (305.0), chronic liver disease and cirrhosis (571), toxic effect of alcohol (980) and the supplementary diagnostic category of accidental poisoning by alcohol (E860).

In 1980/1 in Canada, there were 44,021 cases treated on an in-patient basis in general hospitals for alcohol psychoses, alcohol dependence syndrome, non-dependent abuse of alcohol, chronic liver disease and cirrhosis, and toxic effect of alcohol. An additional 4,172 were treated on an in-patient basis in mental and psychiatric hospitals for alcohol psychoses and alcohol dependence syndrome. Finally, 3,477 persons died of the five alcohol diagnoses in 1981 (Adrian 1985: Tables 45, 52 & 63).

If we restrict our definition of casualty to encompass violence, injury and poisonings only, there were 885 general hospital discharges for toxic effects of alcohol in 1980/1 and no cases treated in mental hospitals. There were 167 deaths in 1981 due to toxic effects of alcohol in terms of nature of injury and 95 due to accidental poisoning by alcohol in terms of external cause, consisting of some deaths also classified under toxic effects of alcohol and some other diagnostic categories. However, the figures 167 and 95 should not be summed because of the double supplementary classification of the cause of death.

Unpublished Data

There are a number of other non-alcohol-related principal diagnoses, to which alcohol diagnoses are contributing, underlying or complicating secondary diagnoses. These secondary diagnoses are generally available only in unpublished data which make provision for noting the secondary diagnoses on the patients' medical report.

For instance in 1981/2 in Ontario, there were 15,055 cases treated for primary alcohol diagnoses and 16,348 treated for secondary alcohol diagnoses on an in-patient basis in general hospitals. Mental and psychiatric hospitals accounted for 2,991 cases treated for primary alcohol diagnoses and 603 cases for secondary alcohol diagnoses in 1979/80 (Adrian 1985: Tables 87-88).

Similarly, coroner's statistics for Ontario in 1981 identified 1,245 deaths in which alcohol played a role; this corresponds to 28.8 per cent of all deaths dealt with by the coroner's office (Chief Coroner for Ontario 1982).

However, not all of these hospitalised cases or deaths passed through the hospital casualty department. The question then is to find out how many cases did go through the casualty department.

Dimensions of Alcohol-Related Casualties

Number of Casualties Treated in Hospital

It is possible, through statistical manipulation of existing data bases, to estimate the number of alcohol casualties seen in emergency departments.

In Ontario, provincial regulations require that all public general hospitals report their operating statistics to the Hospital Medical Records Institute (HMRI). These statistics cover all hospital in-patient cases and make provision for recording the principal diagnosis as well as up to 15 secondary, contributing, underlying or complicating diagnoses, including the supplementary external injury diagnoses (E-codes in the ICD-9). An extract data tape, with patient, physician and hospital identifiers deleted, is provided to the Addiction Research Foundation for all cases having a primary or secondary alcohol or drug diagnosis.

In 1983/4, which is the latest year for which we have data, there were a total of 13,139 cases with primary alcohol diagnoses and 20,445 who had secondary alcohol diagnoses. These cases were all treated on an in-patient basis. Like all hospital cases, alcohol cases may be admitted to hospital directly or through the emergency (casualty) department.

The HMRI data base provides information on hospital method of entry (direct or through the emergency department). Of the 13,139 cases with primary alcohol diagnoses, 8,083 (or 61.5 per cent) were admitted through the emergency room and, of the 20,445 cases with secondary alcohol diagnoses, 14,080 (or 68.9 per cent) were admitted through this route (Table 12.1). Over the last five years, a majority of all cases with primary or secondary alcohol diagnoses have been admitted to hospital through the emergency department, in contrast to admission procedures for all cases with all types of diagnoses (where only about 35 to 40 per cent are admitted to hospital through the emergency department) (Adrian *et al.* 1982).

Kinds of Health Problems in Alcohol Patients

While one might expect that most alcohol cases treated in casualty or emergency departments have traumatic injury diagnoses, this is not always the case.

The kinds of health problems associated with alcohol diagnoses for all in-patients were first described for Ontario for the year 1979/80 (Adrian and Layne 1984). More up-to-date data have now become available and are reported here for 1983/4 for cases admitted through the emergency department. Data are based on all alcohol cases treated on an in-patient hospital basis and admitted through the emergency department (60 per cent for primary and 70 per cent for secondary alcohol diagnoses) (Table 12.1). Diagnoses were grouped in terms of the 17 chapter headings of the

Table 12.1: *Number of cases with primary and secondary alcohol diagnoses and number and percentage admitted to hospital through the emergency department; Ontario, 1979-80 to 1983-84*

Year	Total cases	Entry emergency department	Percentage emergency relative to total
		Primary Alcohol Diagnoses	
1979/80	16,129	8,967	55.7
1980/1	11,320	6,505	57.5
1981/2	15,044	8,677	57.7
1982/3	14,130	8,379	59.3
1983/4	13,139	8,083	61.5

Year	Total cases	Emergency department	Percentage entry relative to total
		Secondary Alcohol Diagnoses	
1979/80	21,674	13,960	64.4
1980/1	14,974	10,025	66.9
1981/2	21,182	14,087	66.5
1982/3	20,655	14,131	68.4
1983/4	20,445	14,080	68.9

Source: HMRI data analysed by the author

International Classification of Diseases (see Appendix 2 for list of ICD diagnostic codes in each category).

When alcohol was one of the secondary diagnoses, the diagnosis most responsible for hospitalisation was injury, reported by 20.2 per cent of all cases.

When the five alcohol diagnoses were the primary diagnoses, injury diagnoses were again reported by about 17 to 20 per cent of all patients — 20.1 per cent for supplementary external cause of injury and 16.6 per cent for nature of injury diagnoses. However, they were in fifth and seventh rank, respectively, after mental disorders (33.4 per cent), other alcohol diagnoses (29.4 per cent), digestive disorders (26.8 per cent), circulatory problems (21.3 per cent) and ill-defined conditions (18.8 per cent) (Table 12.2).

Table 12.2: *Health problems[a] found in association with alcohol diagnoses[b] for cases admitted through the Emergency Department, Ontario, 1983/4*

Primary health problems with secondary alcohol diagnoses, by type of problem		Secondary health problems with primary alcohol diagnoses by type of health problem	
	(%)		(%)[c]
Injury	20.2	Mental	33.4
Mental disorders	15.8	Alcohol	29.4
Digestive disorders	15.4	Digestive disorders	26.8
Alcohol diagnoses	11.2	Circulatory disorders	21.3
Circulatory system disorders	10.8	Supplementary injury diagnoses (E-Codes)	20.1
		Ill-defined conditions	18.8
		Injury	16.9
		Infectious diseases	14.7
		Endocrine	14.1
		Respiratory disorders	12.9
		No secondary diagnoses	23.9
Total number of cases	14,012	Total number of cases	6,149

[a] Diagnoses have been grouped into ICD-9 chapter headings
[b] Includes alcoholic psychoses (ICD-9, Code 291); alcohol dependence syndrome (303); non-dependent abuse of alcohol (305.0); chronic liver disease and cirrhosis (571); and toxic effect of alcohol (980)
[c] Due to multiple secondary diagnoses per case, percentages do not add up to 100%

Source: HMRI data analysed by the author

Kinds of Injury Diagnoses

Most injuries, whether reported as primary or secondary diagnoses, consisted of poisonings (38.6 per cent of primary injury diagnoses and 54 per cent of secondary injury diagnoses), fractures (24.8 per cent of primary and 15.7 per cent of secondary injury diagnoses), intracranial injuries (16.1 per cent of primary, 10.5 per cent of secondary), open head wounds, more likely to appear as secondary (10.2 per cent) than primary diag-

Table 12.3: *Injury diagnoses with primary or secondary alcohol diagnoses[a] for cases admitted through the Emergency Department, by type of primary and secondary injury diagnoses, Ontario, 1983/4*

	Percentage of cases with primary injury diagnoses[b] (%)	Percentage of cases with secondary injury diagnoses[c] (%)
Skull fracture	4.7	2.5
Spine and trunk fracture	5.9	5.8
Upper limb fracture	3.4	4.3
Lower limb fracture	10.8	3.1
Dislocations	0.8	0.6
Sprains/strains	0.6	1.0
Intracranial injury	16.1	10.5
Chest/abdomen, pelvis	1.6	0.6
Open head wound	4.5	10.2
Open upper limb wound	2.6	5.3
Open lower limb wound	0.3	0.9
Blood vessel injury	0.3	-
Late effects of injury	0.3	1.4
Superficial injury	1.1	4.3
Contusions	4.6	13.4
Crushing injury	0.2	-
Foreign body in orifice	0.3	0.5
Burns	1.1	1.0
Nerves/spinal cord	0.4	0.6
Traumatic complications	1.8	3.6
Poisoning	38.6	54.0
Total number	2,783	813

[a] Includes alcoholic psychoses (ICD-9, Code 291); alcohol dependence syndrome (303); non-dependent abuse of alcohol (305.0); chronic liver disease and cirrhosis (571); and toxic effect of alcohol (980)
[b] Includes all cases with alcohol secondary diagnoses and primary injury diagnoses
[c] Includes all cases with alcohol primary diagnoses and secondary injury diagnoses

Source: HMRI data analysed by the author

noses (4.5 per cent), and contusions, again more often as the secondary (13.4 per cent) than the primary (4.6 per cent) diagnosis (Table 12.3).

Most injuries were reported for males, cases being about two-thirds male and one-third female, whether reported as primary or secondary diagnoses. Males had slightly higher rates of skull, and spine and trunk fractures, open head wounds and intracranial injuries, traumatic complications and late effects of injury, whereas females had more poisoning diagnoses (Tables 12.4 and 12.5).

Table 12.4: *Sex differences in injury secondary diagnoses with alcohol primary diagnoses[a] for cases admitted through the Emergency Department, by sex and type of injury, Ontario, 1983/4*

Type of injury	Male (%)	Female (%)	Total[b] number
Skull fracture	80.0	20.0	20
Spine and trunk fracture	76.6	23.4	47
Upper limb fracture	60.0	40.0	35
Lower limb fracture	40.0	60.0	25
Dislocations	60.0	40.0	5
Sprains/strains	62.5	37.5	8
Intracranial injury	80.0	20.0	85
Chest/abdomen, pelvis	40.0	60.0	5
Open head wound	77.1	22.9	83
Open upper limb wound	65.1	34.9	43
Open lower limb wound	85.7	14.3	7
Blood vessel injury	-	-	-
Late effects of injury	72.7	27.3	11
Superficial injury	74.3	25.7	35
Contusions	62.4	37.6	109
Crushing injury	-	-	-
Foreign body in orifice	75.0	25.0	4
Burns	50.0	50.0	8
Nerves/spinal cord	40.0	60.0	5
Traumatic complications	82.8	17.2	29
Poisoning	59.9	40.1	439
Total number	66.2	33.8	813

[a] Includes alcoholic psychoses (ICD-9, Code 291); alcohol dependence syndrome (303); non-dependent abuse of alcohol (305.0); chronic liver disease and cirrhosis (571); and toxic effect of alcohol (980)

[b] Totals do not add up due to multiple diagnoses per case

Source: HMRI data analysed by the author

Table 12.5: *Sex differences in injury primary diagnoses with alcohol secondary diagnoses[a] for cases admitted through the Emergency Department, by sex and type of injury, Ontario, 1983/4*

Type of injury	Male (%)	Female (%)	Total[b] number
Skull fracture	84.6	15.4	130
Spine and trunk fracture	77.4	22.6	164
Upper limb fracture	60.6	39.4	94
Lower limb fracture	63.8	36.2	301
Dislocations	76.2	23.8	21
Sprains/strains	55.6	44.4	18
Intracranial injury	77.7	22.3	448
Chest/abdomen, pelvis	81.8	18.2	44
Open head wound	75.4	24.6	126
Open upper limb wound	68.5	31.5	73
Open lower limb wound	77.8	22.2	9
Blood vessel injury	71.4	28.6	7
Late effects of injury	100.0	-	7
Superficial injury	67.7	32.3	31
Contusions	70.5	29.5	129
Crushing injury	100.0	-	5
Foreign body in orifice	66.7	33.3	9
Burns	87.1	12.9	31
Nerves/spinal cord	91.7	8.3	12
Traumatic complications	75.5	24.5	49
Poisoning	53.8	46.2	1,075
Total number	66.0	34.0	2,783

[a] Includes alcoholic psychoses (ICD-9, Code 291); alcohol dependence syndrome (303); non-dependent abuse of alcohol (305.0); chronic liver disease and cirrhosis (571); and toxic effect of alcohol (980)
[b] Totals do not add up due to multiple diagnoses per case

Source. HMRI data analysed by the author

External Circumstances Leading to Injuries

Information on the external circumstances leading to injury is available from the supplementary external cause of injury, or E-Code diagnoses in the ICD-9. The most frequent external circumstances were divided between suicide (28.6 per cent), falls (24.0 per cent), injury (23.8 per cent) and other accidents (6.8 per cent).

Transportation or motor vehicle accidents were barely reported in 3 per cent of all cases treated in hospital (Table 12.6). On the basis of HMRI data, the alcohol traffic accident statistics reported by police

Table 12.6: *External cause of injury diagnoses (E-codes) for cases with alcohol primary diagnoses[a] for cases admitted through the Emergency Department, by type of injury, Ontario, 1983/4*

External cause of injury	Percentage of cases (%)
Railway accident	-
Motor traffic accident	2.5
Motor non-traffic accident	0.2
Other road vehicle accident	0.2
Water transport accident	-
Poisoning	17.6
Falls	24.0
Fires and flames	0.5
Natural factors	2.1
Suffocation	0.4
Other accidents	6.8
Suicide	28.6
Homicide	5.0
Injury	23.8
Total number	1,037

[a] Includes alcoholic psychoses (ICD-9, Code 291); alcohol dependence syndrome (303); non-dependent abuse of alcohol (305.0); chronic liver disease and cirrhosis (571); and toxic effect of alcohol (980)

Source: HMRI data analysed by the author

forces, Ministries of Transport and Statistics Canada represent only a small percentage of all alcohol casualties.

Most injuries were reported for males, cases being about two-thirds male and one-third female. Males had higher rates of homicide and other accidents, while females had higher rates of suicide and injury (Table 12.7).

Estimated Total Alcohol Casualties

Studies have shown that about 20 per cent of all cases (with all types of diagnoses) seen in emergency departments are admitted to hospital (Owens 1985). On the basis of this figure, cases with alcohol diagnoses would account for about 100,000 emergency department visits annually in Ontario, with about 22,000 admitted to hospital on an in-patient basis. Assuming that extrapolation on the basis of population size is appropriate, the corresponding estimates for Canada would be 300,000 emergency room visits with alcohol-related diagnoses and 60,000 in-patient admissions.

Table 12.7: *Sex differences in injury secondary supplemetary external causes of injury diagnoses (E-codes) with alcohol primary diagnoses[a] for cases admitted through the Emergency Department, by sex and type of injury, Ontario, 1983/4*

Type of injury	Male (%)	Female (%)	Total[b] number
Railway accident	-	-	-
Motor traffic accident	88.5	11.5	26
Motor non-traffic accident	100.0	-	2
Other road vehicle accident	50.0	50.0	2
Water transport accident	-	-	-
Poisoning	67.6	32.4	182
Falls	68.7	31.3	249
Fires and flames	40.0	60.0	5
Natural factors	68.2	31.8	22
Suffocation	75.0	25.0	4
Other accidents	67.1	32.9	70
Suicide	62.3	37.7	297
Homicide	76.9	23.1	52
Injury	57.5	42.5	247
Total number	65.9	34.1	1,037

[a] Includes alcoholic psychoses (ICD-9, Code 291); alcohol dependence syndrome (303); non-dependent abuse of alcohol (305.0); chronic liver disease and cirrhosis (571); and toxic effect of alcohol (980)

[b] Totals do not add up due to multiple diagnoses per case

Source: HMRI data analysed by the author

If we consider that injury diagnoses are reported by only about 20 per cent of all hospitalised alcohol cases, the revised estimates of all alcohol casualties having injury diagnoses seen in emergency departments in Ontario is about 20,000 (equals 20 per cent of 100,000 emergency department visits annually) and about 60,000 for Canada (the latter extrapolated on the basis of population).

Another consideration is the estimated number of cases with injury and a hidden alcohol component seen in emergency departments. Previous studies at the Addiction Research Foundation have shown that HMRI figures would put the percentage of all hospital cases with an alcohol component at about 5 per cent, whereas special in-hospital surveys which identify all hospital cases with an alcohol component, whether so noted in the medical record or not, have put the percentage as high as 15 or 20 per cent (Adrian 1982). If the same percentage applies to injury diagnoses, the 'real' alcohol burden on emergency departments may be as high as 300,000 or 400,000 for Ontario with about 60,000 to 80,000 having injury or violence diagnoses. This burden may reach one million to 1.2 million for the country annually, with about 100,000 to 240,000 having injury or violence diagnoses. However, these figures include only injury and violence in which the patient himself had alcohol involvement.

It is also possible to estimate the number of injury cases in patients without alcohol involvement whose injury or illness is due to the action of another person who is under the influence of alcohol, e.g., a sober wife injured by a drunken husband. If the extent of drunken violence resulting in death is similar to the extent of non-lethal alcohol-related violence resulting in treated injury, then it may be estimated that the proportion of physical injury in the general population is similar to the 40 per cent proportion of murders due to alcohol. Therefore, about 40 per cent of all injuries treated in hospital may be alcohol-related. It is debatable whether the injury sustained from an alcohol-related aggressor is less severe than if aggressors are sober — since the former would lack the physical coordination to accurately land blows — or if the injury would be more severe, as inebriated aggressors would be less subject to the restraints of social mores which codify fights to reduce extremely severe or lethal outcomes.

Of the 100,000 patients treated in hospital on an in-patient basis for injury primary diagnoses in Ontario in 1980/1 (Statistics Canada n.d.), about 40 per cent, or 40,000, would have received their injury as the result of another person under the effect of alcohol. Of these, about 40 per cent, or 16,000 would have been admitted through the emergency department. Since about 20 per cent of all emergency cases are admitted to hospital, those 16,000 emergency injury cases admitted to hospital would correspond to a total of about 80,000 cases with a primary diagnosis of injury seen in emergency departments consisting of victims of persons who had been drinking. The corresponding figures for Canada would be about 250,000, with a primary diagnosis of injury cases seen in emergency departments, of which about 50,000 would be admitted to hospital. For every case with primary alcohol diagnoses, there are about two cases with at least one secondary alcohol diagnosis. Should this same 1:2 ratio of primary to secondary diagnoses hold for other diagnostic categories, there may be as many as 250,000 injury cases seen in emergency departments in Ontario and about 750,000 in Canada whose injury results from the action of other alcohol-involved persons.

Discussion and Conclusions

In Canada, there is an abundance of statistics regarding alcohol-related casualties. Some relate to the death and injury aspect of the problem, some relate to the emergency department treatment aspect and, finally, some relate to both combined.

Statistics based on published data cover traffic accidents, fires, murders, morbidity and mortality. These statistics relate to events (accidents, cases treated, murders) and to persons (deceased or injured drivers or pedestrians, and persons whose principal cause of death was an alcohol diagnosis), but generally they do not always allow a count of injured passengers, bystanders or other victims of drunk drivers or murderers, for instance, or of friends or family victimised by persons under the influence of alcohol problems.

By statistical manipulation of data bases, it is possible to identify all cases with an alcohol problem treated as hospital in-patients and entering the hospital through the emergency department, and to identify, along with the major alcohol diagnoses, a broad spectrum of other health problems present, with diagnoses of injury and accident being made in about 20 per cent of all patients. However, almost 30 per cent of all cases with primary alcohol diagnoses have no secondary diagnosis, while most cases have a non-injury-related concomitant diagnosis. In Canada, certainly, most of the burden on casualty departments identifiably due to alcohol problems is not due to classic casualties or the results of short-term violence, but rather to longer-term mental or digestive disorders.

Finally, it is possible to estimate the total burden placed on emergency departments by all alcohol casualties. Diagnoses are to some extent affected by physicians' biases in terms of training and fashions in medical diagnosis. The accuracy and completeness of medical diagnoses entered into hospital medical files by treating physicians and transcribed by medical record librarians is an important element which has not been fully investigated and published thus far.

There are good reasons to believe that, in general, the data closely reflect reality. Ontario medical staff and others involved in recording and processing patient data are highly trained and all hospitals have internal mechanisms for monitoring the quality of medical records. In most hospitals, HMRI forms are completed by Health Records Technicians with one to two years of training in health records sciences. HMRI also provides ongoing training to all hospital staff involved with the HMRI system. Spokespersons for HMRI and the Ontario Ministry of Health have indicated that internal simulations show that the coding of data from medical records to HMRI forms is at least 95 per cent accurate.

The estimated numbers of treated casualties depend on the assumption that the average likelihood of entering the health care system through different streams is applicable for specific diagnosis. Until the relevant diagnoses-specific information becomes available or special investigations for special disease conditions in selected treatment facilities are undertaken, we assume that the 20 per cent of all emergency department cases who are admitted as in-patients to hospitals is applicable for all alcohol-related diagnoses.

The mix of alcohol disorders, other health problems and injuries may differ somewhat at different levels of the health care system, for example, cases admitted to hospital may be more severely ill or injured than cases treated only in emergency departments. It would be useful if the extent and mix of injury in all cases in emergency departments versus hospital in-patients, and in all patients without alcohol diagnoses injured through the action of an alcohol-involved person, were to be investigated by special surveys conducted in emergency departments.

There is a tendency to assume an increased risk of injury among alcohol-involved persons. It is estimated that patients with alcohol diagnoses have between 200 to 500 per cent greater rate of injury than all treated Ontario cases. However, in some cases an injured person may take or be given a 'stiff drink' prior to coming to the hospital and this practice may contribute to inaccurate estimates of alcohol-related casualties.

The number of casualties are likely to be conservative relative to all alcohol casualties, as a number of casualties may be treated outside the hospital medical environment, such as physicians' offices, employee health units, first aid stations, by friends, family or the injured person himself. Some alcohol casualties may not be treated at all. Whether a casualty is treated at all or by whom may depend not only on availability of care, but also on actual or perceived seriousness of injury.

It is hoped that an estimate of alcohol casualties and a delineation of their types may be used to alert casualty officers to the alcohol problem in the presence of other injury diagnoses, as well as to provide an early warning of other health casualty problems likely to be found in the presence of alcohol. In addition, some of these results could be used in prevention programs aimed at preventing alcohol accidents on the job or in the home, similar to current drunk-driving awareness programs. Finally, some of the results and estimation methods described in this paper may be applicable in other jurisdictions.

References

Adrian , M. (comp.) (1979) *Statistical supplement to the annual report 1977-78,* Alcoholism and Drug Addiction Research Foundation, Toronto

— (1985) *Statistics on alcohol and drug use in Canada and other countries, data available by September 1984, volume I: statistics on alcohol use,* Alcoholism and Drug Addiction Research Foundation, Toronto

— (1982) Hospital beds occupied by patients with alcohol-related problems, Kingston, 1964 and 1975, Ontario, 1964, 1977 and 1978-79, and Canada, 1977. In M. Adrian, P. Jull, B. Yeh and L. Jellinek (eds), *Statistics on alcohol and drug users, treatment, labour, unemployment and costs,* Alcohol and Drug Addiction Research Foundation, Substudy No. 1222, pp. 13-24

Adrian, M., M.L. Halliday and M.J. Ashley (1982) Epidemiological uses of management information systems: a pilot study for Ontario. Paper presented to the 110th Annual Meeting of the American Public Health Association, Montreal, P.Q., Canada, November 14-18, 1982

Adrian, M. and N. Layne (1985) Alcohol-associated morbidity. In A. Carmi and S. Schneider (eds), *Drugs and Alcohol,* Springer-Verlag, Berlin, pp. 166-83

Chief Coroner for Ontario (1982) *Metropolitan Toronto coroners' office statistical report,* Ministry of the Solicitor General, Chief Coroner for Ontario, Toronto

Department of Health and Human Services (1983) *Drug use motivation differentials in hospital emergency room episodes 1981: data from the drug abuse warning network, statistical series, series H, no. 2,* U.S. Dept. of Health and Human Services, Public Health Service, Alcohol, Drug Abuse, and Mental Health Administration, National Institute on Drug Abuse, Division of Epidemiology and Statistical Analysis, DHHS Publication No. (ADM) 83-1272, Washington, DC

Government of Canada (1883) *Criminal statistics for the year 1882 appendix to the report of the Minister or [sic] Agriculture for the year 1883.* Printed by order of Parliament, MacLean, Roger & Co., Ottawa [Statistics Canada Catalogue No. 85-201, pp. 98-107, 116-123, 174-175]

Hospital Medical Records Insitute (1982) [Hospital separation data by selected diagnostic categories — 1981-2] HMRI special computer data, Toronto

Owens, A. (1985) An up-close look at emergency medicine specialists. *Medical Economics 62,* 5, 188-215

Popham, R.E. and W. Schmidt (1958) *Statistics of alcohol use and alcoholism in Canada 1871-1956,* University of Toronto Press, Alcoholism and Drug Addiction Research Foundation, Toronto

Statistics Canada (undated) Total number of hospital separations by ICDA chapter, age group and sex, Canada [by province], 1980-81, Statistics Canada, Special Tabulation, Ottawa

World Health Organization International Classification of Diseases (1978) *Manual of the international statistical classification of diseases, injuries, and causes of death.* [Based on the recommendations of the Ninth Revision Conference 1975, and adopted by the Twenty-ninth World Health Assembly] World Health Organization, Geneva

13

Casualties in Poland: Focus on Alcohol

Jacek Morawski and Jacek Moskalewicz

Pathology was not seen in Poland as a phenomenon permanently connected with public life, following World War Two. It was treated by the authorities of the time as a relic of capitalism where 'drunkenness among workers was equally unavoidable a result of their life situation as is typhus, crimes, vermin, bailiffs and other social ailments' (Engels 1949).

With the establishment of a new political system and the new socialist social relations, social problems were to disappear the way they did in Owen's settlement, 'originally consisting of the most diverse and, for the most part very demoralized elements', and later transformed 'into a model colony, in which drunkenness, police, magistrates, lawsuits, poorlaws, charity were unknown. And all this simply by placing the people in conditions worthy of human beings, and especially by carefully bringing up the rising generation' (Engels, 1945).

If pathology was mentioned at all it was generally situated peripherally to social structure, among the petty bourgeoisie and lumpen proletariat. At the same time, government-controlled mass media, literature and film propagated a 'marble' image of the working-class man — representing high moral standards and free from pathologies.

Pathological phenomena were discovered on a wider scale around the mid-1950s, in a period of growing public openness and deep political changes. At that time, it was acknowledged that such phenomena were present in the working class and were most intensive in new industrial centres. These phenomena, delinquency of aggressive character in particular, often brought about tragic consequences. Numerous cases of assault and battery, mugging and accidents were recorded. It turned out that various social ailments apparently inherent to capitalist production

245

relations did not vanish in spite of the change in the socio-political system. Reality, far from optimistic expectations, had to be re-interpreted. For doctrinal reasons, it was difficult to analyse it in Marxist terms and seek the cause of evil in the ruling production relations.

In this socio-political climate, alcohol came to serve as the way of accounting for social problems, as a source of all evil. Alcohol became more and more often the scapegoat in the official propaganda. Thus the blame was not put on the far-from-perfect system nor on the working classes, but on ethyl alcohol whose detrimental influence on man had been known for centuries. This peculiar reification of the causes of social problems tended to obscure systemic sources of pathologies, an obvious price to be paid by any society subject to an abrupt social overhaul.

This function of alcohol in propaganda was denounced by the poets of the time. One of the best poems is by Adam Ważyk—'It's Alcohol That Demoralizes Youth' [To alkohol demoralizuje młodzież]. Painting a black picture of the prospects of the younger generation, it ended with the following lines:

> *Singing parrots neck-tied in sham*
> *People growing hoarse to keep in the game*
> *A magic poster lisping on the tram*
> *That it's alcohol, alcohol is to blame...*
> (Ważyk 1956)

Some propaganda slogans were paradoxically adopted by subculture associated with alcohol use. A drinking song fashionable at that time had this sarcastic refrain:

> *Alcohol is the ruin of mankind*
> *Alcohol is the opium for the masses.*

In spite of the relatively narrow social appeal of the official propaganda over-rating alcohol as the source of social problems, what is remarkable was the imprint it left on many activists in the decades that followed. Its traces are found more than once in the analysis of statistics on alcohol-related casualties.

An overall tendency to amplify alcohol problems in the post-war period prior to the 1970s gave way to a change in emphasis with regard to alcohol and social pathology. The 1970s were a period of relatively fast economic growth accompanied by a noisy propaganda campaign later described as a 'propaganda of success'. Information on social problems was censored in order to prevent spoiling a rosy picture or rapid and harmonious development. For several years the word 'alcohol' was practically barred from the papers and special statistical and scientific reports on alcohol consumption and related problems were limited to confidential documents designated for official use only.

It was not until the Solidarity period of the 1980s that alcohol again became a public issue, with authorities being accused of pro-alcohol policies (Moskalewicz 1981). Alcohol-related problems were either presented as a consequence of the encouragement of alcohol consumption or as an effect of social disorganisation and demoralisation.

In this climate the amplification of alcohol problems could not be a surprise. However, some statistics did not reflect this trend. Alcohol consumption dropped suddenly in 1981 and 1982, which may be attributed to a decrease in supply (25 per cent drop in alcohol production) and restricted availability (limitation in alcohol outlets, high price increases, rationing) (Wald and Moskalewicz 1984). The drop in alcohol consumption was followed by decreasing numbers of hospitalisations due to alcoholic psychoses and alcoholism, as well as by a slight drop in deaths due to cirrhosis of the liver (Morawski 1983).

Reporting Systems

This paper does not apply any formal definition of casualty as there is no word in Polish—the language of the authors—equivalent to the meaning and scope of the English term. Thus the notion requires circumscription, using a number of terms. In translation, the scope of the English word 'casualty' covers at least two clearly different categories of incidents in Polish: unintentional incidents/accidents, and intentional incidents/violent offenses and suicides. The Polish term suggests the analysis of causes and perpetrators while the English one draws more attention to the victim and his condition.

However, these linguistic differences do not preclude a comparative analysis. The paper will present statistical data on casualties related to delinquency, traffic accidents and labour accidents. It will also present data related to poisonings and suicides.

Though statistical sources used here sometimes include data on alcohol, long-range analyses often run into serious obstacles. The data for particular years are not always comparable because of changes in reporting systems, legislation, methods of defining events as casualties, the ways of establishing the condition of victims and the way of establishing sobriety or intoxication.

Data on the involvement of alcohol in casualties are not always published, even if they are aggregated in an appropriate statistical system. Statistical yearbooks which are the universally available source of statistical information include data on alcohol-related traffic accidents and labour accidents only.

Other kinds of statistics, even if they include data on alcohol, are not compiled or may be prepared for the exclusive use of institutions concerned.

Crime and Casualties

No statistics on victims of crimes are compiled in Poland. The prevalence of casualties due to criminal offences can be inferred from data or crimes against life and health. These include such categories of crime as manslaughter, bodily harm, participation in fighting or beating. The relationship between the number of crimes and the number of victims is not clear. A crime may be associated with one person causing bodily harm to several persons; the reverse is possible as well. Assuming, however, that these relationships do not change annually, criminal records can serve as a reliable source for the analysis of long-range trends in prevalence of casualties.

Unfortunately, the analysis of Polish data is also complicated by an abrupt change in the reporting system in the mid-1960s which replaced the publication of statistical data on the number of 'crimes reported to the Public Militia' with the number of 'crimes established in the course of preliminary criminal procedure'. The disparities are well illustrated for the years 1965 to 1967, when two kinds of data were published (Table 13.1).

The differences between the two reporting systems range from 72,000 to 100,000 in crimes and from 50 to 140 in manslaughter. This means that no coefficient can be employed to compare these data. The situation is further complicated by the change introduced to the Polish Penal Code in 1969, which brought about overhauls in the classification of offences.

Table 13.1: *Reported crimes and established crimes*

	1965	1966	1967
Crimes reported to the Public Militia and Attorney's Office	414,007	452,257	409,614
including: manslaughter	439	442	398
Crimes established in preliminary procedure	486,007	525,540	498,027
including: manslaughter	488	542	541

Sources: *Statistical Yearbook* 1961, Fig. 1, 923
Statistical Yearbook 1972, Fig. 2, 893

Thus, the first comparable data appear in the 1971 to 1983 period. The data shown in the table are not fully coherent. After a noticeable decline between the years 1971 and 1976, the total number of crimes started to grow, particularly in the last four years (Table 13.2). A different tendency is seen in crimes against life and health, which usually result in casualties. Their number continued to decline almost steadily, beginning from 1971 until 1983, which saw a 10 per cent rise in the number of offences involving assault causing bodily harm, participation in fights or beatings. The number of cases of manslaughter changes from year to year in a very irregular way and no clear tendency can be identified.

It would be worthwhile at this point to see how these tendencies tie in with trends in alcohol consumption (Figure 13.1). The alcohol consumption curve clearly indicates that its greatest increase (1970-7) coincided with the period of decline in the number of crimes. The greatest slump in alcohol consumption in Poland's post-war history occurred in 1981, but

Table 13.2: *Crimes established in preliminary criminal procedure by category of crime, 1971-1983*

		Category of Crime			
Year	Total	Crimes against life & health	Manslaughter[a]	Assault with bodily harm[b]	Participating in fighting & beating[c]
1971	475,411	26,737	552	18,308	6,400
1972	379,086	23,933	566	16,032	6,023
1973	335,125	23,604	673	14,971	6,217
1974	339,542	20,910	685	13,002	5,599
1975	340,423	19,974	605	12,770	5,448
1976	324,182	17,293	519	11,113	4,568
1977	344,507	17,642	528	11,268	4,823
1978	355,493	15,695	464	10,114	4,222
1979	337,301	14,444	498	9,317	3,876
1980	337,935	14,710	589	9,415	3,840
1981	379,762	14,389	493	9,104	3,986
1982	436,206	13,587	472	8,434	3,752
1983	466,205	15,256	478	9,546	4,104

[a] Penal code, Article 148
[b] Penal code, Articles 155, 156
[c] Penal code, Articles 158, 159

Sources: *Statistical Yearbook* 1984 Fig. 9, 781
Statistical Yearbook 1975 Fig. 1, 837
Statistical Yearbook 1972 Fig. 2, 894
Statistical Yearbook 1980 Fig. 1, 758
Statistical Yearbook 1973 Fig. 2, 863
Statistical Yearbook 1978 Fig. 1, 712

was not reflected in the number of crimes against life and health. At the same time, during the years of increased consumption of alcohol the proportion of offenders under the influence of alcohol among those suspected of committing crimes was on the rise.

While it is puzzling to see this discrepancy between the aggregate level statistics and more specific data on offenders, some hypotheses may be offered. The relationship between the aggregate level of alcohol consumption and crime is confounded by variation in the extent of police attention to alcohol-related crimes during different periods. Also, the relationship may be obscured at the level of criminal events because the police capacity to deal with crime is limited and they do not detect all crimes. Nevertheless, the growing percentage of alcohol-related crimes can reflect a continuing relationship between alcohol and crime in specific events, and not merely changes in police practices (Table 13.3).

Drunken Driving and Casualties

The Polish statistical reporting system on traffic accidents is relatively well-advanced. Data on both perpetrators and victims are published. Through the introduction of basic changes in the data aggregation system

Figure 13.1: *Per capita alcohol consumption in Poland, 1950-1984*

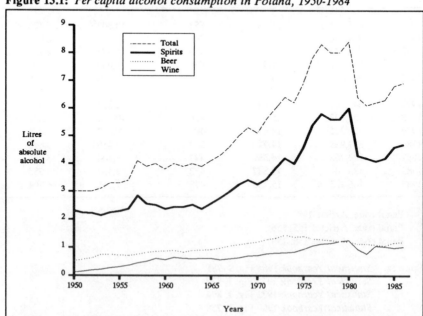

Source: Central Statistical Office

250

Table 13.3: *Persons suspected of committing crimes under the influence of alcohol by selected categories of crimes*

Crime	1965	1970	1975	Percentage 1980	1981	1982[a]	1983	1984	1985
Manslaughter	39.3	53.9	59.4	77.0	75.2		77.5	74.0	75.0
Assault with bodily harm	55.8	56.9	53.3	72.7	67.5		47.3	47.2	56.0
Fighting or beating	49.9	58.3	58.1	79.7	74.3		71.5	71.5	76.5
Rape	32..0	53.2	56.9	82.3	80.5		81.5	79.8	81.9
Tormenting family members	-	55.3	75.2	87.8	85.7		83.9	84.6	85.3
Minor assaults	77.9	80.0	83.6	93.1	93.5		-	-	-

[a] Comparable data for 1982 not available
Source: Public Militia Headquarters

in 1975, the first relatively comparable information refers to the 1975-83 period (Table 13.4). As of 1975, the records cover accidents resulting in death or bodily injury. Victimless accidents are not recorded. It is also the principle to record several causes of an accident (maximum of five) without stating one chief cause.

In spite of an increase in the number of cars, the total number of accidents was relatively stable during the period in question. The number of alcohol-related accidents does not reflect the wide variation in the rate of alcohol consumption. It should be added that drunkenness is registered as a cause of the accident whenever one of the perpetrators is found to be under the influence of alcohol. As a rule, a contributing causal relationship between an accident and inebriation is assumed.

It is noteworthy that the long list of twenty causes does not include causes independent of the persons involved in an accident. In other words, all the causes point to a single individual perpetrator. Also, such causes as poor conditions of roads, lack of separated bicycle ways and lack of pavements for pedestrians — almost a rule in the countryside — go unmentioned.

The number of deaths in road accidents in recent years remained about 6,000, the number of injuries, 50,000. Further details are provided in Table 13.5.

Table 13.4: *Traffic accidents*

Kinds of accidents	1975	1978	1980	1981	1982	1983
Total	39,404	39,181	40,373	43,755	38,832	40,454
Per 10,000 cars	100.6	80.4	73.5	74.8	64.8	63.0
Major causes:						
Infringement of traffic regulations by drivers	26,009	24,974	25,861	29,282	26,254	26,862
Infringement of traffic regulations by pedestrians	13,467	13,786	14,276	14,430	12,459	13,582
Drunken driving or walking:	8,484	9,027	10,432	9,479	9,602	10,084
drunken driving:	4,524	4,379	5,012	5,165	5,844	5,372
passenger cars	1,047	1,454	1,895	2,129	2,592	2,597
motorcycles	1,609	1,247	1,351	1,445	1,480	1,376
bicycles	1,061	907	1,037	932	982	942
trucks	502	481	455	429	507	431
other vehicles	305	290	274	230	283	266
drunken pedestrians	3,682	4,433	5,177	4,050	3,461	4,473
drunken passengers	278	215	243	264	297	239
Faulty technical state of vehicles	1,669	1,363	1,209	1,238	1,163	1,178
Victims:						
Deaths	5,633	5,925	6,002	6,107	5,535	5,561
including juveniles under 14	502	453	470	496	455	428
Injuries	46,385	45,766	46,245	51,365	45,696	47,463
including juveniles under 14	5,388	5,366	5,734	6,644	6,447	6,586

Source: *Statistical Yearbook* 1984 Fig. 40 (521)

Alcohol-related accidents account for 20 to 25 per cent of the total number of road accidents and they more often end with the death of participants (30 per cent of the total of casualty deaths).

Labour Accidents

In recent years, the curtailment of inebriation in the work place has been one of the most important aims of alcohol policy. A new law on alcohol established in 1982 bans consumption of alcohol on work premises under penal sanctions for both workers and their supervisors. An inebriated worker who has an accident is deprived of accident allowance. Official statements and articles in the press concerning this subject seem to create the impression that drinking is one of the major causes of low

Table 13.5: *Victims of traffic accidents on public roads in Poland*

| Year | accidents | Total deaths[a] | injured[b] | Under the influence of alcohol | | |
				accidents	deaths[a]	injured[b]
1979	39,036	5,793	44,975	9,290	1,676	9,662
1980	40,373	6,002	46,245	10,432	1,939	10,875
1981	43,755	6,107	51,365	9,479	1,688	10,640
1982	38,832	5,532	45,696	9,593	1,821	11,020
1983	40,454	5,561	47,463	10,084	1,675	11,134
1984	35,768	4,980	41,325	9,463	1,711	9,907
1985	36,100	4,678	42,290	8,779	1,573	9,534

[a] Death victims are persons who died on the spot or within 30 days as a result of injuries suffered

[b] Injured victims are persons who suffered body injuries and received medical aid

Source: Public Militia Headquarters

labour effectiveness, absenteeism and labour accidents. Data on labour accidents have not been published until very recently.

In recent years, over 200,000 labour accidents involving injuries were being recorded annually, the number of deaths ranging from 1,200 to 1,500. The number of accidents where alcohol was acknowledged as the cause is strikingly low, adding up to some 0.5 per cent of the total accident figure recorded in official reports. It is very likely, however, that their number is lowered on purpose. This has been corroborated by studies carried out in 1970 by the Central Institute of Labour Protection. Although none of the work establishments questioned recorded alcohol as the source of a labour accident, 8 to 15 per cent of all accidents in these work places were found to be alcohol-related, according to these studies. The highest risk of labour accidents was recorded for construction, agriculture and mining (Witkowska 1974). A substantial proportion (8 to 25 per cent) of deaths in labour accidents involve victims with indicators of high inebriation (Raszeja 1976).

The management of work establishments is likely to conceal alcohol-related labour accidents either by recording them as accidents due to other causes or — when minor injuries are involved — not recording them at all. The managers' interest in concealing alcohol as the cause of accidents results from the threat of liability, including penal liability. Thus, the gap between official data and the picture obtained from special studies is corollary to the binding law which also provides that 'a worker who contributed considerably to a labour accident while being in a state of intoxication is not entitled to accident allowance' (Law on Allowances for Labour Accidents and Occupational Diseases 1975). This law, which public opinion regards as too severe and harmful when injury itself is enough punishment, illustrates how legal norms that are not reconciled with a social sense of justice are not respected. It happens sometimes that friends of a labour accident victim help conceal the role of alcohol in the accident by giving their own blood for alcohol measurement tests.

Acute Alcohol Poisonings

Reporting acute poisonings at sanitary-epidemiological stations has been obligatory in Poland since 1973. Information on poisonings is gathered by sanitary-epidemiological stations in the field. Their aggregate records on poisonings with ethanol are included in the broad category of poisonings with chemicals, which makes these data far from complete. According to the Statistical Yearbook of the Main Statistical Office, the number of poisonings with chemicals recorded by these stations totalled 10,740 in 1980; 10,603 in 1981; 13,348 in 1982; 13,536 in 1983. However, there is some evidence from the 1970s that these numbers might be under-estimates. In 1975, the sanitary-epidemiological stations recorded only 5,514 poisonings, while the Institute of Labour Medicine in Łódź estimated the number of acute poisonings in the seventies to reach the level of 30 to 40,000 annually.

Poisonings were more frequent in big cities than in rural areas. More detailed data on acute poisonings were gathered in Łódź in the years 1968 to 1971, covering a typical industrial conurbation with over 750,000 inhabitants and a district with over 2 million inhabitants. These data are acknowledged as characteristic of the whole country. In 1971, 375 poisonings per 100,000 inhabitants were recorded in Łódź, 233 of them suicides. Suicidal poisonings added up to 68 per cent, accidental poisonings to 28 per cent, and occupational poisonings to 1 per cent of all serious poisonings.

Poisonings with ethanol fall entirely into the category of accidental poisonings, accounting for 23.9 per cent of this group. Country-wide, they added up to between 2,000 and 2,700 hospitalised cases of acute poisonings per year. Methanol poisonings accounted for 0.8 per cent of suicidal and 3.1 per cent of accidental poisonings.

According to the Institute of Court Expertise in Kraków, the relationship between acute poisonings and alcohol is manifested in poisonings due to excessive consumption of alcohol, poisoning with substitutes of alcoholic beverages drunk by alcoholics for lack of alcohol, accidental poisonings with carbon dioxide while the victim was intoxicated, and suicides committed in the state of intoxication.

A new phenomenon connected with the economic crisis are sales of strongly poisonous plant protection solutions in vessels provided by customers, usually empty vodka bottles, which are often drunk by mistake during various occasions involving alcohol and adding to a rise in the rate of accidental poisonings (Chłobowska 1984).

Suicides

Polish data on suicides can be drawn from three sources. The first, med-ico-demographic mortality statistics, include data on suicides classified by external causes, injuries and poisonings. These kind of statistics have undergone many changes. The data published in the years 1930 to 1937 are incomplete and cover suicides as the cause of death in cities with over 100,000 inhabitants. At that time, the coefficient of suicides per 10,000 inhabitants ranged from 2.2 to 2.5. The first publication appeared in 1949 and included data from the 1946 to 1948 period, with the coefficient for major cities ranging from 1.2 to 1.5. Since 1950, country-wide statistics have been compiled. The so-called 'National denomination of diseases and causes of mortality' used between 1951 and 1958 was replaced by in-ternational classification in 1959.

Another kind of statistic covers attempted and fatal suicides recorded by the State Police from 1937 — data prior to 1935 are not comparable due to a change in the method of data aggregation — and the Public Militia from 1954. Although these data are relatively complete with regard to suicide fatalities, they only record an estimated one-seventh of non-fatal suicide attempts. Militia statistics from 1970 on include data on the state of intoxication of suicide victims.

Between 1970 and 1977 Poland experienced the largest increase in al-cohol consumption during the post-war era (from 5.2 to 8.3 litres *per capita*). During this time, the proportion of suicides under the influence of alcohol rose from 34 to 46 per cent (Table 13.6).

Further analysis of the period 1975 to 1977 indicates that the rate of suicides immediately following alcohol consumption was, on average, 54.2 per cent for men and 17.3 per cent for women (Table 13.7).

The third kind of statistic covering chiefly non-fatal suicide attempts is the data on acute poisonings, which are not systematic and mostly local. For instance, we only know about the situation in Łódź, where suicidal poisonings accounted for 67.8 per cent of the overall number of poison-ings in that city. Suicide attempts under the influence of alcohol ac-counted for 17.4 per cent, which suggests that alcohol played an important part. However, family and financial problems are considered predominant causes of attempted suicide (Jezierska 1980).

It has been suggested that the most reliable source for the analysis of fatal suicides is provided by medical statistics. This seems to be the case since for many years the total figures of fatal and attempted suicides re-

Table 13.6: *Suicides under the influence of alcohol, 1970-1978*

Year	Total of suicides under the influence of alcohol	Percentage of total suicides under the influence of alcohol
1970	1,490	34.4
1971	1,593	37.7
1972	1,430	36.4
1973	1,599	38.3
1974	1,387	38.4
1975	1,540	41.7
1976	2,104	44.5
1977	2,316	47.0
1978	2,399	46.2

Note: Prior to 1970, statistics on suicide rate did not include alcohol-related figures.
Source: Public Militia Headquarters

corded by the Public Militia were lower than the figures of fatal suicides alone in medical statistics. However, militia statistics have to be consulted as well since medical sources do not include alcohol-related data. A valuable supplement to such analyses is the data on attempted suicides gathered by units that study drug addictions. Relationships between these statistics have not yet been examined but they seem indispensible for the proper interpretation of the findings (Jarosz 1975).

Table 13.7: *Suicides by method and proportion under the influence of alcohol, by gender, 1975-1977*

Suicide Method	Total number and percentage under the influence of alcohol			
	Men		Women	
	N	% inebriated	N	% inebriated
Gas poisoning	777	57.3	597	19.4
Taking poison	152	56.6	88	27.3
Sleeping pills	108	37.0	255	19.6
Cutting veins	154	46.7	57	21.1
Jumping from heights	423	42.1	306	24.2
Drowning	248	48.4	204	9.8
Hanging	7,451	54.8	1,179	14.4
Hurling oneself under vehicle	311	56.6	138	17.4
Shooting	93	59.8	3	33.3
Other	290	60.0	160	16.9
Total	10,007	54.2	2,987	17.3

Source: Hołyst 1983

Conclusions

The basic problem in the study of alcohol-related casualties in Poland is access to adequate information. Published statistical data are scarce, especially where alcohol is involved. Lack of continuity in many statistics makes it impossible to analyse changes in the prevalence of casualties in relation to changes in alcohol consumption figures. This adds considerably to the difficulty of assessing the functioning of a preventive system.

Casualty statistics are not biased by factors of purely technical nature only. Statistical data should be seen as social phenomena which are highly sensitive to the changes in the public presentation of the role of alcohol in various problems and social responses to problems. According to the Polish experience a contribution of alcohol to casualties appears sometimes to be underestimated (e.g., at the workplace, where severe penalties for both victim and management lead to a massive camouflaging of alcohol-related accidents). More often, however, the role of alcohol tends to be exaggerated. Causal links between drinking and casualties are emphasized although the character of this relationship is questionable. Such 'alcoholization' of the causes of casualties results in the perception of their origins being located in the individual instead of on a social or environmental level. This tendency seems to be especially strong when alcohol becomes a public issue and statistical data may serve as an argument in political debate. A low sensitivity of casualty statistics to the changes in alcohol consumption noted in Poland may be attributed to the influence of social and political factors which have tended to either amplify or deflate problems.

Acknowledgements

The authors would like to acknowledge Leszek Stafiej for translation of the manuscript.

References

Chłobowska, Z. (1984) *Niebezpieczne zatrucia* [Dangerous poisonings]. *Problemy alkoholizmu* [*Problems of alcoholism*], *12*, 5-6

Engels, F. (1949) *The housing question.* K.W., Warszawa

Engels, F. (1945) *Socialism: utopian and scientific.* International Publishers, New York

Hołyst, B. (1983) *Samobójstwo* [*Suicide*], PWN, Warszawa

Jarosz, M. (1975) Samobójstwa: statystyczno-socjologiczna charaktery-styka zjawiska [Suicides: statistico- sociological characteristics of the phenomenon]. In GUS, *Statystyka Polski, Wybrane zagadnienia pato-logii spolecznej* [*The Main Statistical Office, Polish statistics, Selected problems of social pathology*], Warszawa, pp. 52-81

Jarosz, M. (1980) *Samozniszczenie, samobójstwo, alkoholizm, narkomania* [*Self-Destruction, suicide, alcoholism, drug addictions*], Ossolineum, Wrocław

Jezierska, A. (1980) Zatrucia samobójcze współistniejace z upojeniem alkoholowym na podstawie materiału kliniki ostrych zatruc w latach 1978-1979 [Suicidal poisonings coinciding with alcohol intoxication based on the materials of the clinic for serious poisonings for the years 1978-1979]. In *VI Konferencja Naukowa Psychiatrów Polskich i Cze-choslowackich, Pamiętniki* [*The 6th Conference of Polish and Cze-choslovak Psychiatrists, Proceedings*], Łódź

Law on allowances for labour accidents and occupational diseases (1975) *Journal of Law, No. 30*, 1983

Moczarski, K. (1970) O konsekwentny rachunek ekonomiczny [For a con-sistent economic calculus]. *Problemy Alkoholizmu* [*Problems of Alco-holism*], 5-6, 1-3

Morawski, J. (1983) Alcohol-related problems in Poland, 1950-1981. In N. Giesbrecht, M. Cahannes, J. Moskalewicz, E. Österberg and R. Room (eds), *Consequences of drinking. Trends in alcohol problem statistics in seven countries*, Addiction Research Foundation, Toronto, pp. 1-24

Moskalewicz, J. (1981) Alcohol as a public issue; recent developments in alcohol control in Poland. *Contemporary Drug Problems*, Spring, 11-21

Raszeja, S. (1976) Przyczyny i mechanizm urazów przy pracy [Causes and mechanisms of labour casualties]. *Archiwum medycyny sądowej i kry-minalistyki* [*Archive of Court Medicine*], 26, 157-64

Wald, I., T. Kulisiewicz, J. Morawski and A. Bogustawski (1981) *Raport o problemach polityki wobec alkoholu* [*Report on alcohol policy*], IWZZ, Warszawa

Wald, I. and J. Moskalewicz (1984) Alcohol policy in a crisis situation. *British Journal of Addiction, 72*, 331-5

Ważyk, A. (1956) *Poemat dla doroslych i inne wiersze* [*An epic for adults and other poems*], PIW, Warszawa

Witkowska, H. (1974) *Analiza różnych źródeł danych statystycznych o wy-padkach przy pracy i poza pracą* [*Analysis of different statistical sources on labour and other accidents*], CIOP, Warszawa, p. 52

14

Alcohol-Related Casualties and Crime in Mexico: Description of Reporting Systems and Results for a Study

Haydeé Rosovsky

Casualties from accidents and violent delinquent behaviour constitute an important problem in Mexican public health. Deaths from accidents and injuries (accidental or intentional) are among the main causes of all deaths and affect age groups considered highly productive (Secretaría de Programación y Presupuesto 1980). Presumably, there are more cases of violent behaviour and accidents that do not lead to death, but which cause disabilities to individuals and considerable losses to society.

The role that alcohol consumption plays as a contributing factor in these types of cases in Mexico is not sufficiently known but there are reasons to assume that the consumption of alcohol constitutes an important risk factor.

This paper will first present some antecedents of the existing information on crimes and accidents in Mexico related to alcohol consumption. Second, it will present a study that has been continuing at the Mexican Institute of Psychiatry since 1984, describe the characteristics of the actual recording of these events, the methods and procedures used in the investigation and, finally, the main results to date, followed by a brief conclusion.

Antecedents

The few official statistics on accidents and violent conduct associated with alcohol in Mexico are consistent in increasing concentration of these cases among traffic accidents and crimes. According to authorities, traffic accidents that occurred under the influence of alcohol rose from 9 per cent to 16 per cent between 1970 and 1983 (Procuraduría General de Justicia del Distrito Federal 1984). It is estimated, according to official information, that about 5 per cent of all traffic accidents on federal highways have taken place under the influence of alcohol (Secretaría de Comunicaciones y Transportes, 1980). Other official information shows that, in convicted delinquents, the percentage that was under the influence of alcohol when the crime was committed has risen from 18.6 per cent in 1973 to 26 per cent in 1982 (Mas *et al.* 1985).

It is fair to say, however, that there are limitations in the information obtained from the authorities: the presence of alcohol is not recorded in other types of accidents and, in the case of crimes, it is not explained in which crimes alcohol has been present.

Through several surveys made in Mexico on alcohol consumption and associated problems, we know that a considerable percentage of the population over 14 years of age does not drink alcohol while, among the consumers, only a small percentage drink, following a continuous and excessive pattern. Nevertheless, a much higher percentage of drinkers consumes infrequently but in great amounts, thus making each drinking occasion one of drunkenness (Calderón *et al.* 1981, Medina-Mora *et al.* 1980, Medina-Mora 1984, Natera *et al.* 1983). This pattern of drinking seems more closely related to social problems than to chronic health problems such as cirrhosis, which is more often associated with a heavy and continuous ingestion.

This assessment is corroborated in that while there has been an increase in the *per capita* consumption of alcohol through the years, it has not been reflected in concomitant changes in the mortality rates of hepatic cirrhosis. The mortality rate due to this illness, though high in comparison to other countries (20 of every 100,000 inhabitants), has remained quite constant at least for the last 20 years (Lopez and Rosovsky 1986).

This situation seems to corroborate a tendency in the rising role that alcohol plays in social problems such as accidents and violent and delinquent behaviour.

Objectives of the Study

The rise in the *per capita* consumption of alcohol and in the accidents and crimes related to it, added to the limitations of the registry system for estimating adequately the magnitude and characteristics of this phenomenon, has aroused the interest and concern of both health authorities and researchers in Mexico.

Because of this, a line of investigation was initiated at the Mexican Institute of Psychiatry to cover the following objectives:

1. To describe the actual procedures of determination and registration of the role that alcohol consumption plays in accidents and crimes that reach the knowledge of the medical and justice authorities of the Federal District.

2. To develop and test a methodology to evaluate in a more adequate form the role that alcohol consumption plays in those cases.

3. To obtain and analyse information pertaining to the socio-demographic characteristics of the involved population, their predominant drinking patterns and previous problems related to alcohol consumption.

The main idea and objective of this study is to improve the registration of alcohol-related casualties and crimes by proposing the strategy of 're-peated sampling' which seems to be a viable alternative in a country like Mexico, whether it be substitution for or improvement of the existing register system (Room 1982).

Characteristics of the Existing Register

The State Attorney's office is the institution in Mexico that prosecutes crimes. It is responsible for the records of proceedings of accusations presented either by the public or by the police. Through the police, arrested suspects are taken to the police headquarters where most of the Public Ministry agencies are located. An investigation is then made that serves as a legal basis for prosecution. Misdemeanors or infractions are only punishable by fine or temporary detention. It is necessary to mention that because of persisting corruption among some of the police, many cases do not become known by the authorities.

At the investigating agencies of the Public Ministry of the Federal District there is a resident doctor from the Federal District's Medical Services who is in charge of determining the physical state of subjects immediately after their arrest or upon the request of the Public Ministry Agent. Alcoholic breath and complete or incomplete drunkenness are the categories used to indicate the presence of alcohol and are registered on the official record. The physical examination the physician performs on the arrested person is purely clinical, lacking laboratory tests that could provide greater objectivity in observation.

Of the many Public Ministry agencies in the Federal District, some of them are located at emergency hospitals that are part of the Federal District's Direction of Medical Services. It is there that people involved in crimes and casualties are taken.

Only casualties that involve a claim against someone become known to the Public Ministry in these emergency hospitals. Some of these cases are examined to determine the presence of alcohol and even though the psycho-physical examination is more complete than at the police headquarters, the basic procedures are the same. The State Attorney's office considers both accidental and criminal offenses as crimes. The grade of responsibility or intention is determined only after the pertinent investigations are made.

Of the complaints filed at the Public Ministry agencies, some are used in the corresponding cases for trial procedures. The rest are sent from the agencies of the Federal District to the main office of the State Attorney's office for their internal use and special official reports, but there is no system for filing information about the presence of alcohol in all reported crimes.

Methods and Procedures of the Study

A search for documentary information from official statistics on accidents and crimes was conducted at the start of the study. The State Attorney's office supplied valuable information as to the incidence, frequency and distribution of crimes in the different city agencies on a monthly, weekly and daily basis.

It was decided to work in two of the agencies. One was located in a police headquarters and the other in an emergency hospital. The criteria for the selection of these two agencies was based on the fact that both offered a balanced representation of the incidence of different crimes and accidents, which vary according to the city area in which such agencies are located. It was decided to work for a period of one month at both agencies with an additional week used for the testing of instrumentations and procedures prior to the investigation.

The fieldwork was done with a team of interviewers (psychologists) that had been previously trained. The team worked two shifts from Monday to Thursday and three shifts from Friday to Sunday because, according to the authorities, those were the times when there is a higher incidence of events.

The design of the study presented a series of obstacles as there were no precedents for this type of research in Mexico, because of the nature of the problem itself and the conditions under which the study had to be conducted.

Sample

It was decided, initially, to take as cases the subjects detained during the month of the project that, according to the criteria of the authorities, were under the influence of alcohol. Nevertheless, it was observed that on many occasions at the police headquarters, the physician in charge of determining the presence of alcohol was not present. Even when the doctor was at the agency, the determination of the presence of alcohol was made only on those people brought in immediately after the crime or accident had happened and when the Public Ministry agent requested it.

For these reasons, it was decided to question all the subjects brought in, both the ones that were examined by the physician and those that were not, to determine if they had consumed alcohol on the day of the event. The subjects that had not been to the doctor were added to the sample of cases if they admitted consuming alcohol the day of the crime or accident. A comparison group was chosen from people detained for similar offenses but without presence of alcohol. The procedure included matching the first subject brought in, after a case was chosen, with a similar cause of attendance where no alcohol was involved. This criterion later proved to be a methodological error. It would have been preferable to draw a systematic sample of the people without alcohol. Therefore, we had situations in which some cases could not be compared since the offense was 'drunken driving' or 'public drunkenness'.

Instruments

The instruments used were a registration form and a questionnaire. The registration forms were completed on people that arrived at the agencies during the month of the fieldwork and contained information on sociodemographic variables, type of event (crime or accident) and the notation of the presence or absence of alcohol in one of the mentioned categories as used by the authorities: 'with alcoholic breath', 'complete' or 'incomplete drunk'. It was also indicated by whom this determination was made, the physician or the interviewer. This registration form, apart from giving general information about the population and type of events, permitted the selection of the sample.

The second instrument used was a questionnaire applied through a direct interview with the sample, which contained the following information: demographic characteristics, type of crime or accident, regular pattern of alcohol consumption, alcohol consumption on the day of the event and previous alcohol related problems. This questionnaire was administered to the sample of cases with the presence of alcohol as well as to the comparison group without the presence of alcohol.

Results

Table 14.1 shows the distribution by sex of the sample in both agencies. Of the people registered during the month of observation at the emergency hospital, 430 (61 per cent of the 708) were examined by the physician to determine if they were under the influence of alcohol; in 51 cases (7 per cent of the 708), doctors found that alcohol was present and scored one of the mentioned categories used in the official registration system.

Table 14.1: *Distribution of the population in both agencies, per cent and number by sex and agency*

Agencies	Male		Female		Total		
Emergency Hospital	70.0	496	30.0	212	100.0	708	68.0
Police Agency	82.0	274	18.0	60	100.0	334	32.0
Total	73.9	770	26.1	272	100.0	1,042	100.0

The interviewers asked all 708 people if they had consumed alcohol on the day of the event. In the 51 cases that doctors detected presence of alcohol, interviewers also obtained an affirmative answer.

Of the 278 people for whom the physician did not determine the presence of alcohol, 71 (25.5 per cent) reported to the interviewers that they consumed alcohol on the day of the event and, together with the 51, made up the sample of 122 cases with alcohol in the emergency hospital; 67 people with similar causes of attendance, but where alcohol was not found, constituted the comparison group.

Of the 334 people registered during the month of observation at the police agency, only 129 (39 per cent of the 334) were examined by the physician to determine whether or not they were under the influence of alcohol. Of these subjects, the physician detected the presence of alcohol in 52 cases (15.5 per cent of the 334). The presence of alcohol was registered in accordance with the mentioned categories. Here too, the interviewers asked all 334 people if they had consumed alcohol on the day of the event. Of the 52 cases the physician had detected, 51 answered affirmatively and the remaining case did not; this was a case of intoxication by inhalant (thinner) which was also the cause of his detention. Of the 205 people that were not examined by the physician, 80 people (39 per cent) reported having consumed alcohol on the day of the event and, together with the 51 people where alcohol had been detected by the doctor and the interviewers, they made up the sample of 131 cases with alcohol in this agency; 27 with no alcohol present constituted the comparison group (Table 14.2).

There were 47 cases (24 at the emergency hospital and 23 at the police agency) among both agencies which were excluded from the sample because a) at the emergency hospital some cases were seriously injured; b) some of those arrested for drinking in the streets or other minor offenses were able to pay the fines immediately and left; or c) others arrested for

Table 14.2: *Sample of the population studied via a questionnaire in both agencies*

Agencies	Cases with alcohol the day of the event		Comparison group without alcohol the day of the event		Total	
	%	N	%	N	%	N
Emergency Hospital	47.5	98	71.0	67	55.0	165[a]
Police Agency	52.5	108	29.0	27	45.0	135[b]
Total	100.0	206	100.0	94	100.0	300[c]

[a] 93% males
[b] 98.5% males
[c] 95% males

crimes had been transferred to other detention centres. Finally, the complete sample of cases with and without alcohol was 300 (Table 14.2); the questionnaire was administered to them in both agencies.

It is important to state that through existing procedures only 7 per cent and 15 per cent of cases under the influence of alcohol were registered in each agency respectively. However, 17 per cent and 39 per cent were detected through the application of this study. This difference can be attributed to the fact that the interviewers were present at both agencies most of the time, and that when the doctor was present he only examined those people brought in immediately after the event. Many subjects were arrested several days after their crimes and thus were not checked by the physician, whereas the interviewers did question them. This permitted a greater number of cases to be identified.

It is important to point out that in the emergency hospital a larger proportion of people were examined by a physician in comparison to the police agency (61 per cent and 39 per cent respectively). This can be explained by the fact that at the hospital there were many doctors present at all times. However, the proportion of cases with alcohol detected by the physician was larger at the police headquarters. It seems that in the hospital more attention is paid to the injuries of the people than to the presence of alcohol.

With regard to the socio-economic characteristics, the following were found of the population observed and of the sample obtained.

The population of 1,042 people (Table 14.1) which was observed in both agencies through the registration forms can be described as having a low educational level, with occupations and salaries corresponding to middle-low and low social classes. The majority were male and 50 per cent were under 25 year of age; the mean age was 28.

Reasons for attendance depended on the type of agency. At the emergency hospital, injuries were due to a variety of causes: casualties at home (17 per cent), on the streets (16 per cent), at work (16 per cent); people who had been involved in quarrels (13 per cent) or had been victims of assault (10 per cent); casualties due to the collision of vehicles (8 per cent) and people who had been run over by a car (7 per cent). In the sample of cases with alcohol at this agency, the main causes were claims of injuries inflicted in quarrels, assaults, family disputes, collisions or having been run over by a car (Figure 14.1). There were no significant differences in the type of casualties among age groups.

At the police agency there were different reasons for attendance: drinking of alcohol on the street (11 per cent), traffic accidents (10 per cent), robbery (10 per cent), street disturbance (8 per cent), quarrels resulting in injuries (8 per cent), drunk driving (6 per cent). In the sample of cases with alcohol at this agency, the main causes were: being arrested for drinking alcohol on the street, inflicting injuries, drunk driving, robbery, street disturbance and damaging others' property (Figure 14.2). There were some age differences at this agency in the type of arrests: people under 25 years of age presented a higher incidence of drinking on

Figure 14.1: *Types of events: cases with alcohol at the emergency hospital (N = 98)*

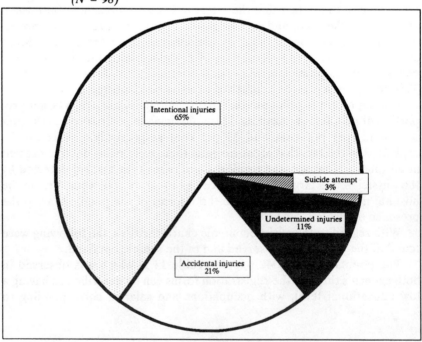

the street, causing injuries and theft. People over 25 years were arrested in a higher proportion for drunk driving.

Patterns of Consumption

The questionnaire included information on regular pattern of alcohol consumption and its ingestion on the day of the event.

The regular pattern of consumption of the interviewed sample in both agencies was similar in respect to the main alcoholic beverages consumed: distilled beverages, beer and *pulque* (Figure 14.3).

Figure 14.2: *Types of events: cases with alcohol at the police agency (N = 98)*

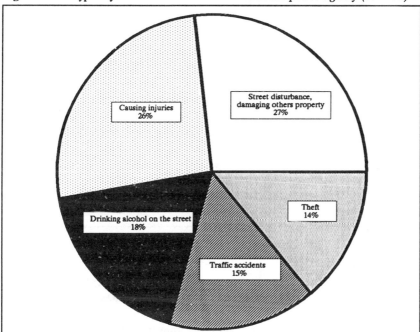

The consumption was categorised in three groups: low, moderate and high, combining quantity, ethanol concentration of the beverages and frequency of consumption. Statistically significant differences ($\chi^2 = 11.57$; $p < .01$) were found between the cases with alcohol and the comparison group in relation to distilled beverages: high consumption prevailed in the alcohol cases and moderate consumption in the comparison group, while with beer and *pulque* no statistically significant differences were found.

Interestingly, in the cases with alcohol, 8 per cent of consumption of pure alcohol was reported, mainly with a higher pattern of ingestion. In

Figure 14.3: *Regular pattern of consumption of the sample by type of beverage (N = 300)*

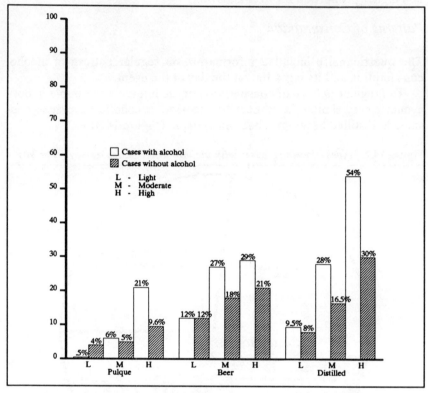

contrast, in the comparison group, no consumption of this type of beverage was reported.

In relation to the frequency of consumption, the sample of cases with alcohol reported, mainly, consuming 'one to three times a month' (57 per cent) and 'two to three times a week' (20 per cent). In the comparison group, the consumption of 'one to three times a month' (48 per cent) also prevailed. However, the second frequency of consumption reported was 'at least once a year' (29 per cent).

Some differences were found between people under 25 years of age and older people in the reported ingestion of *pulque* (22 per cent and 32 per cent, respectively) and of table wines (9 per cent and 2 per cent, respectively) (Table 14.3).

The drunkenness frequency in the cases with alcohol was higher than in the comparison group (Figure 14.4). Only 2 per cent of the cases with alcohol in the sample reported 'not getting drunk' when they drink, while 39 per cent of the group without alcohol were in this category.

Table 14.3: *Regular pattern of consumption of beverage by age group*

	(N = 300)							
	15-25 years old				over 25 years old			
	Cases with alcohol N = 98		Comparison group N = 51		Cases with alcohol N = 108		Comparison group N = 43	
	%	N	%	N	%	N	%	N
Distilled beverage	75.5	(77)	60	(30)	79	(85)	7.7	(33)
Beer	69	(68)	66	(71)	66	(71)	49	(21)
Pulque	22	(22)	12	(6)	32	(35)	28	(12)
Table wine	9	(9)	8	(4)	2	(2)	2	(1)
Pure alcohol	8	(8)	--	--	8	(9)	2	(1)

No differences were found between the two groups regarding their regular pattern of consumption and the pattern on the day of the event; still, 60 per cent of the cases with alcohol reported to have been drunk or intoxicated at the time of the event. Forty-five per cent had been drinking for one to three hours, and 41 per cent more than three hours.

Previous Problems Related to Alcohol Consumption

The sample of cases with alcohol presented consistently higher percentages of problems with alcohol consumption than the comparison group in the areas examined; these include health and social problems, and trouble with the authorities (Table 14.4).

Statistically significant differences were found between both groups in 'having problems with the family' ($x^2 = 13.45 \ p < .01$) and 'having received a warning from a physician of damaging consequences of drinking' ($x^2 = 7.06 \ p < .01$).

Conclusions and Comments

The actual registration system of alcohol-related accidents and crimes in Mexico has significant limitations at the present time. In those agencies charged with the responsibility of generating the data base, one finds that the criteria and categories for collecting data on the alcohol dimension are not adequate.

Other factors mentioned in this paper seem to indicate that under-registration is a problem. This appears to be due to the lack of uniform-

Figure 14.4: *Drunkenness frequency of the sample (N = 300)*

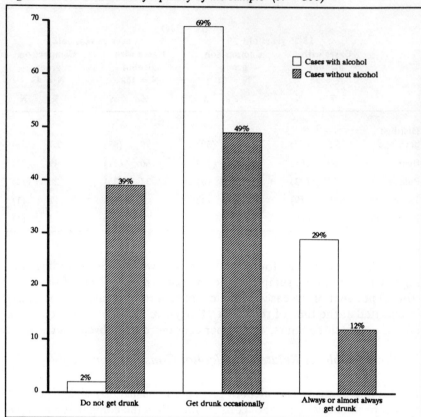

ity in applying the procedures to determine alcohol presence in many cases. The lack of precise and objective assessment procedures, such as laboratory test, also contributes to the limitation of the system. Additional information on the drinking history of the people involved in the events is not gathered.

Though Mexico has an ample sub-structure of data reporting systems, the normative and organisational actions are still in a developing phase; therefore, an improvement in the statistical information system on the alcohol problem is still to be attained. To implement, for example, a blood alcohol content measurement system (BAC) requires that not only the proper judicial frame exist but also that the necessary reagents unavailable in Mexico have to be imported.

Although the present conditions are not ideal, these could be improved if a systematic examination, using the existing procedures, were carried out. It would also be useful if additional information on previous drinking patterns could be obtained. The data that are generated are not

Table 14.4: *Previous alcohol-related problems of the sample*

Type of problems	Cases (with alcohol) (N = 206) %	Comparison group (without alcohol) (N = 94) %
Has been informed by a physician of damaging effects of drinking	24	11
Has considered drinking in smaller amounts or stop drinking	73	37
Has been drinking during several days	32	11
Cannot remember the next morning what has been done the previous night	39	17
Has been drinking at work	34	10
Having difficulties with the family	41	19
Having fights while under the influence of alcohol	34	11
Feeling the effects of drinking in his work	41	18
Having had difficulties with the police related to alcohol consumption	13	7

readily available; only part are disseminated and are not always relevant to the alcohol problem.

The study population in the Public Ministry agencies was predominantly representative of the largest social sector in Mexico; these arc also the most vulnerable and prone to be detected by these authorities. This socio-economic group has a low income and educational level.

Under the present conditions of the administration of justice in our country, the groups with higher socio-economic levels, although also involved in casualties and crimes, can more easily avoid being detained by the police authorities through the use of their economic or social power, or by attending private health services. The unemployment and under-employment conditions of significant portions of the population seem to favour the occurrence of many of the events observed at the agencies. Therefore, the conditions of life of these people play an important role. Unfortunately, this is difficult to modify. The pattern of alcohol consumption predominant in this population coincides with the findings of other studies in the Mexican general population. Alcohol ingestion is reported to be, in a substantial proportion, infrequent but excessive, with more numerous episodes of drunkenness than in the general population. It is important to point out that distilled beverages were most often consumed by those participating in the study, while in the general population the highest reported use was beer. Further research is required to assess whether this pattern is only present in the population involved in crimes and casualties or if this is a new trend of consumption of the general population.

Previous problems related to alcohol consumption that were reported by the sample appear to be similar to other studies where the family and physician are the ones who primarily indicate problems related to alcohol. Other social settings such as work and friends seem to be less sensitive in Mexico to the problem and show more tolerant attitudes.

Finally, in regard to the method that was used in this study, it can be said that it proved to be useful in obtaining the research objectives. However, in the second phase of the study, further refinement of the method will be carried out to overcome the deficiencies in the design and sample selection. It is expected that a methodology based on the experiences from this research endeavour will result which will have applicability in repeated sampling in other geographic areas of the country, and with long term continuity. This strategy could be useful in achieving a more thorough understanding of alcohol-related problems.

© 1989 Haydeé Rosovsky

References

Calderón, G., C. Campillo and C. Suárez (1981) Respuestas de la comunidad ante los problemas relacionados con el alcohol. International Report. Instituto Mexicano de Siquiatria, World Health Organization

Lopez, J.L. and H. Rosovsky (1986) Estudio epidemiologico sobre los accidentes y delitos relacionados con el consumo de alcohol. *Salud Publica 28*, 5, 515-20

Mas, C., C. Varela and A. Manrique (1985) Indicadores médicos y no médicos del problema del alcohol en México. IMP, en prensa

Mas, C., C. Varela and A. Manrique (1986) Variables medicas y sociales relacionadas con el consumo de alcohol en Mexico revista. *Salud Publica de Mexico, 28*, 5, 473-9

Medina-Mora, M.E., A. de la Parra and G. Terroba (1980) El Consumo de alcohol en la población del DF. *Revista de Salud Pública de México, 22*,281-288

Medina-Mora, M.E. (1984) Factores sociales relacionados con el consumo de alcohol en México y EEUU. Trabajo presentado en la 2a. Reunión de Investigación del Instituto Mexicano de Psiquiatría, Octubre-Noviembre, México

Natera, G., M. Renconco, R. Almendares and H. Rosovsky (1983) Comparación transcultural de las costumbres y actitudes asociadas al uso de alcohol en las zonas rurales. *Acta Psiquiatría América Latina, 29,* 116-127

Procuraduría General de Justicia del Distrito Federal (1984) Dirección General de Organización y Métodos

Room, R. (1982) Alcohol statistics project. World Health Organization Annex 4 – MNH 82.7

Rosovsky, H. (1986) Indicadores para la evaluacion epidemiologica del alcoholismo. Paper presented at the meeting of the National Epidemiology Association, Zacatecas, Mexico

Secretaría de Comunicaciones y Transportes (1980) *Anuario estadístico de accidentes viales en caminos de jurisdiccion federal*

Secretaría de Programación y Presupuesto (1980) Anuarios Estadísticos de los Estados Unidos Mexicanos, Instituto Nacional de Estadística, Geografía e Informática.

Section IV:

EXEMPLARY ANALYSIS

15

Biological Markers of Alcohol Intake Among 4,796 Subjects Injured in Accidents[*]

**Laure Papoz, Jacques Weill, Claude Got,
Jean L'Hoste, Yvon Chich and Yves Goehrs**

Introduction

Traffic accidents are known to be strongly associated with alcoholic intoxication, so many countries enforce a legal limit on the blood alcohol concentration of drivers. Epidemiological studies have so far been mostly based on blood- or breath-alcohol values measured at the time of the accident (Kastrup *et al.* 1983, McDermott and Hughes 1982, Vine and Watson 1983, Woodward 1983, Blanc *et al.* 1980, Got *et al.* 1984). Only a few authors have tried to evaluate to what extent the presence of alcohol in the blood might be related to chronic heavy drinking (Pikkarainen and Pentilla 1980, Murat *et al.* 1980, Murat and Weill 1985, Dunbar *et al.* 1985).

Nevertheless, the knowledge of this relation, if any, might be of paramount importance in optimising preventive action against accidents. This is particularly true in France, where alcohol consumption remains one of the highest in the world (Haut Comité d'Etude et d'Information sur l'Alcoolisme 1984) and where traffic accidents are the major cause of premature death, leading to about 11,000 deaths each year (INSERM 1977). Furthermore, alcohol consumption is likely to play a part in other kinds of accidents occurring at home, at work or during leisure or sports activities.

---

[*] This paper first appeared in the *British Medical Journal, 292,* 1234-1237 (10 May 1986). Permission to reprint the paper was granted by the authors and the journal.

To tackle these problems a nationwide epidemiological survey was started in 1982, at the Prime Minister's request, to assess the proportions of occasional and chronic heavy drinkers concerned in accidents. It was decided to measure systematically, in addition to blood-alcohol concentration, the γ-glutamyltransferase activity and the mean corpuscular volume, both of which, alone (Rosalki and Rau 1972, Unger and Johnson 1974) and in combination (Papoz *et al.* 1981), correlate reasonably well with usual alcohol intake.

Population and Methods

Population

The subjects were recruited from October 1982 to March 1983 in the emergency units of 21 hospitals, two in Paris and the other 19 in towns all over France. In each centre the study schedule was planned so that each day of the week and each hour of the day were equally represented.

The criteria for inclusion were: (a) that the subject presented, with or without apparent injury, after an accident of any kind, including traffic accidents, accidents at work, in the home or during leisure or sporting activities and fights; (b) that the subject or family member gave consent for blood sampling; (c) that the blood was sampled within three hours of accident; and (d) that the subject was aged 15 or over.

In the case of car accidents, any passengers were assumed not to have been responsible and were excluded from the study.

Data Collection

The main characteristics of the subject (sex, age and socioeconomic status) and circumstances of the accident (time, place, kind, vehicle and severity) were obtained in an interview performed by a senior medical student assigned to the study and specifically trained over several sessions.

Laboratory Measures

The blood alcohol concentration and mean corpuscular volume were determined locally by routine methods. Measurement of γ-glutamyltransferase activity was performed centrally under the supervision of one of us and estimated at 37°C on a reaction rate automated analyser using a method derived from that of Szasz (1979).

Statistical Analysis

Data processing, including strict control of the values, was conducted by the National Road Safety Agency and the National Institute for Health and Medical Research.

Classic methods were used for comparisons (χ^2 test and Student's t test) and correlations (Pearson's r coefficient). Logarithmic transformation was applied to the individual γ-glutamyltransferase values before calculation.

The subjects were classified as 'chronic heavy drinkers' on the sole basis of their γ-glutamyltransferase activities and mean corpuscular volume according to the discriminant functions established for both sexes in another study (Papoz *et al.* 1981). This study included 995 healthy adults (604 men and 391 women), who were taken as a reference population for the present study. In addition to giving blood samples for γ-glutamyltransferase and mean corpuscular volume determination, these 995 adults have been systematically interviewed on their usual dietary habits,

Figure 15.1: *Classification of subjects according to their mean corpuscular volume and γ-glutamyltransferase values*

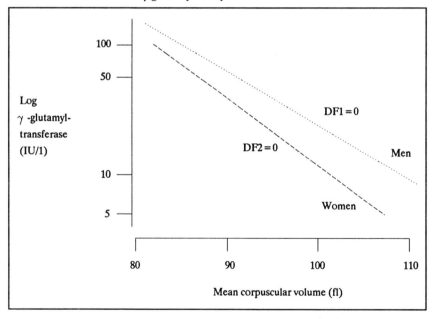

Men: DFI = log γ-glutamyltransferase + 0.043 mean corpuscular volume -5.67. Women: DF2 = log γ-glutamyltransferase + 0.048 mean corpuscular volume -5.85. Light drinkers were those falling below and heavy drinkers those falling above the corresponding straight lines (DF1 = 0 for men or DF2 = 0 for women).

279

Table 15.1: *Characteristics of injured subjects compared with those of total French population*

	Men Casualties (n=3427) %(No)		French population %	Women Casualties (n=1369) %(No)		French population %
Age:						
15-24	32	(1081)	20	25	(346)	18
25-34	28	(952)	21	22	(310)	20
35-44	18	(602)	16	13	(175)	14
45-54	12	(412)	16	12	(156)	14
≥ 55	11	(380)	27	28	(378)	34
Socio-economic status:						
Farmers	2.4	(80)	1.2	10.0	(14)	0.5
Managers	6.7	(227)	11.7	6.1	(83)	5.7
Middle managers	6.7	(228)	8.5	3.5	(48)	4.2
Employees	17.3	(589)	5.8	26.2	(357)	17.2
Workers	33.6	(1145)	20.2	5.3	(72)	5.4
Army, artists, police	2.4	(82)	1.6	0.6	(8)	0.2
Students, retired, non-workers	18.8	(643)	44.8	52.1	(709)	61.9
Unemployed	7.3	(249)	4.2	4.7	(63)	4.9
Professional drivers	4.8	(163)	2.0	0.6	(8)	<0.1
Accident:						
Traffic	38	(1313)		43	(578)	
Work	26	(882)		8	(111)	
Home	17	(580)		35	(483)	
Sport	7	(230)		5	(70)	
Fight	12	(420)		9	(123)	
Admitted to hospital after accident	37	(1281)		42	(573)	

including alcohol consumption. Those men who usually drank more than 80 g of pure alcohol daily and those women who drank more than 30 g were considered as heavy drinkers and all others as light drinkers. The equations of the corresponding discriminant functions given in Figure 15.1 were estimated on the basis of this classification. These functions were linear combinations of γ-glutamyltransferase activities and mean corpuscular volume, in which the coefficients were calculated to maximise the difference between heavy and light drinkers. The constant term was adjusted so that the specificity of the method would be theoretically 90 per cent. Heavy drinkers were then defined by a positive score and light drinkers by a negative one. Finally, each equation resulted in a straight line, allowing a simple graphic method for the individual allocation of the casualties. Acute intoxication was assessed on the basis of a blood-alcohol concentration exceeding 80 mg/100 ml which is the legal upper limit for drivers in France. Age was not taken into account since its coefficient was not significant in the reference population, either for men (mean age (SD) 41.8 (12.0) years, range 19 to 75) or for women (39.8 (13.1) years, range 18 to 76).

Results

Characteristics

A total of 4,796 subjects of both sexes were included in the study. The baseline characteristics are given in Table 15.1 and compared with those of the total population according to the 1982 French national census (Institut National de la Statistique et des Etudes Economiques 1984). Compared with the national data, the sample of casualties included an excess of men (72 per cent) and of young active people (mean age 34.5 in men and 42.2 in women). Traffic accidents accounted for about four cases out of ten in both men and women. Not surprisingly, men were more often the victims of occupational accidents (26 per cent), whereas women were more often victims of accidents occurring at home (35 per cent). Overall, about four subjects out of ten remained in hospital after their admission to the emergency unit.

Biological Markers

The distribution of γ-glutamyltransferase and mean corpuscular volume values showed considerable differences between injured subjects and the reference population (Table 15.2). The mean values as well as the proportions of subjects with a γ-glutamyltransferase value higher than 40 IU/l or mean corpuscular volume higher than 97 fl were all significantly higher among injured subjects, especially among men. A blood-alcohol concentration greater than 10 mg/100 ml was found in 41 per cent of the men and in 25 per cent it was over 80 mg/100 ml. In both sexes alcoholic intoxication was commonly associated with fights — more often than with traffic accidents in men and more often than with domestic accidents in women (Table 15.3).

Significant correlations were found between each of γ-glutamyltransferase and mean corpuscular volume values and the blood-alcohol concentration. Blood-alcohol concentration seemed poorly related to age, but this lack of correlation was probably due to the non-linearity of the relation; a detailed analysis showed that blood-alcohol concentration

Table 15.2: *Biological results of the injured subjects compared with reference population.*

	Men		Women	
	Casualties (n = 3427)	Reference population (n = 604)	Casualties (n = 1369)	Reference population (n = 391)
Blood-alcohol concentration:				
Mean (mmol/l)	12.6		5.2	
Range (mmol/l)	0-113.3		0-104.5	
% (No) ≥17.4 mmol/l	25 (868)		11 (146)	
γ-Glutamyltransferase:				
Mean (IU/I)	53	28	37	17
Range (IU/I)	4-1428	4-174	3-1038	3-132
% (No) >40 IU/I	30 (102)	17 (104)	17 (228)	6 (22)
Mean corpuscular volume:				
Mean (fl)	92	91	91	90
Range (fl)	66-123	79-110	71-120	76-104
% (No) >97 fl	17 (594)	10 (60)	12 (164)	4 (17)

Conversion: *SI to traditional units* — Blood alcohol: 1 mmol/l = 0.046 g/l

Table 15.3: *Biological results in injured subjects according to type of accident*

Type of accidents (and No of subjects)	Blood alcohol ≥17.4 mmol/l % (No)	γ-Glutamyltransferase >40 IU/I % (No)	Mean corpuscular volume >97 fl % (No)
Men:	(n = 868)	(n = 1012)	(n = 594)
Traffic (1313)	30.9 (406)	30.1 (395)	18.1 (237)
Work (882)	8.3 (73)	27.0 (238)	13.0 (115)
Home (580)	25.0 (145)	35.3 (205)	22.4 (130)
Sport (230)	3.0 (7)	12.6 (29)	4.8 (11)
Fight (420)	56.4 (237)	34.5 (145)	24.0 (101)
Women:	(n = 146)	(n = 228)	(n = 164)
Traffic (578)	8.5 (49)	14.5 (84)	9.2 (53)
Work (111)	0.9 (1)	8.1 (9)	4.5 (5)
Home (483)	12.4 (60)	22.0 (106)	16.8 (81)
Sport (70)	1.4 (1)	4.3 (3)	1.4 (1)
Fight (123)	28.5 (35)	21.1 (26)	19.5 (24)

Conversion: *SI to traditional units* — Blood alcohol: 1 mmol/l = 0.046 g/l

increased with age up to 45, then remained more or less stable up to 65 and decreased afterwards.

Classification of the Subjects

Among men, 27 per cent of the accident victims were classified as chronic heavy drinkers according to equation DF1 (positive score). This means that their γ-glutamyltransferase and mean corpuscular volume values were at least equal to those of the men in the reference population who reported a daily consumption of 80 g or more of pure alcohol. For women the figure was 32 per cent according to equation DF2, which referred to a limit of 30 g of pure alcohol (Table 15.4).

Table 15.4: *Classification of the injured subjects according to their γ-glutamyltransferase and mean corpuscular volume values using discriminant functions assessed in reference population*

	Casualties		Reference population	
	Men (n = 3427)	**Women** (n = 1369)	**Men** (n = 604)	**Women** (n = 391)
Alcohol consumption:				
Mean (g pure alcohol/day)	Unknown		43	13
% (No) >80 g/day	Unknown		11 (64)	
% (No) >30 g/day	Unknown			14 (56)
Classification according to discriminant functions:				
Chronic drinkers (DF1>0)	27 (934)		12 (75)	
Chronic drinkers (DF2>0)		32 (434)		13 (51)
Specificity (%)*		Unknown	90	90
Sensitivity (%)†		Unknown	33	28

* Percentage of subjects not classified as chronic drinkers among those declaring less than 80 g/day (or 30 g/day)
† Percentage of subjects classified as chronic drinkers among those declaring more than 80 g/day (or 30 g/day)

It was then possible to estimate the proportion of occasional drinkers defined by a blood-alcohol concentration greater than 80 mg/100 ml associated with a negative DF1 (or DF2) score. Overall 11 per cent (390) of men and 2 per cent (32) of women fell into this category. All subjects not recognized as chronic or occasional drinkers on these criteria were classified as 'non-drinkers'. The breakdown by kind of accident showed that occasional drinking was frequent in fights (men 29 per cent, women 6 per cent) and in traffic accident for men (15 per cent) but very rare in accidents occurring at work or at home. Subjects injured in fights and in domestic accidents were more often classified as chronic heavy drinkers, whatever their sex (Table 15.5). In addition, chronic drinkers were on average 10 years older than occasional drinkers or non-drinkers (42 years versus 32 years, $p < 0.001$ in men; 49 years versus 39 years, $p < 0.001$ in women). Among chronic drinkers, the proportion of divorced subjects was significantly higher (14 per cent versus 4 per cent, $p < 0.001$ in men; 26 per cent versus 14 per cent, $p < 0.001$ in women). Another striking result was that the percentage of unemployed people was at least twice as high in the groups of occasional drinkers as in the rest of the casualties (14.5 per cent versus 6.8 per cent, $p < 0.001$ in men; 9.4 per cent versus 4.5 per cent in women, where the sizes of the groups were too small to reach statistical significance).

Table 15.5: *Comparison of non-drinkers, occasional drinkers, and chronic drinkers according to type of accident. Values are percentages and numbers*

Type of drinkers (and no. of subjects)	Traffic	Work	Home	Sport	Fight
Men:					
Non-drinkers (2103)	58 (760)	75 (656)	57 (328)	90 (208)	36 (151)
Occasional drinkers (390)	15 (192)	2 (22)	8 (46)	2 (4)	29 (124)
Chronic drinkers (934)	27 (361)	23 (203)	35 (206)	8 (18)	35 (145)
Women:					
Non-drinkers (903)	71 (411)	81 (90)	59 (283)	86 (60)	45 (46)
Occasional drinkers (32)	2 (13)	1 (1)	2 (10)	1 (1)	6 (7)
Chronic drinkers (434)	27 (154)	18 (20)	39 (190)	13 (9)	49 (60)

Discussion

This study was designed to avoid the main bias generally encountered regarding the time and place of accidents. The sample taken was as large as possible and was taken in 21 centres from all parts of France to achieve representativeness. Nevertheless, it is impossible to assess its representativeness in the absence of reliable exhaustive statistics for all kinds of casualties. The possibility that some selection affected recruitment cannot be excluded since the subjects were admitted only to public hospitals with an emergency unit which had agreed to participate in the study. Obviously some accidents occurring far from the hospital centre or casualties admitted to private clinics were missed. This was more likely to happen for accidents at home or during sport, since the legal aspects of the other accidents generally led to police intervention and thus to the use of the public care system. Nevertheless, this possible bias could not explain the strong relations found between blood-alcohol concentration and γ-glutamyltransferase activity or mean corpuscular volume, which provide the basis for our conclusions.

Another weakness of the study was the lack of a control group of non-injured subjects investigated in similar conditions (except for the accident itself) — that is, during driving, working, fighting and so on. This was not even considered for obvious reasons of feasibility. Nevertheless, in a study that was performed in 1977 on 3,040 non-injured drivers, the blood-alcohol concentration was more than 80 mg/100 ml in 4.1 per cent of men and 0.2 per cent of women (Biecheler *et al.* 1985). The corresponding figures among the casualties from traffic accidents were 30.9 per cent and 8.5 per cent, representing odds ratios equal to 10.4 in men and 46.4 in women. The original finding in our study lies in the very important proportion of chronic drinkers among the casualties, shown by, first, the high percentage of subjects with increased values of γ-glutamyltransferase or mean corpuscular volume, or both; second, the strong correlation coefficient of those markers with the blood-alcohol concentration; and third, the results of the discriminant analysis. In addition, we analysed the differences between the various kinds of accidents.

The method of classification used, based on γ-glutamyltransferase and mean corpuscular volume values, was a substitute for the actual daily consumption of alcohol, which could not be obtained reliably under the conditions of the study. In fact, in relation to the true prevalence of heavy drinkers in the population, several subjects were misclassified because of the sensitivity and specificity of the particular test we used. For this reason we chose a specificity of 90 per cent so that errors of classification were mainly due to false negative subjects. Thus the final proportions of chronic drinkers were probably underestimated. We must emphasise that the method used in this study is appropriate for describing a population, or comparing different groups, but is unreliable for assessing accurately the alcohol consumption of individuals.

The cut-off points chosen to classify subjects as chronic heavy drinkers (80 g of pure alcohol in men and 30 g in women) are also debatable. They do not correspond to the concept of a threshold in alcohol consumption but rather to the usual values considered in France. A similar analysis performed with other cut-off points would also yield a greater prevalence of heavy drinkers among casualties. It is important to keep in mind the fact that the reliability of our results lies in the comparative approach adopted in this study. This approach was made possible by the systematic measurement of γ-glutamyltransferase activities (performed centrally) and mean corpuscular volume and the availability of epidemiological data previously collected in a healthy population.

Clearly these results do not allow us to conclude that alcohol consumption has a causal role in accidents. Among chronic drinkers it is not known whether abstinence contributes to greater vigilance or not.

Nevertheless, the particularly high proportion of chronic drinkers found among drivers suggests that the parallelism between alcohol consumption and the incidence of fatal road accidents in France is probably not the effect of chance alone. Previous national campaigns for road safety have been directed at occasional drinkers. The low percentage of this kind of intoxicated driver indicates that a more thorough preventive policy must now address the major problem of chronic consumers of alcohol.

Acknowledgements

This work was supported by grants from the French Ministry of Health and Social Affairs (Direction of Health) and the Haute Comité d'Etude et d'Information sur l'Alcoolisme. We thank E. Garat-Lesieux and S. Cenee-Prod'Homme for their technical assistance.

References

Biecheler, M.B., H. Duval, C. Filou, S. Lassarre and J. L'Hoste (1985) Alcool, conduite et insécurité routière. *Cahiers d'Etudes de l'ONSER*, 65

Blanc, J.L., A. Genot, M. Lyoen and H. Vignon (1980) Alcoholemia and traumatology in SAMU 42. *Annales d'Anesthésiologie Françaises, 21*, 165-9

Dunbar J.A., S.A. Ogston, A. Ritchie, M.S. Devgun, J. Hagart and B.T. Martin (1985) Are problem drinkers dangerous drivers? An investigation of arrest for drinking and driving, serum gamma-glutamyl-transpeptidase activities, blood alcohol concentrations, and road traffic accidents: the Tayside Safe Driving Project. *British Medical Journal, 290*, 827-30

Got, C., G. Faverjon and C. Thomas (1984) Alcool et accidents mortels de la circulation. *Bulletin du Haut Comité d'Etude et d'Information sur l'Alcoolisme, 1-2*, 38-60

Haut Comité d'Etude et d'Information sur l'Alcoolisme (1984) *La consommation des boissons*, La Documentation Française, Paris

INSERM [Institut National de la Santé de la Recherche Médicale] (1977) *Statisiques des causes médicales des décès, Tome I: Résultats France*, Editions INSERM, Paris, pp. 141-53

Institut National de la Statistique et des Etudes Economiques(1984) *Recensement général de la population de 1982*, INSEE, Paris, Collections de l'INSEE, Série D. 98

Kastrup, M., A. Dupont, M. Bille and H. Lund (1983) Drunken drivers in Denmark: A nationwide epidemiological study of psychiatric patients, alcohol and traffic accidents. *Journal of Studies on Alcohol,* *44*, 47-56

McDermott, F.T. and E.S. Hughes (1982) Compulsory blood alcohol testing of road crash casualties in Victoria: the second three years (1978-1980). *Medical Journal of Australia, i,* 294-6

Murat, J.E. and J. Weill (1985) Alcoolisme et urgences chirurgicales. *Lyon Chirurgical, 81,* 262-6

Murat, J.E., J. Weill, J. Lamy and G. Leroy (1980) Incidence de l'alcoolisme sur le nature des lésions traumatiques des accidentés de la route. *Annales de Médecine des Accidents et du Trafic, 26,* 14

Papoz, L., J.M. Warnet, G. Péquignot, E. Eschwege, J.R. Claude and D. Schwartz (1981) Alcohol consumption in a healthy population. *Journal of the American Medical Association, 245,* 1748-51

Pikkarainen, J. and A. Pentilla (1980) Screening of arrested drunken drivers for alcoholism. In L. Goldberg (ed), *Proceedings of the 8th International Conference on Alcohol, Drugs and Traffic Safety, Volume 1,* Stockholm, pp. 288-99

Rosalki S.B. and D. Rau (1972) Serum gamma-glutamyltranspeptidase activity in alcoholism. *Clinica Chimica Acta, 39,* 41-7

Szasz, G. (1979) A kinetic photometric method for serum gamma-glutamyltranspeptidase. *Clinical Chemistry, 15,* 124-36

Unger, K.W. and D.J. Johnson (1974) Red blood cell mean corpuscular volume: a potential indicator of alcohol usage in a working population. *American Journal of Medical Science, 267,* 281-9

Vine, J. and T.R. Watson (1983) Incidence of drug and alcohol intake in road traffic accident victims. *Medical Journal of Australia, i,* 612-5

Woodward, A. (1983) Motorcycle accidents in Nottinghamshire. *Public Health, 97,* 139-48

16

A Study of Alcohol Use and Injuries Among Emergency Room Patients

Cheryl J. Stephens Cherpitel

Although a large amount of literature exists on alcohol's role in various casualties (reviewed in Aarens *et al.* 1977, Roizen 1982), the usual focus of most studies has been specific areas such as motor vehicle accidents and fatalities rather than injuries (for example, Haberman and Baden 1978). It has been suggested that a number of both fatal and non-fatal casualties are more likely to arise among alcoholics or heavy drinkers than among other persons (US Department of Health and Human Services 1983), and the potential for some of these problems to occur may be heightened by even moderate consumption (Moore and Gerstein 1981). Much of the data linking alcohol consumption to fatal and non-fatal events has been derived from reports of trauma histories among alcoholics or heavy drinkers and case series reports for various types of casualties. Good epidemiologic studies in this area are largely lacking, with a few exceptions.

Klatsky *et al.* (1981), reporting prospective data on 8,060 Kaiser Permanente plan members, found those who averaged six or more drinks daily were three times more likely to die in a traffic accident and 2.7 times more likely to die in other kinds of accidents in the subsequent ten years when compared with lighter drinkers matched on age, sex, race, cigarette use and city. Case-control studies have been reported for both fatal motor vehicle accidents and fatal pedestrian injuries. Cameron (1977) reported drivers with blood-alcohol concentrations (BACs) above 100 mg/ 100 ml percent to be three to 15 times more likely to be involved in fatal crashes than non-drinking drivers not involved in accidents in similar locations at similar times. Studies comparing fatally injured pedestrians with site- and time-matched non-injured pedestrians found alcohol

288

involvement significantly greater in cases compared to controls (Haddon *et al.* 1961, Honkanen *et al.* 1976; Blomberg *et al.* 1979).

The role of alcohol in non-vehicular accidents has not been well studied because on-the-scene investigations are less frequently conducted and most studies are undertaken in hospital emergency rooms or casualty departments (US Department of Health and Human Services 1983). These studies have shown considerable variation in the proportion of casualty cases including vehicular accidents in which alcohol was present, due to varying study methodologies and the time lapsed between injury occurrence and when care was sought in non-fatal cases. Holt *et al.* (1980), reporting from Edinburgh, found positive breath alcohols in 49 per cent of 702 casualty patients seen on 17 different evenings (ten of which were weekends) compared to 32.5 per cent of other emergency department patients. Honkanen and Visuri (1976), reporting from Helsinki, found 37 per cent of 1,012 victims needing blood grouping on admission to have positive BACs. One would expect to find higher BACs among those seeking emergency care on weekend evenings or those whose conditions were serious enough to require blood grouping on admission.

There has been only one previous large-scale study of alcohol in the whole range of emergency room cases in the US (Wechsler *et al.* 1969). This study, which was based on a probability sample of those seen over a one-year period in the emergency room at Massachusetts General Hospital, found 22 per cent of the injury patients to be positive for breath alcohol.

Because of the lack of large-scale epidemiologic studies concerning the role of alcohol in various casualties, and because casualties are relatively rare events and emergency rooms are the primary source of treatment for such events, a study of alcohol use among emergency room patients was undertaken at San Francisco General Hospital (SFGH). San Francisco General Hospital was chosen because of its being the major trauma center serving the San Francisco Bay Area.

This emergency room sees about 220 adult patients daily. Specifically, the study sought to examine the prevalence of alcohol use among patients seeking treatment for injuries and illnesses by both using a breath test to estimate blood alcohol level at the time of emergency room admission and obtaining a patient's self-report of alcohol consumption six hours prior to the injury or illness. The nature of emergency room visits often creates circumstances under which data collection may prove to be difficult. Therefore, the SFGH study had a second agenda, which was to serve as a pilot study for refining methodology for a larger emergency room study to be carried out in four hospitals at a later date. This second agenda will also be addressed in this paper.

Methodology

The study design was cross-sectional, with data being collected via a 15 to 20 minute interviewer-administered questionnaire and a breath sample to estimate blood-alcohol level in the emergency room at the time treatment was sought.

A probability sample of every fifth person over the age of 18 was drawn on a 24-hour basis from those admitted to the emergency room. Sampling around-the-clock over a two-month period yielded 2,516 screened patients. Patients who were in police custody at the time of emergency room admission were included as part of the study population, but were not breathalyzed or interviewed. Patients with psychiatric problems only were not part of the study population as they were seen by the psychiatric emergency service. The 60-day sampling period included the Christmas and New Year holidays as well as the Super Bowl football game which was held 30 miles from the hospital.

The Alco-Sensor III breathalyzer was used to estimate blood-alcohol level. This machine provides estimates of blood-alcohol which have a Pearson's correlation coefficient as high as .963 for oral exhalation with cooperative patients (Gibb *et al*. 1984) when compared to chemical analysis of blood. Patients were interviewed regarding the injury or illness which brought them to the emergency room, alcohol use during the six hours prior to the injury or illness, whether they were feeling drunk at the time of the event and demographic characteristics.

Procedures

The sample was drawn from admission forms which reached a central location anywhere from ten minutes to an hour after the patient had arrived at the emergency room. This time differential was dependent upon the severity of injury or illness, with the most serious cases receiving highest priority for processing. Since around-the-clock sampling was carried out, this differential was not expected to create any sampling bias, although given levels of severity of cases may have been clustered. To maintain integrity of the sample, 24-hour-a-day vigilance was required as it was not infrequent for over 100 patients to be admitted during an eight-hour shift.

Breath tests and interviews were carried out with informed consent as soon as possible after a patient had been selected for the study. Patients were interviewed either prior to treatment, as in the case of low priority patients who remained in the waiting room, or after treatment, when the patient was able to respond. Occasionally, patients were followed into hospital and interviewed on the ward if they had been admitted. Because of the nature of the study, some subjects were either admitted to the emergency room with a condition or under treatment which interfered with their understanding of the study and their ability to respond. In such cases, clearance was obtained from the attending physician or nurse that the patient was able to respond coherently prior to being approached. If a patient had been selected for the study, but was unable to be interviewed at the time sampled, the attending physician, at his or her own discretion, obtained a breathalyzer reading. This reduced the potential problem of deflated breathalyzer readings as an indicator of alcohol use at the time of emergency room admission for those patients who could not be interviewed immediately. Breathalyzer results were not obtained for 5 per cent of those interviewed. Each shift was staffed with a Spanish speaking interviewer to handle the Spanish language interviews (10.7 per cent of all those interviewed). On some shifts, a Spanish speaking interviewer was not available, in which case, with the patient's permission, a home visit was made within two or three days to obtain the interview. Home visits were made for 30 patients.

Obtaining patient interviews became difficult for reasons other than those anticipated (refusals, patient conditions which prohibited the interview and language barriers other than Spanish). Over 60 per cent of patients seeking care in the emergency room had non-emergency problems, not unlike other emergency rooms in the United States. Consequently, many patients remained in the waiting room for some time but, unfortunately, the waiting room was not the most advantageous place for conducting interviews because of the frequently crowded conditions. Patients could not be removed from within 'hearing distance' when their names were being called, as the interview was not to delay treatment, so finding a place to interview patients was often problematic. Interviews were not infrequently conducted in treatment rooms but, again, care was not to be delayed, so many interviews were carried out piecemeal, between treatment procedures and patient trips to the x-ray department and laboratory. Due to these constraints, some sampled patients were not interviewed because they could not be located (although they did receive treatment) or they were discharged before the interview could be completed and, in some cases, before they were even approached to be interviewed.

Another group from which obtaining interviews was problematic was those who registered in the emergency room but were never seen. A majority of this group in all likelihood did not come to the emergency room for treatment, but rather for one of a number of other 'services' provided by the emergency room. Patients who are actually seen by a physician may be provided with a free bag meal (on a limited basis) upon request or free bus tokens. Facilities for showers and cots for sleeping may be made available regardless of whether a patient is seen. During a time of shrinking voluntary services available to the 'socially least fortunate groups of drunkards' (Mäkelä and Room 1985), a number of these individuals may find their way to major metropolitan emergency rooms when such services are provided, despite the possibility of increasing discrimination in providing medical services against those perceived as drunkards, as suggested by Mäkelä and Room (1985).

Sample

Three-fourths (75.4 per cent) of the sample selected resulted in completed interviews. Table 16.1 shows the reasons why completed interviews were not obtained. Only 9 percent of the sample refused interviews and of these, 10 percent (n = 21) were because the patient had participated at least once already in the study and did not wish to be interviewed again. Sampling the same individual more than once was not a surprising finding as a number of patients use the emergency room as their primary source of medical care for chronic health problems. Additionally, as discussed above, some individuals use the emergency room for non-medical services and a number of these were actually sampled and interviewed but were not seen by a physician. Those who were not interviewed because of failure to locate, regardless of whether they were seen, accounted for 15 per cent of the non-interviews. Another 15 per cent of the non-interviews were due to patient condition and of these 18 per cent were deceased (n = 16). Language barriers also accounted for another 15 per cent of those not interviewed, with Asian languages predominating. Almost 10 per cent in this group were Spanish speaking, however, but failed to be contacted by a Spanish speaking interviewer.

Demographic characteristics on all interviewed, all non-interviewed and refusals (as a separate group of non-interviewed) are shown in Table

Table 16.1: *Reasons for non-interviews*

	Percentage of sample (n = 2516)	n
Refusals	9.1	230
Not treated (55)		
Unable to locate but treated (36)	6.9	173
Discharged prior to interview (82)		
Patient condition prohibited interview	3.5	89
In police custody	1.4	34
Language barrier	3.7	94
	24.6%	620

16.2. Refusals were looked at separately as it was thought they might be a different group from the others not interviewed.

Two-thirds of all three groups were male, a percentage which has been found elsewhere in major metropolitan emergency rooms. Among those interviewed, whites accounted for slightly more than blacks with

Table 16.2: *Characteristics of interviewed, all non-interviewed and refusals (in per cent)*

		Interviewed 1896	Non-interviewed 620	Refusals[a] 230
Sex	Male	65.8	66.1	70.0
	Female	34.2	33.9	30.0
Race	White	36.1	17.6	34.8
	Black	30.8	17.9	32.6
	Latino	21.0	9.2	11.7
	Asian	2.2	9.0	.4
	Other	9.4	5.3	1.8
	Missing	.5	41.0	18.6
Age	18-29	39.6	32.6	35.7
	30-39	29.7	28.5	31.3
	40-49	13.9	12.7	14.8
	50-59	8.2	10.8	10.0
	60-69	4.2	6.3	3.0
	70 +	4.3	6.4	3.9
	Missing	.1	2.3	1.3

[a] Subset of 620 non-interviewed

Latinos contributing 21 per cent. Because of the large amount of missing data on race for both non-interviewed (41 per cent) and refusals (18.6 per cent), an accurate estimate of the actual demographic composition of these two groups could not be made. However, the data available suggest that Latinos may be significantly under-represented among both non-interviewed and refusals, while Asians may be under-represented among all the non-interviewed.

Almost 70 per cent of those interviewed were under 40 years of age with 40 per cent being under 30. No significant difference in age between interviewed and non-interviewed was found for any age groups except those between 18 and 29, and no significant differences were found between those interviewed and refusals. A larger proportion of those over 60 were not interviewed for reasons other than refusals. These individuals may likely have had conditions which prohibited being interviewed. They may also have had language barriers of primarily Asian origin, as suggested by the over-representation of this ethnic group among the non-interviewed.

Results

Of the entire sample interviewed, 29.3 per cent were admitted to the emergency room for injuries. Thirty-one per cent of the males and 24 per cent of the females reported injuries. Table 16.3 gives breathalyzer results for the 1,807 patients on whom both breathalyzer and interview data were obtained (89 patients were interviewed but not breathalyzed with 37 of these refusing to be breathalyzed).

As seen in Table 16.3, Part A, almost twice the proportion of injury patients had positive (.01%; or 10 mg/100 ml or more) breathalyzer readings (23.1 per cent) compared to non-injury patients (12.1 per cent). This association remained for readings at both 50 mg/100 ml and above and at 100 mg/100 ml and above. All of these differences were statistically significant ($p < .05$). It should be noted here that the non-injury category includes 3 per cent ($N = 63$) of the sample who were admitted to the emergency room because of either alcohol intoxication or poisoning, or

Table 16.3: *Breathalyzer reading for injured and non-injured for total interviewed and by sex (in per cent)*

A. Total	Total (n = 1807)	Injured (n = 523)	Non-injured (n = 1284)
Positive[a]	15.3	23.1	12.1
$\geq$.05	12.5	19.3	9.8
$\geq$.10	9.8	15.7	7.5
$p < 0.05$[b]			
B. Males	**Total (n = 1191)**	**Injured (n = 374)**	**Non-injured (n = 817)**
Positive[a]	18.8	27.3	15.0
$\geq$.05	15.4	23.0	12.1
$\geq$.10	12.1	18.7	9.3
$p < 0.05$[b]			
C. Females	**Total (n = 616)**	**Injured (n = 149)**	**Non-injured (n = 467)**
Positive[a]	8.4	12.8	7.0
$\geq$.05	6.8	10.1	5.7
$\geq$.10	5.3	8.1	4.4

[a] Positive is greater than or equal to .01, or 10 mg of alcohol per 100 ml of blood
[b] Significant differences were found between injured and non-injured at all three levels of breathalyzer readings for the Total and Males

for detoxification. Fifty-three per cent of this group had positive breath-alyzer readings while 41% had readings at 100 mg/100 ml and above.

As seen in Part B of Table 16.3, the relationship between positive breathalyzer readings and injuries continued for males and was statistically significant ($p < .05$) at all three levels of breathalyzer readings. Among females (Table 16.3, Part C), however, although the proportion of positive breathalyzer readings at all three levels was almost twice as great for injuries compared to non-injuries, none of these differences were statistically significant. Males reported twice the proportion of positive breathalyzer readings at all three levels for both injured and non-injured compared to females.

Non-Interviewed and Refusals

Breathalyzer readings were obtained on 13 per cent (n = 81) of the non-interviewed and 14.8 percent of the refusals (n = 34) among the non-interviewed. These readings were obtained in situations where patients either began the interview and then decided not to participate or could not be re-located to complete the interview after treatment. Forty per cent of those non-interviewed had positive breathalyzer readings and 32 per cent had readings at 100 mg/100 ml and above. Among the refusals, 44 per cent had positive readings with 38 per cent at 100 mg/100 ml and above. These proportions of positive breathalyzer readings for both the non-interviewed and the refusals were significantly higher than the 15 per cent positive and 9.8 per cent at 100 mg/100 ml and above found among the interviewed.

Drinking Six Hours Before the Event

Patients were asked whether they had been drinking within six hours of having their accident or noticing their medical problem, and whether they were feeling drunk at the time of the event. Forty per cent of males and 20 per cent of females reported drinking before their injury and close to a third of both sexes who had been drinking reported feeling drunk at the time of injury: 35 per cent of males (n = 54) and 31 per cent of females (n = 9). Only about half this proportion of males and females, however, reported drinking prior to noticing their medical problem: 20 per cent of males and 8 per cent of females. Compared to positive breathalyzer readings, a significantly larger proportion of both sexes reported drinking six hours prior to the injury. However, compared to breathalyzer readings at 100 mg/100 ml and above, a smaller, but not significant, proportion of all injured for both sexes reported feeling drunk at the time of injury: 15 per cent of males and 6 per cent of females.

Type and Cause of Injury

Breathalyzer results were next examined among those injured by type and cause of injury. As seen in Table 16.4 over a third of those with head injuries had positive breathalyzer readings and 23.5 per cent had readings at 100 mg/100 ml or above. The smallest proportion of positive breathalyzer readings was found among those with 'other injuries', the category which included injuries of lesser severity than those found in the other categories. Chi-square tests of statistical significance were performed for all three levels of breathalyzer readings, with no significant differences found.

Table 16.4: *Breathalyzer reading by type of injury (in per cent)*

Type of injury	No.	Breathalyzer positive[a]	.05	.1
laceration/abrasion	(184)	28.3	25.0	19.6
contusion	(119)	21.8	17.6	14.2
fracture/dislocation	(69)	24.6	20.3	18.9
sprain/strain	(97)	15.5	12.4	9.3
burn	(11)	18.2	18.2	18.2
head injury	(17)	35.3	29.4	23.5
other injury	(26)	11.5	3.8	3.8
		$\chi^2 = 7.38$ (df = 6)	$\chi^2 = 9.89$ (df = 6)	$\chi^2 = 7.7$ (df = 6)

[a] Positive is greater than or equal to .01, or 10 mg of alcohol per 100 ml of blood

Table 16.5 shows breathalyzer readings by cause of injury. The largest proportion of positive readings was found for those injured in fights or assaults (37.1 per cent) with falls ranking second (25.2 per cent). Again, the category of 'other cause', which included injuries of lesser severity, ranked lowest for positive breathalyzer readings. A statistically significant difference ($p < 0.001$) was found for all three levels of breathalyzer readings by cause of injury, using chi-square tests.

Discussion

Patients interviewed in the emergency room at San Francisco General Hospital were predominately male and under 40 years of age. Fifteen per cent of the sample had positive breathalyzer readings. This reached 23 per cent among those reporting injuries, which was similar to that found by Wechsler *et al.* in their 1969 study of emergency room patients. The

Table 16.5: *Breathalyzer reading by cause of injury (in per cent)*

Cause of injury	No.	Breathalyzer positive[a]	.05	.1
fall	(123)	25.2	21.1	18.7
cutting or piercing object	(66)	12.1	10.6	9.1
motor vehicle collision	(74)	20.3	14.9	12.2
other collision	(40)	17.5	10.0	7.5
fire or explosion	(8)	12.5	12.5	12.5
fight or assault	(143)	37.1	34.3	26.6
other cause	(69)	8.7	4.4	3.0
		$\chi^2 = 22.9^b$	$\chi^2 = 30.0^b$	$\chi^2 = 22.8^b$
		(df = 6)	(df = 6)	(df = 6)

[a] Positive is greater than or equal to .01, or 10 mg of alcohol per 100 ml of blood
[b] $p < .001$

15 per cent positive breathalyzer readings for those interviewed may be an underestimate of blood alcohol at the time of emergency room admission, suggested by the fact that among the limited number of those who were not interviewed, but on whom breathalyzer data were available, 40 per cent had positive readings. However, it should also be remembered that the 60 days of data collection included three different occasions in which alcohol is traditionally used to celebrate (Christmas, New Year, Super Bowl) which may have produced a seasonally inflated prevalence of positive breathalyzer readings. Additionally, drinking after the event which brought the patient to the emergency room was not controlled in this analysis and may have inflated the number of positive breathalyzer readings.

The proportion of positive breathalyzer readings was twice as great for injury patients compared to non-injury patients and this difference continued at each level of breathalyzer reading for both males and females, although these differences were not significant among females. The consistency of this difference, however, suggests this as a real finding and not just the result of multiple comparisons. The lack of a significant difference among females may be due to the small number of females with positive breathalyzer readings who reported injuries (n = 19). The observed difference in breathalyzer readings between injury and non-injury patients may be a conservative estimate because the non-injury category included 63 patients who were admitted to the emergency room for alcohol ingestion or for detoxification and 53 per cent of this group had positive breathalyzer readings. Males had a larger proportion of positive breathalyzer readings at each level among both injured and non-injured compared to females, which was not a surprising finding.

A significantly larger proportion of both sexes reported drinking six hours prior to the injury compared to positive breathalyzer readings. However, since length of time lapsed from the injury occurrence to arrival at the emergency room was not controlled, self-reported alcohol consumption and breathalyzer readings are not comparable.

Positive breathalyzer readings were associated with cause of injury but not with type of injury. This finding suggests that alcohol consumption may be a better predictor of the circumstances around which an injury occurs than of the actual outcome of the injury sustained. The proportion of positive breathalyzer readings by injury type was surprisingly similar to that found by Wechsler *et al.* (1969) in their analysis of home accident patients, with head injuries having the highest alcohol involvement. The group with the largest proportion of positive breathalyzer readings (37%) were those who had been injured in fights or assaults, which was also similar to Wechsler *et al.*'s findings.

Findings from this study, based on both breathalyzer readings at the time of emergency room admission and self-reports of alcohol consumption prior to injury, suggest that alcohol is associated with injuries for which treatment is sought in an emergency room, particularly among males. Additional analysis must include, in relation to body weight, the length of time lapsed between injury occurrence and arrival at the emergency room, and alcohol consumption following the injury event. Further work on alcohol's involvement in injury occurrence by type and cause of injury will require a much larger number of cases, particularly for an analysis within age and sex specific categories. Additionally, the severity of injury may vary with blood-alcohol level, and this also needs to be examined. Future studies of emergency room patients should take special account of those who are not interviewed, particularly those who refuse, as these study findings suggest a much greater involvement of alcohol, based on admission breathalyzer readings among this group.

© 1989 Cheryl J. Stephens Cherpitel

References

Aarens, M., T. Cameron, J. Roizen, R. Roizen, R. Room, D. Schneberk and D. Wingard (eds) (1977) *Alcohol, casualties and crime.* Alcohol, Casualties and Crime Project Final Report, Report No. C-18, Social Research Group, University of California, Berkeley

Blomberg, R.D., D.F. Preusser, A. Hale and R.G. Ulmer (1979) *A comparison of alcohol involvement in pedestrians and pedestrian casualties.* Report No. DOT HS-805 249, National Highway Traffic Safety Administration, NTIS No. PB80-166275, Washington, D.C.

Cameron, T. (1977) Alcohol and traffic. In M. Aarens, T. Cameron, R. Roizen, R. Room, D. Schneberk and D. Wingard (eds), *Alcohol, casualties and crime*. Alcohol, Casualties and Crime Project Final Report, Report No. C-18, Social Research Group, Berkeley, pp. 120-288

Gibb, K., A. Yee, C. Johnston, S. Martin and R. Nowak (1984) Accuracy and usefulness of a breath alcohol analyzer. *Annals of Emergency Medicine, 13*, 516-20

Haberman, P.W., and M.M. Baden (1978) *Alcohol, other drugs and violent death*. Oxford University Press, New York

Haddon, W., P. Valien, J.R. McCarroll and C.J. Umberger (1961) A controlled investigation of the characteristics of adult pedestrians fatally injured by motor vehicles in Manhattan. *Journal of Chronic Diseases, 14*, 655-78

Holt, S., I. Stuart, J. Dixon, R. Elton, T. Taylor and K. Little (1980) Alcohol and the emergency service patient. *British Medical Journal, 281*, 638-40

Honkanen, R., L. Ertama, P. Kuosmanen, M. Linnoila, and T. Visuri (1976) A case-control study on alcohol as a risk factor in pedestrian accidents. In R. Honkanen (ed), *Alcohol involvement in accidents*, Department of Public Health, University of Helsinki

Honkanen, R., and T. Visuri (1976) Blood alcohol levels in a series of injured patients with special reference to accident and type of injury. In R. Honkanen (ed), *Alcohol involvement in accidents*, Department of Public Health, University of Helsinki

Klatsky, A., G. Friedman and A. Sieglaub (1981) Alcohol and mortality: A ten-year Kaiser Permanente experience. *Annals of Internal Medicine, 95*, 139-45

Mäkelä, K., and R. Room (1985) Alcohol policy and the rights of the drunkard. *Alcoholism: Clinical and Experimental Research, 9*, 2-5

Moore, M.H., and D.R. Gerstein (eds) (1981) *Alcohol and public policy: beyond the shadow of prohibition*. National Academy Press, Washington, D.C., p. 463

Roizen, J. (1982) Estimating alcohol involvement in serious events. In National Institute on Alcohol Abuse and Alcoholism, *Alcohol consumption and related problems*, Alcohol and Health Monograph No. 1 DHHS Pub. No. (ADM) 82-1190, Superintendent of Documents, US Government Printing Office, Washington, DC, pp. 179-219

US Department of Health and Human Services (1983) *Fifth Special Report to the U.S. Congress on Alcohol and Health*. NIAAA, DHHS Pub. No. (ADM) 84-1291, Superintendent of Documents, US Government Printing Office, Washington, DC

Wechsler, H., E. Kasey, D. Thum and H. Demone (1969) Alcohol level and home accidents. *Public Health Reports, 84*, 1043-50

17

Accidents and Injuries Among Treated Alcoholics and Their Families

Harold D. Holder

Alcohol is a significant contributing factor in injuries and accidents in general and among alcoholics in particular (Honkanen *et al.* 1983, James *et al.* 1984). It is often postulated that alcoholics incur injuries at a higher rate than their age/gender groups, but accurate measurements of the prevalence and incidence of injury-producing accidents in this group have been difficult to obtain (NIAAA, 1983). Injuries related to alcohol misuse have significant social costs in terms of increased medical care, lost production, higher family disruption and premature death.

The most recent estimation of the cost to the United States for alcohol abuse has been set at $89.5 billion for 1980 (Harwood *et al.* 1984). This total includes some $79 billion in 'core costs', including medical treatment for a specific diagnosis of alcoholism as well as medical treatment for illnesses and accidents related to drinking. The total 1980 estimated cost for medical treatment of alcoholism including administrative costs was over $10.5 billion (Harwood *et al.* 1984).

In general, alcoholics and their family members are significantly higher consumers of health care services than non-alcoholics. It has been shown that prior to alcoholism treatment for the alcoholic, the total family (including the alcoholic) uses health care at a rate which is two to three times higher than comparable families of similar size, ages and gender mix (Becker and Sanders 1984, Plotnick *et al.* 1982, Holder and Hallan, 1976; Holder, Blose and Gasioroski 1985). Alcoholics account for the majority of this difference but non-alcoholic family members are also above-average health care consumers.

In a study of repeated hospitalization for the same disease, Zook, Savickis, and Moore (1980) found that patients with a history of chronic

300

alcoholism had a ratio of repeated-to-first hospitalisations that ranged from 1.9 to 3.6. Persons with no alcoholism noted ranged from only 0.6 to 2.2. Zook and Moore (1980) also found that alcoholism was one of six diagnostic categories which contained two-thirds of the most costly 20 per cent of patients but only one-third of the other 80 per cent of patients.

Overview of the Paper

The purpose of this paper is (1) to evaluate the usefulness of health insurance records as a source of data concerning alcohol-related casualties, (2) to discuss the causal inference concerning the impact of alcoholism treatment on the reduction of injuries and accidents, and (3) to present findings from two studies of enrollees with the public employee health insurance plans of the State of California and of the US Government.

Health Insurance Records as Data Sources

Most US citizens have at least partial coverage of their medical expenses from some form of public and/or private health insurance. Medical charges for injuries resulting from accidents are 100 per cent covered by most insurance policies. As such, the health insurance records of an individual and his or her family represent a potentially valuable and reliable source of data concerning injury-producing accidents. The following discussion reviews some of the advantages and limitations of health insurance records as data sources for research.

Advantages

1. Completeness: Health insurance claims are usually systematically filed by health care providers as a means to recover medical treatment charges and can represent a generally complete record of the health care activity of an individual and the entire family. It is possible that certain types of care such as cosmetic surgery or other forms of elective surgery may not be covered; no health insurance claim is filed and a record of the care lost. However, providers are more likely to err on the side of filing a claim in hopes of obtaining full or partial payment. This is particularly true for medical treatment for injuries, for health insurance claims for injuries are less likely to be denied by carriers and are thus more likely to be contained in a family health claim history.

2. Longitudinal data: If an individual retains his or her coverage with a particular carrier, then longitudinal studies of that individual are possible. This enables a study of injuries over a longer period of time to determine prevalence and incidence rates.

3. Identification: With the increased specific coverage of alcoholism treatment and the recent increases in mandated health insurance coverage for alcoholism in individual states, the use of surrogate diagnoses for alcoholism treatment has decreased. In addition, there has been a substantial increase in the number of specialty treatment facilities for alcoholism, both public and private, such that any admitted patient is a diagnosed alcoholic.

4. Accuracy: Medical care treatment is more accurately recorded with greater detail and precision in health insurance claims than self-reports by patients. While self-reported injuries could be accurate over a relatively short period of time, a longer longitudinal study based on self-report only is problematic.

5. Surrogate Diagnoses: Even when there is denial of a drinking problem, it is possible to use alternative diagnoses or health care patterns to identify potential problem drinkers even without a specific alcoholism diagnosis.

6. Costs: Use of the medical care charges and benefits paid by health insurance carriers permits a direct measurement of costs associated with injuries for heavy drinkers. Most studies to date of cost estimates associated with alcohol misuse have employed indirect, estimating techniques.

7. Confidentiality: An individual's records with a health insurance carrier are confidential and when used in a research project all personal identification is removed by the insurance company. Data provided in such an anonymous manner protects the identity and rights of the individual better than personal interviews.

8. Practicality: Most large insurance companies process health insurance records on computers. Consequently, a file of health care claims can be conveniently developed for research purposes with no breach of personal identities via computer analysis.

Limitations

1. Drinking History: Since health insurance records reflect medical treatment, no information about current drinking (e.g. prior to an injury) or drinking history is available.

2. Limits on Available Data: As the health insurance company controls the distribution of data for research purposes, the company can limit the types of data made available.

3. Identification: The identification of problem drinkers is dependent upon the medical care provider who files the claim. If the provider is reluctant to identify the patient as an alcoholic or fears denial of the claim, alternative diagnoses may be used.

4. Influence of Insurance Benefits: While not necessarily a problem in identification of injuries, patterns of treatment and diagnosis of alcoholism are influenced with the benefits provided under the health insurance policy.

5. Self-Selection: Patients, identified as alcoholics via health care diagnosis on health insurance claims, must have sufficient motivation or personal difficulties to come to the attention of a treatment provider. These patients may or may not be representative of other alcoholics in an enrolled population.

Like other sources of data, health insurance records are not mutually exclusive of other sources. Such records do provide unique data, particularly longitudinal, and should be used with an awareness of their limitations (*see* Gertman and Restuccia 1981).

Alcoholism Treatment and Reduction and Prevention of Injuries

With the increased prevalence and use of alcoholism treatment services, the question of cost and cost savings has been raised. Many US health insurance companies see alcoholism treatments as 'add-on' to existing general health costs. An alternative perspective is that alcoholism treatment serves two positive functions: (1) it serves as an appropriate primary diagnosis other than 'surrogate diagnoses' and (2) provides rehabilitation and thus contributes to overall patient health and the reduction of injury.

As a more appropriate diagnosis, alcoholism is being treated under a diagnosis based on the condition. Treatment is more appropriate than under a surrogate diagnosis which often only treats physical injury as a consequence of heavy drinking but does not prevent future accidents. Alcoholism services have the capability to improve the health and well-being of alcoholics and thus lower their future need for medical care. If alcoholism treatment can contribute to lower frequency of injury and associated medical costs, then one can conclude that some alcoholism treatment costs can be 'offset' by lower medical care costs for treatment of injuries and physical rehabilitation (*see* Saxe *et al.* 1983). In this paper such a cost savings will be called 'offset', i.e. reduction of the costs of medical care.

Causation and Alcoholism Treatment

One of the important issues involving offset costs is whether to attribute 'cause' to alcoholism treatment for observed changes in injuries. A concern about cause in this context is a concern for a 'necessary and sufficient' condition to use the words of philosophy of science. A lengthy discussion of causation is not needed here, but some basic points are important.

There exists no common agreement among behavioural scientists as to what constitutes causation or under what exact conditions causation can be unequivocally determined. The operational meaning of causation can depend upon the type of research design employed, the subject matter being investigated, and the measurements obtained. In other words, causation is situation specific.

Whether a controlled experiment or a quasi-experimental approach is employed, we simply cannot infer with total confidence that alcoholism treatment 'causes' a change in injury-producing accidents. This results from two sources of potential variance: (1) variance in the alcoholism treatment method (both quality and type) employed, and (2) variance in the treated population including personal motivation, life difficulties, and level of emotional support. We are left only with the option to assess the potential contribution of alcoholism treatment to changes in accident and injury levels, given that other factors can also contribute to changes in accidents and injuries.

Any inference of a contribution by alcoholism treatment is based on observed changes in injury frequency. The null hypothesis is 'no contribution'. Basic research designs are usually a 'before' and 'after', or one with a control group of alcoholics or both. The classic experimental design requires a random selection of an untreated control group of alcoholics and a comparison of the mean number of injuries of the control group to the mean of the treated group, which is also randomly selected from the same population. This ideal design is unlikely in practice due to ethical considerations of systematic denial of treatment to an identified 'control group'. In addition, diagnosis which requires personal contact with the patient is obtrusive and thus produces a form of intervention. An alternative is a pre/post design where the injury rate for the treated group before alcoholism treatment began is compared with the rate after treatment is initiated, i.e. the treated group serves as its own control.

The absence of a randomly-selected control group presents special problems for inferring causation (contribution) to injuries. This occurs because there is no opportunity to assign subjects to either a treatment or no-treatment condition. People have self-selected alcoholism treatment and no information about an equivalent no-treatment group is available.

In this situation, inferring causal relationships is problematic because of the difficulty of ruling out a number of plausible alternative interpretations (*see* Cook and Campbell 1979). Such alternatives include: (1) testing, (2) instrumentation, (3) history, (4) maturation, and (5) statistical regression. Of these, testing and instrumentation are least likely to present problems. Testing is only a problem if obtrusive measures are used such that subjects change performance in response to being questioned or tested. Instrumentation is only a problem if the type of measurement is changed or the basis of data collection is altered during the period of the study.

History becomes a problem in causal interpretation if other events occurred during the study period which affected the outcome measure. This could include a change in health care benefits under an insurance program (such as a new benefit, e.g. dental coverage) or if a major change in available health care services occurred (such as opening a new hospital in the area).

Maturation is a problem if people systematically alter their health care patterns during the study. This could occur in response to increased awareness of available care or reduced health care use in response to organisational (employer or health insurance company) efforts to control costs. Aging can also contribute to any changed pattern of injury (and thus medical costs).

The most serious problem to causal inference is likely to be statistical regression. This occurs as a result of the natural cyclical pattern or random behaviour of a time series. Over time, a high level for a measure will naturally be followed by a lower level or vice versa. For example, above-average injury rates can be followed by below-average rates, such that on the long term, injury levels are at the average. This 'regression to the mean' makes interpretation difficult because of the rapid increase in health care use which usually occurs prior to alcoholism treatment and the rapid fall in health care use following treatment initiation.

What support exists for assigning some of the change in general health care patterns to alcoholism? First, if the post-treatment initiation pattern of injuries is lower than the pre-treatment levels, then improvement can be inferred. However, the definition of the pre-treatment level is critical such that the length of time over which measures are taken is the major issue.

While data are most readily available for the twelve-month period prior to and following treatment initiation, the most marked changes in health care cost usually occur during these periods. Pre-treatment costs are highest over this period, and this twelve-month period is most likely to show statistically significant reductions in injuries and care costs following treatment initiation.

The next longest period is 24-months pre- and post-treatment. Use of this time period evens out the sharp increases which occur over the twelve-month period just prior to treatment and gives a long post-treatment initiation period for follow-up. In general, the longer the post-treatment period, the longer the time available for injury patterns to stabilise or even out.

Injuries and Accidents for Alcoholics and Their Family Members

Results of two research studies are described here in terms of patterns of injuries and accidents requiring medical treatment. The source of the data in each was a complete history of medical care claims for the alcoholic and the entire enrolled family over a specific time.

Enrollees of the State of California Employee Health Benefits Plan

In 1974, the State of California undertook a pilot program to test the feasibility of providing health insurance coverage for alcoholism for all employees of the state and their dependents, as well as employees of some public and county municipalities which contract with the state for health insurance benefits. About 337,000 beneficiaries (employees, retirees and family members) were covered by the health insurance benefits. The pilot program benefits were offered by several different insurance carriers, including four pre-paid group practices, two service types, two indemnity type carriers and one individual practice. However, three carriers — Blue Cross/Blue Shield, California Western Occidental and the Kaiser Foundation Group Plan — provided coverage for more than 90 per cent of the state employees. As part of the evaluation of this program, the entire health care records for any enrollee who received alcoholism treatment during the period July, 1974 through October, 1975, as well as other enrolled family members, were collected for the period twelve months before initial alcoholism treatment and for a follow-up period. Follow-up data were collected on two study groups: Group 1 — all alcoholics and their families before treatment and up through March, 1976 and Group 2 — Blue Cross/Blue Shield enrollees only for an additional 36-months post-treatment along with a matched comparison group. Injury patterns for both study groups are described below.

While Group 1 contained all alcoholics in the pilot program as part of the program evaluation, Kaiser, as a pre-paid health maintenance organisation (HMO), did not provide diagnosis and medical procedure information to the study. Therefore, the analysis of accidents and injuries for Group 1 could only be based on the data provided by Blue Cross/Blue Shield and California Western Occidental. All results shown below are for enrollees from these groups.

The characteristics of Group 1 are shown in Table 17.1. There were 122 alcoholics and 166 other family members on the study. The alcoholics were mainly male (58 per cent), as expected, but a surprising number were female (42 per cent). This unexpected number of female alcoholics in treatment was likely the result of a special effort to get supervisory personnel to identify and refer problem drinking employees to treatment during the pilot program. Over 85 per cent of the alcoholics were in the 35 to 70-year-old age group. The average family size was 2.36 persons. The initial study found an average of $46 per month reduction per alcoholic treated in total health care costs, including the cost of alcoholism treatment over all health insurance plans in the study. This is primarily the result of fewer in-patient admissions as both charges per stay and

Table 17.1: *Description of State of California (USA) Public Employees health insurance enrollees, two study groups*

| | Group 1, 1973-1975 | | | Group 2, 1977-1979 | |
	Alcoholics	**Other family members**		**Alcoholic families**	**Non-alcoholic comparison families**
			Total Families 76		83
Total Persons	122	166	Total Persons 162		244
Male	58%	51%	Male 50%		50%
Female	42%	49%	Female 50%		50%
Ages	**%**	**%**	**Ages**	**%**	**%**
18	0.0	23.9	18	22.2	27.4
18-20	1.8	4.6	18-20	3.0	2.4
21-24	3.5	8.0	21-24	0.6	3.3
25-34	8.8	4.5	25-34	3.7	11.4
35-44	10.5	8.0	35-44	9.3	12.3
45-54	33.3	22.7	45-54	33.9	20.0
55-64	38.6	20.4	55-64	23.4	18.9
65-70	3.5	3.4	65-70	1.9	1.6
71 +	0.0	4.6	71 +	1.8	2.4
	100.0	100.1		99.3	99.7

x̄ persons per family = 2.36   x̄ persons per family = 2.13   2.9

Source: California Public Health Employees Health Insurance System

length of stay increased during the follow-up period compared with the twelve-month pre-treatment period (*see* Holder and Hallan 1976).

Using the *International Classification of Diseases* (ICDA), Edition 8, annual rates per 100 persons for specific types of injuries can be developed. These estimates are shown in Table 17.2. The number of events for each type of diagnosis (along with the range of ICDA codes used) and the estimated annual rates (incidents) per 100 persons are shown. The most striking difference between alcoholics and their family members is the rate of fractures. Alcoholics incurred fractures at a rate over five times that of other family members. (However, as other family members have a substantially higher rate after treatment, this difference could be a random variation.) While the rate of internal injuries for other family members is close to zero, alcoholics have such injuries at an annual rate of 5 per 100 persons. One can infer that alcoholics have more serious injuries than other family members in that other family members have superficial injuries (small cuts, bruises, etc.) at a rate of 16 per 100

Table 17.2: *Injuries and accidents: alcoholics and their families, State of California (USA) Public Employees, Group 1, 1973-1975—before and after initiation of alcoholism treatment*

International classification of diseases (ICDA, Edition 8)	Estimated annual rates per 100 persons					
	Pre-treatment			Post initial treatment		
	Alcoholics	Other family members	Total family	Alcoholics	Other family members	Total family
Fractures	27.90	4.8	14.0	22.2	19.8	16.2
Dislocation, sprains strains (830-849)	3.3	6.0	4.9	6.5	4.9	5.1
Internal injury (850-869)	4.9	.0	2.1	.9	0.0	0.3
Lacerations (870-909)	9.0	7.2	7.9	8.3	9.2	8.6
Superficial injury (910-929)	4.1	16.3	11.1	8.3	5.0	5.7
Foreign bodies in body openings (930-939)	0.0	0.6	0.3	0.0	0.5	0.3
Burns (940-949)	0.0	0.0	0.0	0.0	0.0	0.0
Injury to nervous system (950-959)	0.0	0.0	0.0	0.0	0.0	0.0
Toxic effects (960-989)	4.1	0.6	2.1	1.9	0.6	1.0
Other injuries (unspecified) (990-999)	2.5	0.0	1.0	1.9	0.2	1.6

Source: California Public Employees Health Insurance System

persons while alcoholics incur superficial injuries at an annual rate of only 4 per 100. While both alcoholics and their families have similar low rates for burns, injury to the nervous system or foreign objects in body openings, alcoholics have higher rates for 'toxic effects' including ingestion of alcohol.

These rates are based on the twelve-month period before initial alcoholism treatment and provide a baseline for documenting changes (if any) in such injury rates following initiation of alcoholism treatment. After treatment begins, there is a decrease in fractures for alcoholics but an increase for other family members. Alcoholics may be incurring less serious accidents as superficial injuries increase in frequency (4.1 pre-treatment to 8.3 post-treatment initiation). There is essentially no change for lacerations, burns, foreign objects in body openings and nervous system injuries.

Table 17.3 shows the estimated annual rates per 100 for the pre-treatment diagnostic groups by age groups for alcoholics. While small cell size reduces generalisation and increases the variance of these rates, the table does show that fractures tend to occur in the older (45 and older) age groups while lacerations and internal injury tend to occur in the younger (less than 35) age groups. Pre- and post-treatment rates are shown in Table 17.3 by gender. In Group 1, male alcoholics showed greater change in injury rates than females. Males had a pre-treatment

Table 17.3: *Estimated annual rate per 100 persons for accidents and injuries by age group and sex of alcoholics, State of California (USA) Public Employees, Group 1, 1973-1975*

| | Pre-treatment only events | | | | | | Pre and post treatment | | | |
| | | | | | | | Male | | Female | |
	25	25-34	35-44	45-54	55-64	65-70	Pre	Post	Pre	Post
Fractures	0.0	9.1	0.0	58.0	17.0	0.0	32.0	16.8	21.6	19.8
Dislocations, sprains	0.0	0.0	0.0	4.9	4.3	0.0	4.2	1.3	2.0	10.8
Internal injury	0.0	18.2	0.0	0.0	8.5	0.0	8.5	0.0	0.0	0.0
Lacerations	0.0	45.5	0.0	7.3	6.4	0.0	14.1	5.2	2.0	9.0
Superficial injury	0.0	0.0	0.0	9.8	2.1	0.0	1.4	7.8	7.8	5.4
Toxic effects	0.0	0.0	15.4	0.0	6.4	0.0	2.8	0.0	5.9	3.6
Other injuries	0.0	0.0	0.0	0.0	6.4	0.0	0.0	0.0	5.9	4.3
N =	6	11	13	41	47	4		71		51

Source: California Public Employees Health Insurance System

rate of fractures of 32 compared to a post-treatment rate of 16.8 while females only dropped from 21.6 (pre) to 19.8 (post).

The description of Group 2 families with alcoholics is shown in Table 17.1. It was not possible to identify the alcoholics from the data provided by Blue Cross/Blue Shield and therefore the entire family (N = 76) is used in the analysis and per person (N = 162) rates are calculated. In addition, a comparison group of families without any alcoholic members (N = 83) which were matched (but not perfectly) in family size and family composition (ages and gender) to the alcoholic families were randomly selected from the total Blue Cross/Blue Shield enrolled population. There were 244 individuals in the comparison families. These families provided a benchmark for injury rates by diagnostic group to the families with alcoholic members (hereafter called the 'alcoholic families').

Table 17.4 shows three-year average rates for those 35 years and older as well as for those in the comparison families with similar ages. The estimated rates suggest that alcoholics may account for more of the differences between the families in fractures or at least that family member over 35 in alcoholic families have higher fracture risks. The other injury categories are similar.

The Federal Employee Health Insurance Plan with Aetna Insurance Company

As part of the continuing national interest in the costs and benefits of alcoholism treatment, the National Institute on Alcohol Abuse and Alcoholism sponsored a study of the health care patterns of treated alcoholics and their families who were federal employees enrolled with the Aetna Life and Casualty Company. Membership in the study group was defined as an enrollee who received alcoholism treatment anytime during 1980-3 and the family was continuously enrolled during this four-year period. An additional age-stratified group of families was randomly selected as a comparison group.

Descriptions of both family groups (alcoholic and non-alcoholic) are shown in Table 17.5. There are 1,645 alcoholic families and 3,598 non-alcoholic families in the study with an average family size of 2.55 to 2.47 respectively. The mean family age for both groups is 50 and the distribution of age groups is comparable. In short, for all practical purposes, these families are the same, based on the descriptive data available to the study. Holder *et al.* (1985) analysed the annual total health care use and costs of both family groups. Alcoholic families had total health care costs per month per family member which was almost twice that for the comparison families. In-patient days per year per person were three times that of the members of non-alcoholic families.

Table 17.4: *Injuries and accidents: persons 35 and older. Families with alcoholic members and comparison families with no alcoholic members, State of California (USA) Public Employees, Group 2, 1977-1979 — after alcoholism treatment*

	Families with alcoholic members		Families without alcoholic members	
	3-year total events	Estimated annual rate* per 100 persons	3-year total events	Estimated annual rate* per 100 persons
Fractures	43	12.57	22	5.42
Dislocations, sprains, and strains	11	3.21	10	2.46
Internal injury	1	0.28	0	0.00
Lacerations	4	1.15	5	1.22
Superficial injury	4	1.16	2	1.48
Foreign bodies in body openings	0	0.28	0	0.00
Burns	0	0.00	0	0.00
Injury to nervous system	0	0.00	0	0.00
Toxic effects	1	0.28	1	0.24
Other injuries	9	2.63	3	0.74
	N = 114		N = 135	

* Based on 3-year average
Source: Aetna Life and Casualty Company

A description of treated alcoholics is shown in Table 17.6. They were mainly male (64.5 per cent) with a mean age of around 53 and most were enrollees (64.2 per cent).

The Aetna Insurance Co. did not record diagnoses by ICDA codes, but rather according to a set of general categories of 'cause'. Therefore, medical care resulting from accidents was coded 'accidents'. Medical procedure codes (CPT-4) were reported for all accident-related claims if the provider was a surgeon, which gives additional information about the location of injuries. Table 17.7 shows the percentages of injuries requiring surgical care by type of procedure over the four years of the study. Little or no differences in the types of procedures is shown. As with the California study groups, there were essentially no burns recorded.

The estimated annual rates for injury-producing accidents per 100 alcoholics was 63.6 before treatment and 42.6 after treatment began. These

Table 17.5: *Demographic profile: alcoholic and non-alcoholic family study group. Federal employee health insurance enrollees, Aetna Life and Casualty Company—1980-83*

Group characteristics	Alcoholic group	Non-alcoholic group
Number of families	1,645	3,598
Average family size:		
Mean	2.55	2.47
Percent distribution		
1	21.8	23.0
2	38.2	39.2
3-4	30.7	30.0
5 +	9.4	7.8
Total	100.1	100.0
Average family age[a]:		
Mean 49.7	50.3	
Percent distribution		
18	1.2	1.2
18-20	1.9	1.9
21-24	3.7	3.7
25-34	18.7	18.7
35-44	15.9	15.9
45-54	12.1	12.1
55-64	22.2	22.2
65-70	13.6	9.4
71 +	10.7	14.8
Total	100.0	99.9
Type of plan:		
Percent distribution		
High option only	79.9	78.0
Low option only	11.9	13.7
Both	8.1	8.3
Total	99.9	100.0
Type of family:		
Percent distribution		
Enrollee only	21.8	22.3
Enrollee and spouse	35.1	33.7
Enrollee and child(ren)	7.5	7.8
Enrollee, spouse, and child	31.2	28.3
Enrollee, spouse, child and other	.5	.2
Enrollee and other	0	.1
No enrollee[b]	4.0	7.7
Total	100.1	100.1

a As of 1-1-84
b Refers to families in which no claims for enrollee were filed over the four-year period
Source: Aetna Life and Casualty Company

averages have been adjusted for differences in the mean number of months before treatment per person (20.71 months) and after treatment initiation (23.64 months).

Table 17.8 shows the annual injury-producing accident rates per 100 by age and by gender for alcoholics, other family members, and members of the comparison families. Within each group, rates are shown for the total, by gender and then further developed by age group. It should be noted that members of the male and female groups for the 'other family members' include both spouses of the alcoholics in group 1 as well as other members of the alcoholic's family. For the alcoholics, the age/gender categories for those under 35 have small cell sizes, consequently the results are less conclusive than for the age groups 35 and older. For alcoholics 35 and older, the accident rates for females are slightly higher than males between 35 and 64 and significantly higher during the retirement ages, 65 and older. These rates for these age/sex groups are substantially higher than the comparable members of non-alcoholic comparison families as well as the other (assumed to be)

Table 17.6: *Demographic profile of individual alcoholics: composite, 1980-1983. U.S. federal employee health insurance enrollees*

Enrollee characteristics		Continuous Aetna coverage
Number		1,697
Sex	Male	64.5%
	Female	35.5%
Age[a]	18	2.9%
	18-20	4.2
	21-24	3.9
	25-34	3.9
	35-44	11.0
	45-54	19.3
	55-64	29.2
	65-70	14.9
	71 +	10.7
		100.0%
Mean age[a]		52.8 years
Enrollment status	Enrollee	64.2%
	Spouse	24.4
	Dependent Child	11.3
	Other	.1
		100.0%

a As of 1-1-84
Source: Aetna Life and Casualty Company

Table 17.7: *Accidents: surgical procedures and/or injury location.[a] Federal employees (USA) health insurance enrollees with Aetna Life and Casualty Company — 1980-1983*

Surgical procedures and/or injury location	Members of alcoholic families (%)	Members of non-alcoholic families (%)
(A) General lacerations/wound repair (12000-13000)	25	28
(B) Burns (1600-16035)	0	**[b]
(C) Musculoskeletal system – general (20000-20999)	3	4
(D) Head (21010-21499)	3	2
(E) Neck and thorax (21501-21899)	**[b]	**[b]
(F) Spine (22010-22899)	**[b]	0
(G) Abdomen (22900-22999)	0	0
(H) Shoulder (23000-23929)	5	2
(I) Upper arm and elbow (23930-24999)	2	2
(J) Forearm and wrist (25000-25999)	9	9
(K) Hand and finger (26010-26989)	8	7
(L) Pelvis and hip joint (26990-27299)	4	6
(M) Femur and knee joint (27301-27599)	3	7
(N) Leg and ankle joint (27600-28899)	7	5
(O) Foot (28001-28899)	4	5
(P) Casts and strapping (29000-29799)	4	5
(Q) Other - general and miscellaneous	20	17

a Based on *Physicians' Current Procedural Terminology*, 4th Edition, 1985
b Less than 1%
Source: Aetna Life and Casualty Company

Table 17.8: *Estimated annual injury producing accidents per 100 persons by age and gender: U.S. federal employees health insurance enrollees, Aetna Life and Casualty Company—1980-83*

	All ages	18	18-20	21-24	25-34	35-44	45-54	55-64	65-70	71 +
I Alcoholic										
All N = 1645	50.0	92.85	40.07	89.53	71.77	42.69	39.57	43.95	30.19	46.73
Male N = 1070	44.5	125.00	57.05	85.29	76.87	41.94	38.17	41.19	24.84	32.32
Female N = 575	51.6	58.82	12.50	105.55	62.50	44.33	42.30	48.75	39.67	71.34
II Other family members										
All N = 2550	28.3	48.86	22.58	43.43	21.07	30.83	21.36	24.75	28.20	19.32
Male N = 1061	34.7	38.32	33.47	59.52	26.66	30.62	26.14	18.53	19.49	18.30
Female N = 1489	23.7	36.61	11.87	27.66	17.76	30.89	19.07	28.30	33.50	20.35
III Families without alcoholic members										
All N = 8887	25.98	52.68	23.57	39.94	17.57	24.84	20.88	22.79	19.67	20.88
Male N = 4725	25.97	62.01	30.65	61.29	19.20	35.27	22.56	20.42	15.45	17.61
Female N = 4162	25.63	42.08	15.41	21.75	16.66	18.49	19.43	24.72	24.66	23.69

Source: Aetna Life and Casualty Company

non-alcoholic members of their own families. Over all ages, alcoholic males have higher accident rates (44.5) than non-alcoholic males from alcoholic families (34.7) and the non-alcoholic males in the comparison families (25.97). Likewise, female alcoholics are higher (51.6) than non-alcoholic female members from alcoholic families (23.7) and the non-alcoholic females in comparison families (25.63). It should be noted that the purpose of this is a gender comparison, therefore some of the males and females in the 'other family member' category were spouses of alcoholics in category II. As a comparison, for the entire family with an alcoholic member, the four-year annual average rate per 100 persons is 40.1 and about 26 for the families with no alcoholic members, as shown in Table 17.8.

Summary and Conclusions

With a clear recognition of limitations, the value of health insurance claims as a source of data for research into the accident and injury rates of alcoholics can be demonstrated with the studies summarised here. All of these data are limited to treated alcoholics, their family members and randomly selected comparison families, but do provide insights into the differences in accident and injury rates of the three groups, as well as the changes in rates which correspond to the initiation of alcoholism treatment by the alcoholic family member.

Overall, alcoholics appear to have injury-producing accident rates which are from two to three times that of non-alcoholics. This difference is less after alcoholism treatment initiation but does not converge to the level of the non-alcoholics until three years (possibly more) after treatment initiation. These injuries appear to be primarily the result of a greater risk of fractures than any other type of injury. Alcoholics do not appear (at least in these two study groups) to have higher rates of burns than non-alcoholics.

When differences in injury rates by gender and by age group are examined (to the degree that the cell sizes are sufficient to permit reasonable inference), female alcoholics have higher injury rates than males in general and by age group. These results suggest that while some of the injury rates for alcoholics are a function of age, the observed differences in rates appear to be more the consequence of the alcoholism condition.

In each study, the lower rates of injuries for alcoholics following treatment lend support to the hypothesis that treatment for alcoholism is a means of reducing the risk of accidents. However, as the post-treatment risk rates are not equal to the rates for non-alcoholics, additional risk reduction measures and interventions should be considered.

References

Becker, F.W. and B.K. Sanders (1984) The Illinois Medicare/Medicaid Alcoholism Services demonstration: Medicaid cost trends and utilization patterns — managerial report, report prepared under contract with the Illinois Department of Alcohol and Substance Abuse, Center for Policy Studies and Program Evaluation, Sangamon State University.

Cook, T. and D. Campbell (1979) *Quasi-experimentation: design and analysis issues for field settings.* Houghton Mifflin, Boston

Gertman, P.M. and J.D. Restuccia (1981) The appropriateness evaluation protocol: a technique for assessing unnecessary days of hospital care. *Medical Care*, 19, 8, 855-71

Harwood, H.J., D.M. Napolitans, P. Kristiansen and J. Collins (1984) Economic costs to society of alcohol and drug abuse and mental illness, report for the Alcohol, Drug Abuse and Mental Health Administration, US Department of Health and Human Services, Research Triangle Institute, Research Triangle Park, NC

Holder, H.D. and J.B. Hallan (1976) A study of health insurance coverage for alcoholism for California State employees: two year experience summary, report prepared under contract with the National Institute on Alcohol Abuse and Alcoholism, H-2, Inc., Raleigh, NC

— (1978) The California pilot program to provide health insurance coverage for alcoholism treatment — one year after, report prepared under contract with the National Institute on Alcohol Abuse and Alcoholism, H-2, Inc., Chapel Hill, NC

— (1981) Medical care and alcoholism treatment costs and utilization: a five-year analysis of the California pilot project to provide health insurance coverage for alcoholism, report prepared under contract with the National Institute on Alcohol Abuse and Alcoholism, H-2, Inc., Chapel Hill, NC

Holder, H.D., J.O. Blose and M.J. Gasioroski (1985) Alcoholism treatment impact on total health care utilization and costs: a four-year longitudinal analysis of the Federal Employees Health Benefit Program with Aetna Life Insurance Company, report prepared for the National Institute on Alcohol Abuse and Alcoholism, H-2, Inc., Chapel Hill, NC

Honkanen, R., L. Ertama, P. Kuosmanen, M. Linnoila, A. Alha and T. Visuri (1983) The role of alcohol in accidental falls. *Journal of Studies on Alcohol, 44*, 231-45

James, J.J., D. Dargon and R.G. Day (1984) Serum vs breath alcohol levels and accidental injury: analysis among US army personnel in an emergency room setting. *Military Medicine, 149*, 369-74

Jones, K.R. and T.R. Vischi (1979) Impact on alcohol, drug abuse and mental health treatment on medical care utilization. *Medical Care, 17*, 1-82

National Institute on Alcohol Abuse and Alcoholism (1983) *Alcohol and health*. US Department of Health and Human Services, Rockville, MD

Plotnick, D.E., K.M. Adams, H.R. Hunter and J.C. Rowe (1982) Alcoholism treatment programs within prepaid group practice HMO's: a final report, report prepared under contract with the National Institute on Alcohol Abuse and Alcoholism, Group Health Association of America, Washington, DC

Saxe, L., D. Dougherty, K. Esty *et al.* (1983) The effectiveness and costs of alcoholism treatment, report prepared under contract to the Office of Technology Assessment, Congress of the United States, Washington, DC

Zook, C.J. and F.D. Moore (1980) High-cost users of medical care. *The New England Journal of Medicine, 302,* 996-1002

Zook, C.J., S.F. Savickis and F.D. Moore (1980) Repeated hospitalization for the same disease: a multiplier of national health costs. *Health and Society, 58,* 454-71

18

Trends in Alcohol Consumption and Violent Death[*]

Ole-Jørgen Skog

This paper is dedicated to the memory of Kettil Bruun

During the last decade, there has been a growing interest in the consequences of changes in *per capita* alcohol consumption in relation to the health of the population. So far, attention has mostly been focused on the consequences of long term abuse, such as chronic diseases.

This interest has, *inter alia*, been stimulated by the discovery of regularities in the distribution of alcohol consumption, implying that there is a connection between the general level of consumption in the population and the prevalence of heavy alcohol use (Ledermann 1956, 1964, Bruun *et al.* 1975, Skog 1985a). Therefore, a relationship between *per capita* alcohol consumption and the prevalence of chronic alcohol-related diseases is to be expected. The empirical evidence for this relationship is still very much limited to cirrhosis of the liver, while the importance of *per capita* consumption in relation to other diseases has received much less attention.

This bias does probably not imply that *per capita* alcohol consumption is relevant only in relation to cirrhosis of the liver. Rather, it is in all probability mostly due to methodological difficulties. In periods where alcohol consumption is changing, other etiological factors tend to change as well. Unless the etiological significance of alcohol is large, when compared to other factors, the effect of the former change may therefore be difficult to assess. The fact that there is a (distributed) time-lag between

[*] This paper first appeared in the *British Journal of Addiction, 81*, 365-79 (1986). Permission to reprint the paper was granted by the author and the journal.

changes in alcohol consumption and chronic diseases (Skog 1980a, 1984a, 1985b) increases these problems even further. It may in fact be quite difficult to demonstrate the existence of relationships which are strongly lagged, even when the true relationships are very strong (Skog 1980b).

The aggregate relationship between *per capita* alcohol consumption and acute health consequences, such as violent deaths, has not received very much attention either. At the individual level there exists a large amount of literature, but this is not so at the population level. However, in many countries the number of alcohol-related violent deaths may actually be at least as large as the number of alcohol-related deaths from diseases. One should therefore extend the public health perspective advocated by Bruun *et al.* and investigate more closely the health consequences of acute intoxications in relation to *per capita* alcohol consumption.

It is a well-known fact that alcohol intoxication plays a significant role in the chain of events resulting in violent deaths. In many types of accidents, the causal role of alcohol is reasonably well understood as being due to inhibitory effects on perceptual and motor skills. In other types of violent deaths, such as suicide and homicide, the causal role of alcohol is much more complex. Nevertheless it is generally agreed that alcoholic beverages are frequently involved in the latter type of violent deaths as well.

The relationship between *per capita* consumption of alcohol and rates of violent deaths depends, *inter alia*, on how the individual risk is causally determined by the person's drinking habits. Therefore, we shall start by reviewing some evidence bearing on this issue and formulate some assumptions on the basis of this evidence.

Generally, the risk of violent death due to alcohol within a specified period of time will depend on four basic dimensions of drinking behaviour. First, how often the person drinks during this period. Second, how much he drinks on each drinking occasion. Third, the kind of contexts in which he uses alcohol. And fourth, how he behaves while intoxicated. Since at the moment we are primarily interested in the risk in relation to annual intake, we shall bring the first two dimensions into focus.

Within any given drinking occasion, the risk is likely to be a convex (i.e. curved upwards) function of BAC. This is well established for road casualties (Borkenstein *et al.* 1964, Glad 1983). It probably holds true for many other casualties as well. On the other hand, for fixed BAC, the risk is likely to be approximately proportional to (and hence a linear function of) the frequency of drinking. Other things being equal, a person who drinks four times a week is exposed to increased risk twice as often as a person drinking twice a week. (Tolerance may possibly complicate the latter relationship, at least to some extent.)

Jointly, these two hypotheses imply that risk is only moderately curved, when seen in terms of annual intake. In fact, persons with a high annual intake on the average do not drink very much more on each occasion than persons with a moderate and low annual intake, then the risk will be nearly a linear function of the annual intake. If, however, frequent drinkers also drink heavily on each occasion, a linear approximation may be poor.

Linear risk models may perhaps be more realistic approximations when we turn from interindividual differences to changes over a period of time. In cases where changes in annual intake do not, to any significant extent, affect the drinking pattern, i.e. the relative occurrence of high-intake and low-intake occasions, but mainly reflect changes in the frequency of drinking, then the risk should change in proportion to the change in the annual intake, i.e. linearly.

In terms of relative risks, the differences between moderate consumers and heavy consumers ought to be considerably smaller for casualties than for chronic diseases. The risk seems to be a nearly exponentially increasing function of annual intake for diseases like liver cirrhosis (Skog 1984a, Péquignot *et al.* 1978, Tuyns *et al.* 1984) and oesophageal cancer (Tuyns 1979). An overwhelming majority of those dying from these diseases will be very heavy drinkers (Péquignot *et al.* 1978), and the mortality rate will depend critically on the 'tail' of the distribution of alcohol consumption (*see* Skog 1980b). Hence, the relationship between *per capita* alcohol consumption and mortality rates for these diseases may be fairly sensitive to minor fluctuations in the distribution of alcohol consumption.

If the risk actually is less curved for casualties, as suggested above, then the heavy drinkers should be responsible for a smaller share, and the light and moderate drinkers for a larger share of such consequences. Some empirical data exist corroborating this hypothesis (Moore *et al.* 1981, Skog 1985c). Furthermore, the mortality rate should depend less critically on the tail of the distribution. It is generally true that the less curved the risk function is, the more closely related *per capita* consumption and mortality ought to be. In fact, when the risk is a linear function of annual intake, the distribution pattern is quite immaterial.

The aggregation problem, i.e. the problem of going from the level of individuals to the level of populations, thus seems to be somewhat smaller in relation to casualties, since the risk of experiencing this type of damage within a given period depends on the intake during that period, rather than the whole drinking career. On the other hand, the risk of alcohol-related casualties depends to a much larger extent on other aspects of a person's drinking habits besides the annual intake, when compared to chronic diseases. Chronic diseases do not to any significant extent depend on the context where the drinking takes place, and neither does the drinking pattern seem to h; ve more than marginal effects on the risk of diseases like cirrhosis when long-term level of intake is kept fixed (Tuyns *et al.* 1984, Lelbach 1974). Apparently this is not true for casualties. It is definitely more dangerous to be drunk behind the steering wheel or at the top of a staircase, than in bed, and it is probably more dangerous to be dead drunk (say, BAC of 30 mg/100 ml) ten times a year, than to be only moderately intoxicated (say, BAC of 10 mg/100 ml) 30 times a year. The latter conjecture can be shown to be true if the risk depends on the frequency of drinking and amounts on each occasion as suggested above.

The aggregate relationship between *per capita* consumption and casualties should consequently depend on several aspects of the drinking culture. On the one hand, cross-cultural comparisons involving countries which are very different in terms of contexts and patterns of drinking may show no relationship at all, or very weak relationships, particularly since explosive drinking patterns occur more frequently in low consumption cultures than in high consumption countries (*see* Mäkelä 1978). In longitudinal studies, this problem may be smaller since drinking patterns and modes of behaviour may change more slowly than frequency of drinking. However, contextual changes and preventive efforts aimed at reducing the risk of casualties in general, may sometimes prevent the increasing consumption level from giving rise to higher rates of violent death.

In conclusion, on the basis of existing knowledge and the individual level hypotheses outlined above, there is reason to expect that *per capita* alcohol consumption is significant in relation to rates of violent deaths. Increasing *per capita* consumption would as a rule be expected to lead to elevated mortality rates, particularly if the patterns of drinking, the contexts of drinking and the cultural rules for drunken comportment remain very much the same. In that case one would expect an approximately linear relationship. Needless to say, one should not expect a fixed relationship between aggregate consumption and casualties, since several other factors — including some related to drinking — are also relevant.

In Norway, alcohol consumption has doubled in the post-war period. On the basis of the arguments outlined above one would expect that this increase has had an effect on the rates of violent deaths. There are no signs that the qualitative aspects of Norwegian drinking culture has changed enough to compensate for this alleged effect. In this article we shall analyse the trends in violent deaths in Norway during the period 1951 to 1980 in relation to trends in *per capita* alcohol consumption. We shall test the deduced aggregate level hypothesis that the strong increase in alcohol consumption during this period has had a proportional effect on the rates of violent deaths in Norway. The data to be used do not allow for testing of individual level hypotheses on which the aggregate level hypothesis is based and the former hypotheses are left open for future studies.

Data and Method

Since no specific statistics on alcohol-related violent death exist, we shall have to analyse the overall mortality rates and try to uncover the effect of changing levels of consumption by statistical methods.

The likelihood of being able to uncover such a relationship,if it exists, depends strongly on the absolute magnitude of the mortality figures. If the figures are too small, random fluctuations from one year to the next will seriously reduce this likelihood. In order to get large enough numbers, all causes of violent death have been pooled together. Thus the mortality data cover all kinds of accidents, as well as homicides and suicides. An analysis for separate causes of death may be attempted if the pooled data give significant results. Such analyses have not yet been made, except for motor vehicle accidents , where the numbers turned out to be too small (Skog 1984b).

Mortality figures for each gender in the age groups 15-19, 20-9, 30-9, 40-9, 50-9, 60-9, and 70 years and older were obtained from *NOS Medical Statistical Report (1951-61)*, *NOS Health Statistics (1962-3)* and *NOS Causes of Death (1964-80)*. The age-specific mortality rates were calculated for each gender, as well as the age-adjusted mortality rates for the population of 15 years and older, using a standard population (Lilienfeld and Lilienfeld 1980: 81).

Statistics on the consumption of alcoholic beverages in terms of pure alcohol *per capita* 15 years and older were obtained from *NOS Historical Statistics 1968*, *NOS Historical Statistics 1978* and *NOS Alcohol Statistics* for the remaining years.

Since it is not possible to age-adjust consumption figures, one might ask whether one should age-adjust mortality rates. In the present case the answer is positive due to the fact that demographic changes have opposite effects on the two variables. Among the elderly, alcohol consumption is below the average, while rates of violent deaths are much higher than the average. Increase in the proportion of old people, therefore, has the effect of increasing unadjusted mortality rates, while at the same time decreasing the unadjusted consumption levels, as compared to age-adjusted figures. These opposite effects would deflate a temporal correlation between the variables. Hence, by leaving both variables unadjusted a larger bias would be produced than by leaving only one unadjusted. Furthermore, the resulting 'errors' in the consumption figures are likely to be small when compared with all other kinds of errors in these figures, due to home-production, smuggling, hoarding, etc.

A statistical analysis of temporal covariation can of course neither prove nor disprove a hypothesis about causal relations. Confounding variables may produce a spurious correlation, or prevent a true causal relation from manifesting itself. It is therefore important to use statistical techniques which minimise the risk of spurious correlation, and at the same time maximise the likelihood of identifying a genuine relationship.

Simply comparing the trends for the dependent and the independent variable is not a good strategy. During the post-war period most socio-economic and epidemiological variables have either been increasing or decreasing and there are large temporal correlations (positive or negative) between almost any pair of variables. Coinciding trends are in fact not a good criterion for the validity of our hypothesis.

Violent deaths have a multiplicity of causes, and alcohol intoxication is only one of them. Statistically, one may try to divide the total number of deaths into two classes—those caused by alcohol intoxication and those that are not, calling this group noise. According to the hypothesis the former class is closely related to *per capita* alcohol consumption, while the latter is determined by other causes, which may also change over a period of time.

If violent deaths caused by other factors than alcohol have been increasing in roughly the same way as alcohol consumption, we shall observe coinciding trends, even if our hypothesis is incorrect. If, on the other hand, this noise series has been decreasing at the same or a higher rate than alcohol-related deaths have increased, then we shall observe no correlation at all, or even a negative correlation. Statistically, these problems are due to temporal correlations between alcohol consumption and other etiological factors, i.e. the noise.

One method for removing this confounding effect of trends in the noise series is called *filtering*, and the idea is to remove trends before cross-correlating the two series. The extent to which filtering the data will reduce the problem of confounding variables, will depend on the nature of the temporal correlation between alcohol consumption and other risk factors. If the latter correlation mainly mirrors the fact that both alcohol consumption and other risk factors change systematically over a period of time, rather than resulting from an intimate causal connection, filtering the data may completely remove this disturbing correlation or substantially reduce it. Strictly causal relations will not be removed by filtering, however, so that mortality rates will still correlate positively with genuine risk factors, like alcohol consumption. The general philosophy behind this technique is described by Box and Jenkins (1976). Elsewhere it has been shown that we obtain an adequate filter for the Norwegian data, simply by differencing the series (Skog 1983). This means that we should analyse changes in consumption from one year to the next in relation to changes in violent deaths, instead of using the consumption levels and mortality levels themselves.

The main difficulty with the filtering technique is that much of the systematic variance in the variables is removed, while much of the random variance in the noise remains. In fact, the part of the noise variance which is due to erratic fluctuations from one year to the next, rather than to systematic changes over some time, may increase. This problem may be quite serious if the absolute number of deaths is small, in which case the erratic fluctuations may be fairly large, thus producing a low signal/noise ratio in the filtered series.

One can keep the latter problem at a minimum by using statistical methods with optimum efficiency. This is obtained by fitting parametric models to the data by the method of (conditional) maximum likelihood. If $M(t)$ and $A(t)$ denote mortality rate per 100,000 and *per capita* alcohol consumption in litres per year at time $T = t$, one can estimate the parameters of the model

$$M(t) = a + bA(t) + N(t).$$

The parameter b describes how many deaths per 100,000 which an increase in *per capita* consumption of one litre would produce, while a denotes the expected (or average) rate of violent deaths which are independent of alcohol use. The variable $N(t)$ describes annual variations in death rates which are independent of alcohol use. This noise will normally have temporal structure, i.e. it tends to change systematically from one year to the next.

The temporal structure of the noise series should be taken into consideration when estimating the model, in order to attain optimum statistical efficiency. In the following analyses we shall describe the noise by autoregressive processes, and solve the resulting non-linear equations by the Cochrane-Orcutt algorithm (Cochrane and Orcutt 1949). The standard errors of the estimates are calculated from the estimated information matrix.

In addition to overall mortality rates, we shall also analyse age- and sex-specific mortality. We shall try to estimate the effect of changes in *per capita* alcohol consumption on mortality rates in different demographic strata of the population.

Changes in alcohol-related violent deaths in a specific demographic substratum are, of course, primarily related to changes in consumption level in this substratum. Consumption in one substratum has an effect on mortality in other substrata, only in cases where an alcohol-intoxicated person causes another person's death. Quantitatively, the latter effect is likely to be only marginal, and it may at first sight seem difficult to compare mortality trends in specific substrata with trends in *per capita* consumption.

However, granted that changes in *per capita* consumption have had effects on rates of violent deaths in the population as a whole, it is obviously meaningful to ask in which demographic substrata this effect has occurred. Therefore, it is not illogical to ask to what extent the overall changes in consumption level in the population have affected, say, mortality among middle-aged males. The important point is that the answer to this question depends on two things. First, how the overall changes in consumption in the population have expressed themselves in the specific substratum in question. And second, how the latter change in consumption has affected mortality rates. Hence, in this case we are actually studying the outcome of a two-step process. If the year-to-year changes in consumption level for a specific stratum are strongly correlated with year-to-year changes in *per capita* consumption, then one should expect to find reasonably strong correlation between *per capita* consumption and mortality rates for this substratum. If *per capita* consumption is not a good indicator for this specific substratum, one would expect low correlations.

The alcohol effect parameter obtained when age- and sex-specific mortality rates are regressed on *per capita* consumption figures will depend on both steps in the process mentioned above. When comparing parameter estimates across substrate, one should in fact take into consideration possible differences with respect to consumption levels and trends.

According to available survey data, the ratio of male to female consumption has been fairly stable during the 1960s and 1970s. During the late 1970s there appears to have been a slightly stronger increase among females (Nordlund 1981). However, as a first approximation we may assume that the consumption level of both male and female has changed proportionally with *per capita* consumption.

Norwegian males drink about four times as much as females (Nordlund 1981). Therefore, we should expect about four times as many alcohol-related violent deaths among males as among females. When sex-specific mortality rates are regressed on *per capita* consumption we should consequently expect the alcohol effect parameter for males to exceed the one for females by a factor of about four.

Available evidence suggests a somewhat more complex pattern across age groups. Among the younger age groups (particularly those below 20 years) the rate of increase seems to have been larger than in the rest of the population (Brun-Gulbrandson 1978). Nevertheless, there is no reason to doubt that there is a fairly high correlation between the annual changes in consumption for each age group and the annual changes in *per capita* consumption. Hence *per capita* consumption is a reasonably good indicator. However, the parameter estimates obtained for the younger age groups should be expected to be inaccurately larger when compared with the true value, due to the stronger increase in consumption. A large value does not imply that these groups are particularly accident-prone.

Results

Trends in *per capita* alcohol consumption and rates of violent deaths
among males and females in Norway from 1951 and 1980 are shown in
Figure 18.1. Alcohol consumption was doubled in this period, and the
rate of increase was particularly strong from the middle of the 1960s to
the middle of the 1970s. On the other hand, rates of violent deaths show
no dramatic trends during the same period. Among the males the average annual increase (estimated via regression on time, $r = .66$) amounts to
0.4 per cent, corresponding to an increase of 12 per cent in 30 years. For
females, the corresponding figures are 0.5 and 16 per cent ($r = .64$). A
naive interpretation of this could be that the increase in alcohol consumption has had practically no effect on rates of violent deaths during
this period. However, as was pointed out above, such a conclusion is not
warranted.

Table 18.1:   *Cross-correlations at different lags between per capita alcohol*
consumption 15 years and older, and age-adjusted rates of violent
deaths 15 years and older in Norway 1951-80

Lag		-3	-2	-1	0	1	2	3
Males	Raw data	0.57	0.54	0.57	0.74	0.65	0.56	0.50
	Filtered data	0.10	-0.09	0.04	0.51	0.12	-0.21	-0.12
Females	Raw data	0.31	0.41	0.49	0.60	0.49	0.46	0.41
	Filtered data	-0.31	0.22	-0.15	0.11	-0.13	0.11	-0.14
Both	Raw data	0.55	0.56	0.62	0.78	0.67	0.59	0.53
	Filtered data	-0.09	0.05	-0.05	0.42	0.02	-0.09	-0.16

The cross-correlations at different lags between the consumption series and the mortality series are shown in Table 18.1. At positive lags one
sees present mortality in relation to consumption in the past, while the
order is reversed at negative lags.

In the total adult population, as well as among both males and
females, there are moderately large correlations in the raw data at all
lags, positive as well as negative. The fact that present mortality is positively correlated with future consumption should serve as a warning
against premature causal interpretations of the trends, since these correlations are causally absurd.

In the total adult population significant correlation ($p < .01$) remains
at lag zero after filtering, while all correlations at positive and negative
lags have disappeared. This suggests that there is a simultaneous

Figure 18.1: *Per capita alcohol consumption and age-adjusted rates of violent deaths among males and females 15 years and older in Norway 1951-80*

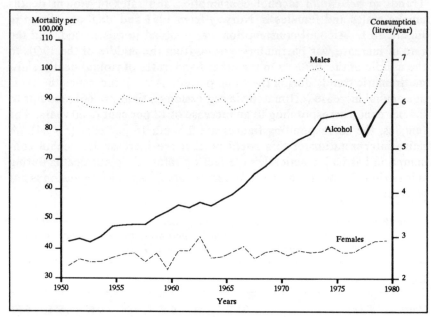

connection between the two variables which is not simply due to coinciding trends. There seems to be no time-lag in this relationship. This means that when alcohol consumption changes from one year to the next, an immediate response to this change can be identified in the mortality series. To put it differently, the two series are synchronised to the effect that in years with strong increase in alcohol consumption one finds a positive change in the mortality series. In years when consumption decreases or increases only moderately, the mortality rate goes down.

Whether this correlation at lag zero is in fact the product of a causal mechanism as outlined above, is of course difficult to decide. A third factor, or set of factors, which influences both mortality rates and alcohol consumption, may exist. However, certain factors of this type would be expected to affect both male and female mortality and one should find correlations for both sexes. If, on the other hand, the correlation is produced by a causal mechanism, one should expect a much higher correlation for males than for females, since males drink much more than females.

Among females the correlations disappear when we filter the data, and the correlations found in the raw data may only be a product of the simple, but insignificant fact that the series are both increasing, albeit slowly in the case of mortality rates. Therefore, no intimate connection between the variables can be demonstrated among alcohol consumption and rates of violent deaths in females.

Among males a highly significant correlation ($p < .01$) remains at lag zero after filtering, while all correlations at positive and negative lags have disappeared. This suggests (see below) that the noise series actually may have a downward trend among males, and hence that the very modest increase in overall mortality is the net result of two divergent trends-- an increasing trend due to alcohol consumption and a decreasing trend in violent deaths due to other causes.

The annual changes in male mortality rates are plotted against the annual changes in alcohol consumption in the scatter diagram in Figure 18.2. There are no signs of curvilinearity, and we shall proceed on the assumption that the relationships are in fact linear.

In order to obtain better estimates of the apparent effect of alcohol consumption on mortality, the model outlined in the preceding section was fitted to the data. The autocorrelation function for the estimated

Figure 18.2: *Scatter diagram for differenced alcohol consumption series and differenced male mortality series (lag zero)*

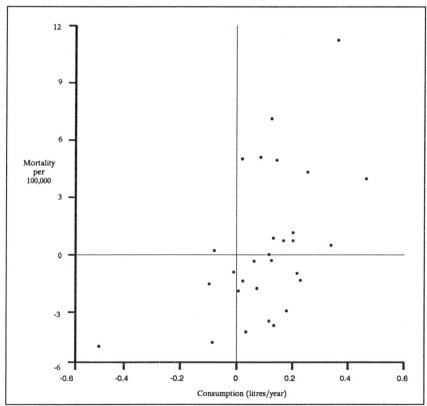

(differenced) noise series suggested a third order autoregressive process for the total adult population, a first order autoregressive process for the male population and a third order process for the female population. None of the estimated differenced noise series had means significantly different from zero. The models were estimated on the differenced series on these presumptions, and the results are reproduced in Table 18.2. Note that when the model is estimated on differenced data the intercept term in the regression equation disappears.

Table 18.2: *Results of model estimation on differenced series for population 15 years and older. Standard errors in parentheses*

Parameter	Males		Estimates Females		Both	
Alcohol effect	9.1	(2.8)	0.9	(1.2)	3.9	(1.5)
Noise lag 1	-0.20	(0.21)	-0.65	(0.18)	-0.31	(0.19)
Noise lag 2			-0.42	(0.21)	-0.09	(0.21)
Noise lag 3			-0.48	(0.18)	-0.50	(0.18)

In the total adult population the estimated alcohol effect parameter (standard errors in parentheses) is 3.9 (1.5), suggesting that an increase in *per capita* consumption of one litre should be expected to lead to an increase in rates of violent deaths of 3.9 per 100,000 inhabitants. For males, an increase in *per capita* consumption of one litre/year should, according to the results, correspond to an increase in rates of violent deaths of 9.1 (2.8) per 100,000 inhabitants.

Among females, the alcohol effect parameter is much smaller and does not reach statistical significance. However, as was pointed out in the preceding section, one would in fact expect a much smaller parameter value among females. Due to differences in consumption level, the parameter value for females ought to be about one-fourth of the value found in the male population. Consequently, one would expect a 'true' parameter value of about two for females, and this is within the confidence limits of the result actually obtained. In fact the data do not permit the rejection of a hypothesis stating that violent deaths among females have been affected by the change in *per capita* consumption in proportion to their level of consumption. We can only conclude that the data have failed to confirm or reject this hypothesis.

The diagnostic tests of the results obtained from the differenced data did not suggest serious discrepancies. The residuals did not show signs of autocorrelation, nor were there any significant cross-correlations between the residuals and prewhitened alcohol consumption.

The model has been fitted to the raw data as well. For males we obtain a substantially smaller estimate for the alcohol effect parameter, namely 3.8. This is probably due to the possibility mentioned above of a downward trend in the noise series. This would lead to underestimation of the alcohol effect parameter, since the trends in alcohol consumption and the noise series would move in opposite directions. The diagnostic checks confirm this interpretation, since it was found that the residuals correlated with prewhitened alcohol consumption ($r(0) = .35$; $p < .10$). The model was also fitted to the data differenced twice, with nearly the same result as on first differences ($b = 11.0$). This corroborates the assumption that opposite and nearly linear trends exist in the two classes of violent deaths.

In order to investigate how the effects of changes in consumption are distributed across different age groups of the population, the same analysis has been made on age-specific mortality rates. The trends in violent deaths in different age groups are shown in Figure 18.3 (males) and Figure 18.4 (females). Except among the oldest, the trends do not seem to be very different across age groups. However, in both sexes there has been a slightly more pronounced increase in younger age groups compared with the middle-aged.

Table 18.3: *Cross-correlations at lag zero and results of model estimation on differenced data in different age groups, standard errors in parentheses — males*

Age	Cross-corr. Raw data	Filt. data	Alcohol effect	lag 1	lag 2	lag 3
15-29	0.58	0.42**	11.5 (3.7)***	-0.47 (0.20)		
30-39	0.49	0.15§	10.4 (5.7)*	-0.51 (0.18)		
40-49	0.64	0.33*	6.7 (3.5)*	-0.61 (0.17)	-0.46 (0.17)	
50-59	0.55	0.42**	9.6 (5.0)*	0.18 (0.20)	0.45 (0.22)	-0.28 (0.22)
60-69	0.02	0.11§	3.7 (8.9)§	-0.57 (0.16)		
70 +	0.42	-0.12§	0.8 (8.7)§	-0.77 (0.12)		

*** $p < .01$ ** $p < .05$ * $p < .10$ § N.S.

Starting with males, we note that in the filtered series there are significant correlations between alcohol consumption and mortality rates in the age groups 15 to 29 and 40 to 59 years. In the age group 30 to 39, the correlation is not significant. Taking into consideration the temporal structure of the noise, however, it turns out that the alcohol effect parameter is at least as high in this group. We find that the parameter estimate is reasonably close to ten in age groups between 15 and 59, except among males 40 to 49 years of age, where it is slightly (though not

Figure 18.3: *Age-specific rates of violent deaths in Norway 1951-80, horizontal lines indicate average levels for the period — males*

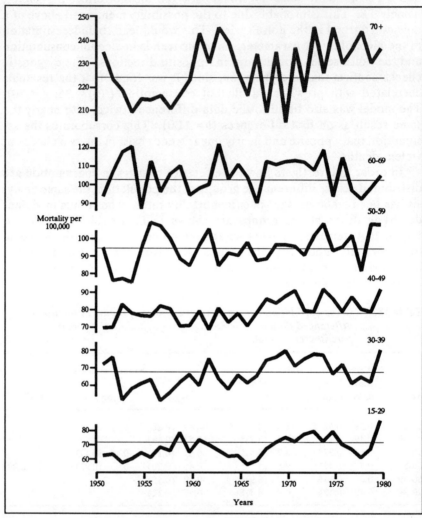

significantly) smaller. For the age groups above 60 years, the estimated values are small and insignificant (Table 18.3).

Among females, none of the cross-correlations between the filtered series are significant. By using the more powerful technique of model fitting, we obtain estimates for the alcohol effect parameter which are fairly stable around two for most age groups, except the oldest (Table 18.4). It is worth noting that this even holds true for the age group 15 to 29, where the cross-correlation actually was negative. Furthermore, the relationship is statistically significant ($p < .01$) in the age group 30 to 39, while the

Figure 18.4: *Age-specific rates of violent deaths in Norway 1951-80, horizontal lines indicate average levels for the period — females*

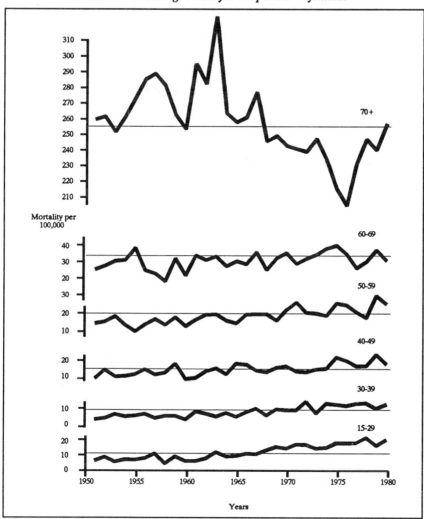

age group 50 to 59 represents a borderline case $(.05 < p < .10)$. When cross-correlations are calculated, these relationships are effectively masked by the strong negative autocorrelation structure of the noise series. Among females 70 years and older, a large negative value is found, but this estimate is far from being statistically significant. However, this large negative value is responsible for the low estimate obtained in the analysis of all females 15 years and older. In fact, the parameter estimate for the latter population is a weighted average of the age-specific parameter estimates, the weights being the ones defining the standard population. When the model is estimated for the age group 15 to 59, the parameter estimate becomes 2.5 (0.9). As was pointed out above, this is approximately the value to be expected on the basis of the result obtained for males, when the differences in consumption level are taken into consideration.

Table 18.4: *Cross-correlation at lag zero and results of model estimation on differenced data in different age groups, standard erros in parentheses — females*

Age	Cross-corr. Raw data	Filt. data	Alcohol effect		lag 1		lag 2		lag 3	
15-29	0.92	-0.11§	2.0	(1.3)§	-0.75	(0.19)	-0.35	(0.21)		
30-39	0.86	0.03§	2.2	(0.7)***	-1.12	(0.13)	-0.72	(0.14)		
40-49	0.66	0.09§	2.1	(1.9)§	-0.49	(0.17)	-0.58	(0.17)		
50-59	0.75	0.22§	2.8	(1.5)*	-0.82	(0.17)	-0.82	(0.21)	-0.55	(0.20)
60-69	0.45	0.12§	2.2	(3.2)§	-0.63	(0.19)	-0.36	(0.22)	-0.39	(0.20)
70 +	0.66	0.01§	-6.8	(11.8)§	-0.35	(0.19)	-0.16	(0.20)	-0.41	(0.19)

*** $p < .01$ ** $p < .10$ § N.S.

The fact that there was no significant relationship for the older age groups is reassuring, since it is well known that alcohol plays a very minor role in relation to violent deaths among the elderly. A prospective study of non-fatal accidents at the Oslo City Casualty Department in 1973 (Reigstad *et al.* 1977) found that ethanol intoxication was most frequent in the age groups 35 to 65. Therefore, the method used here produces significant results where effects are to be expected, but not in age groups where effects should not be expected.

In the prospective study mentioned above it was found that ethanol intoxication occurred less frequently in the age groups 15 to 34 than in the population at large. We obtained fairly high parameter estimates for this age group, however, and this may be related to the fact, mentioned above, that alcohol consumption has increased very strongly among youth and young adults in the post-war period. If consumption has increased, say, twice as fast among adolescents and young adults as in the population at large, then the effect on mortality of an increase in consumption of one litre would be only one-half of the value indicated by our parameter estimate for this group. The large parameter estimate for this group is therefore likely to signify a strong relative increase in alcohol-related violent deaths (due to strong increase in consumption), rather than indicating that a high proportion of such deaths are alcohol-related.

Discussion

While straightforward inspection of trends does not support the hypothesis that increasing alcohol consumption after World War II has had significant effects on violent deaths in Norway, a closer analysis clearly supports this hypothesis. The analysis of the filtered data has uncovered significant relationships between *per capita* alcohol consumption and rates of violent deaths among Norwegian males. This relationship was present in the age groups 15 to 59, but not among older men.

Among females, the results are not so clear. On the one hand, the cross-correlations between the filtered series were not significant. However, this does not necessarily mean that rates of violent deaths among females have been unaffected by changes in the consumption of alcohol. In a series consisting only of 30 observations, a correlation would have to exceed 0.37 in order to be statistically significant at the 5 per cent level. Now, in all age groups except the youngest, the ratio of the standard deviations for the differenced consumption and mortality series are less than 0.1. Hence, the alcohol effect parameter would have to be approximately four if the correlations would be of statistical significance. This seems very unlikely, since it implies that about one-half of violent deaths among females would have to be related to alcohol use during the seventies. In conclusion, a realistic hypothesis about alcohol consumption's effect on mortality rates of females would be very difficult to verify via straightforward cross-correlations in a series of only 30 observations. The standard error of the estimate is simply too large when compared to the expected 'true' value.

The more powerful technique of fitting parametric models to the data while taking the temporal structure of the noise series into consideration, produces surprisingly stable results across age groups in the mortality data of the female. The results (standard errors in parentheses) imply about 2.5 (0.9) violent deaths per 100,000 females per liter alcohol *per capita* in the age span 15-59.

On the presumption that our linear model is correct, we can use this estimate to calculate rates of alcohol-related violent deaths in different years. The results suggest that about 15 (5) per cent of violent deaths among females were alcohol-related in the middle of the 1950s, and about 25 (10) per cent in the middle of the 1970s. The slight increase observed in rates of violent deaths among females would thus seem to be almost entirely due to increased alcohol consumption. Violent deaths due to other causes therefore appear to have been fairly stable among females in the age groups 15 to 59 (but obviously not among the elderly according to Figure 18.4). This would imply that practically the same parameter estimates should be found by fitting the model to the raw data — and, in fact, this is the case.

Among males, the alcohol effect parameter is about ten in the age groups 15 to 59, when estimated on the differenced data. At higher ages the estimates are small and insignificant. Still, presuming that our linear model is correct, these figures would imply that in the total male population 15 years and older, 25 (8) violent deaths per 100,000 were alcohol-related in the early 1950s, or about one-quarter of all violent deaths. By the end of the 1970s the alcohol-related mortality rate should, according to these calculations, have increased to about 50 (15). Since the total rate of violent deaths in this group was close to 100 per 100,000 in the same period, it appears that about one-half (between one- and two-thirds) of these deaths were related to alcohol use. As can be seen from Figure 18.5, this implies a steadily declining trend in violent deaths from other causes. In fact it appears from these estimates that non-alcoholic violent deaths among males have been reduced by as much as one-third during these 30 years.

It is not unlikely that non-alcoholic violent deaths among males have been significantly reduced during the historical period considered here. There have been considerable efforts to make our environment more safe, particularly in relation to industrial accidents. Alcohol is known to be involved in only a very small fraction (5 to 10 per cent) of industrial accidents in Norway (Reigstad 1977). The relative contribution of industrial fatal accidents has gone down from about one-third in the early 1950s to about one-sixth in the 1970s (Reigstad 1978), and this trend alone would explain most of the estimated decline in non-alcoholic violent deaths among Norwegian males. Furthermore, these kinds of accidents may also explain the apparent differences between the genders in trends of non-alcoholic violent deaths.

It thus appears that increasing alcohol consumption has been responsible for an increasing proportion of violent deaths in Norway—in particular among males, but perhaps to some extent also among females. If our results can be trusted, it appears that alcohol is now the most important single factor in relation to violent deaths among Norwegian males. In fact, can this result be trusted? It is a difficult question to which we cannot give a definite answer. However, there are a number of studies of alcohol intoxication among victims in different kinds of accidents, both fatal and non-fatal, in Norway in the post-war period. Most of these studies concern males. By combining the results of these studies we can obtain an independent assessment of the impact of alcohol use on rates of violent deaths among males.

The relative importance of some major causes of violent deaths in Norway can be seen in Table 18.5.

Compared to other countries, both homicide and suicide rates are still low in Norway, in spite of the fact that both have increased substantially during the last decade. Suicides now account for nearly one-fifth of all vi-

Figure 18.5: *Predicted trends in rates of violent deaths related to alcohol use and to other causes, respectively, among Norwegian males (derived from model estimated on differenced data)*

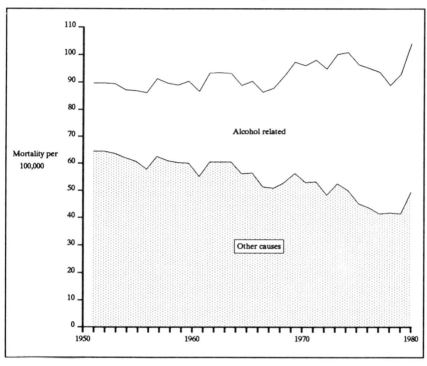

Table 18.5: *Distribution of violent deaths according to major causes among Norwegian males and females 1951-80, based on age adjusted 10 year average rates, %*

Cause	1951-60		1961-70		1971-80	
	Males	Females	Males	Females	Males	Females
Falling	19.9	66.6	19.2	60.2	18.7	50.5
Drowning	8.1	2.3	6.8	2.0	6.0	1.4
Motor vehicle	13.4	7.4	21.9	14.7	20.8	16.3
Marine transportation	16.1	0.8	15.4	1.3	11.8	0.7
Alcohol poisoning	2.5	0.4	2.6	0.7	4.6	1.7
Other accidents	21.9	9.6	16.1	7.4	15.3	9.1
All accidents	81.9	87.1	82.0	86.3	77.3	79.7
Suicide	17.5	11.9	17.2	12.6	21.4	18.8
Homicide	0.6	1.0	0.8	1.1	1.3	1.5
All violent deaths	100.0	100.0	100.0	100.0	100.0	100.0

olent deaths in both genders. One study of suicide (Teige and Fleisher 1981) and two studies of attempted suicide (Berg *et al.* 1978, Dahl *et al.* 1980) report ethanol intoxication in nearly one-half of all the cases. All these studies are from the 1970s. The causal role of alcohol is of course extremely difficult to assess in relation to suicides.

Motor vehicle accidents are now the second largest category among males, accounting for nearly one-fifth of all cases. These accidents have increased strongly, particularly during the first part of the period. Autopsies suggest that at least one-third, and perhaps as many as one-half, are caused by alcohol intoxication (Lundevall and Olaisen 1976, Andenæs and Sorensen 1979). These studies also suggest that the relative importance of alcohol has been increasing.

Falls account for nearly one-fifth of all violent deaths among males, and this fraction has remained fairly stable during most of the period. The quantitative importance of alcohol is not unequivocally documented. Two studies of non-fatal falling accidents in the 1970s (Lereim and Ringkjob [undated], Reikeraas *et al.* 1982) report alcohol intoxication in 56 and 18 per cent of the cases. Since several studies (Honkanen *et al.* 1975, Bjerver *et al.* 1971, Holt *et al.* 1980) suggest that alcohol intoxication occurs more frequently in very serious accidents, it seems likely that at least one-quarter of all fatal falling accidents among males are due to alcohol.

A significant fraction of all violent deaths in Norway occurs among sailors. Although these accidents (mostly drowning) have been declining during the last decade, they still account for more than 10 per cent of all violent deaths. Arner (1970, 1973), analysing data from the late 1950s and early 1960s, found that alcohol was involved in at least one-third of the violent deaths among merchant seamen. More recent studies are not available.

The relative importance of drowning accidents (not including marine transportation) has gone down a little during the period of study. In the 1970s they accounted for 6 per cent of violent deaths among Norwegian males. Studies from the 1970s report alcohol intoxication in two-thirds of the victims (Skulberg 1974). This may indicate an increase, but the studies are not directly comparable.

Alcohol poisoning has increased significantly during the period of observation, and contributed nearly 5 per cent to violent deaths among males in the 1970s.

The importance of alcohol in the remaining causes of violent death is uncertain. However, this residual category includes important causes like fire and hypothermia, where alcohol is known to be of importance.

Summing up these figures, disregarding homicides and the residual category, one finds that alcohol was involved in about 35 per cent of all violent deaths among males during the last decade of the period. This is probably a minimum figure. It is, of course, an open question as to what extent alcohol actually was the crucial causal factor in all these deaths. These figures illustrate, however, that the figures obtained in the preceding sections are not necessarily unrealistic.

The results obtained from the time series analysis are strengthened by the following facts: (1) The point estimate of about 50 per cent for males agrees reasonably well with the results obtained in prevalence studies. The true figure is probably somewhat higher than the estimated lower limit of one-third, while it is probably well below the upper limit of two-thirds. (2) Ignoring the elderly, where the causal importance of alcohol ought to be small, the results for males and females agree with the relative differences in consumption of alcohol between the genders. (3) The strong decline in industrial accidents during the period of observation corresponds reasonably well with the estimated trend in non-alcoholic violent deaths obtained from the time-series analysis of the male data. This factor also explains the estimated differences between the genders with respect to trends in non-alcoholic violent deaths.

Thus, one may conclude that the strong increase in alcohol consumption in Norway after World War II seems to have had negative effects not only in relation to chronic abuse, as witnessed by trends in liver cirrhosis mortality (Skog 1980b, 1979), and deaths from chronic alcoholism (Skog 1985c), but also in relation to acute intoxication and fatal casualties. Although the latter trends are to a large extent counteracted by positive trends in other risk factors, it seems to be true that in the absence of a growing alcohol consumption level, Norway could have experienced a significant reduction, rather than a slight increase, in rates of violent deaths among males. However, as always in this type of analysis, we should remind ourselves that this conclusion is based on certain assumptions which may or may not be fulfilled.

Acknowledgement

This report is part of a joint Nordic study (the SAS-project) of Trends in Alcohol Related Damage, supported by the Nordic Council for Alcohol and Drug Research.

I would like to thank Joan Rambech for correcting my spelling errors and Liv Skog for drawing the diagrams.

References

Andenæs, J. and R.K. Sorensen (1979) Alkohol og dødsulykker i traffikken, *Lov og rett*, 83-109

Arner, O. (1970) *Dødsulykker Blant Sjømenn*, Universitetsforlaget, Oslo
— (1973) The role of alcohol in fatal accidents among seamen. *British Journal of Addiction, 68*, 185-9

Berg, K.J., A.W. Shetelig, S. Jørdstad and T.E. Wideroe (1978) Behandling av akutte intoxicasjoner. *Tidsskrift for den Norske Lægeforening, 98*, 98-9

Bjerver, K., L. Goldberg and U. Rydberg (1971) Alkoholens roll i et ulycksfallsmaterial på en kirurgisk akutmottagning. *Läkartidningen, 68*, 3295-300

Borkenstein, R.F., R.F. Crowther, R.P. Shumate, W.P. Ziel and R. Zylman (1964) The role of the drinking driver in traffic accidents. Mimeograph, Indiana University, Bloomington

Box, G.E.P. and G.M. Jenkins (1976) *Time Series Analysis: forecasting and control*, Revised edition, Holden-Day, London

Brun-Gulbrandsen, S. (1978) Forandringer i den norske ungdommens allkoholvaner. In A.-M. Sindballe *et al.* (eds), *Ungdom og alkohol i Norden. Utviklingen i fem land*, Doxa, Stockholm

Bruun, K., G. Edwards, M. Lumio, K. Mäkelä, L. Pan, R.E. Popham, R. Room, W. Schmidt, O.-J. Skog, P. Sulkunen and E. Österberg (1975) *Alcohol control policies in public health perspective*, Finnish Foundation for Alcohol Studies, Helsinki

Cochrane, D. and G.H. Orcutt (1949) Applications of least squares regressions to relationships containing autocorrelated error terms. *Journal of the American Statistical Association, 44*, 32-61

Dahl, N.H., S. Kornstad and G. Aasen (1980) Observasjoner i et forgiftningsmateriale under streiken ved Vinmonopolet. *Tidsskrift for den Norske Lægeforening, 100*, 98-9

Giertsen, J.C. (1970) Drukning i alkoholpåvirket tilstand. *Nordisk Medicin, 83*, 523-7

Glad, A. (1983) *Promillekjøring i Norge*, Transportøkonomisk Institutt, Oslo

Holt, S., I.C. Stewart, J.M.J. Dixon, R.A. Elton, T.V. Taylor and K. Little (1980) Alcohol and the emergency service patient. *British Medical Journal, 281*, 638-40

Honkanen, R., T. Visuri and J. Kilpiö (1975) Blood alcohol levels in accident victims. *Annales Chirurgiae et Gynaecologiae, 64*, 365-8

Ledermann, S. (1956) *Alcool, alcooolisme, alcoolisation, vol. 1*, Presses Universitaires de France, Paris
— (1964) *Alcool, alcoolisme, alcoolisation, vol. 2*, Presses Universitaires de France, Paris

Lelbach, W.L. (1974) Organic pathology related to volume and pattern of alcohol use. In R.J. Gibbins, Y. Israel, H. Kalant, R.E. Popham, W. Schmidt and R.G. Smart (eds), *Research Advances in Alcohol and Drug Problems, Volume 1*, Wiley, Toronto

Lereim, I. and R. Ringkjob (undated) Hodeskader og alkohol, Mimeograph

Lilienfeld, A.M. and D.E. Lilienfeld (1980) *Foundations of epidemiology*, Oxford University Press, Oxford

Lundeval, J. and B. Olaisen (1976) Alkoholpåvirkning hos motorvognførere drept i trafikkulykker, *Lov og rett*, 271-5

Mäkelä, K. (1978) Levels of consumption and social consequences of drinking. In Y. Israel *et al.* (eds), *Research advances in alcohol and drug problems*, Plenum Press, New York, pp. 303-48

Moore, M.H. and D.R. Gerstein (eds) (1981) *Alcohol and public policy: beyond the shadow of prohibition*, National Academy Press, Washington, D.C.

Nordlund, S. (1981) Alkoholdata 1979, Talbellarisk oversikt over resultater fra en intervjuundersøkelse. *SIFA-Mimeograph No. 50*, National Institute for Alcohol Research, Oslo

— (1985) Norske drikkevaner en beskrivelse på grunnlag av offentlig statistikk og survey-data. In O. Arner, R. Hauge and O.-J. Skog (eds), *Alkohol i Norge*, Universitetsforlaget, Oslo

Péquignot, G., A.J. Tuyns and J.L. Berta (1978) Ascitic cirrhosis in relation to alcohol consumption. *International Journal of Epidemiology, 7*, 113-20

Reigstad, A. (1977) *Ulykker i arbeidsmiljøet: en klinisk epidemiologisk studie*, Universitetsforlaget, Oslo

— (1978) Voldsomme og unaturlige dødsfall i Norge og Oslo 1951-1975. *Tidsskrift for den Norske Lægeforening, 98*, 1072-5

Reigstad, A., J.E. Bredesen and P.K.M. Lunde (1977) *Ulykker, Alkohol og Nervemedisin*, Universitetsforlaget, Oslo

Reikeraas, O., A. Reigstad and P.K.M. Lunde (1982) Vinmonopolstreikens innvirkning på sykehusbehandlede skader. *Tidsskrift for den Norske Laegeforening, 102*, 600-4

Skog, O.-J. (1979) Liver cirrhosis mortality as an indicator of heavy alcohol use: Some methodological problems. *SIFA-Mimeograph No. 22*, National Institute for Alcohol Research, Oslo

— (1980a) Liver cirrhosis epidemiology: some methodological problems. *British Journal of Addiction, 75*, 227-43

— (1980b) Time series analysis of the relation between per capita alcohol consumption and liver cirrhosis mortality: the effect of unsystematic fluctuations in death rates. *SIFA-Mimeograph No. 34*, National Institute for Alcohol Research, Oslo

— (1983) Methodological problems in the analysis of temporal covariation between alcohol consumption and ischemic heart disease. *British Journal of Addiction, 78*, 157-72

— (1984a) The risk function for liver cirrhosis from lifetime alcohol consumption. *Journal of Studies on Alcohol, 45*, 199-208

— (1984b) Økt totalforbruk—flere trafikkulykker? *SIFA-Mimeograph No. 87*, National Institute for Alcohol Research, Oslo

— (1985a) The collectivity of drinking cultures: a theory of the distribution of alcohol consumption. *British Journal of Addiction, 80*, 83-99

— (1985b) The wetness of drinking cultures: a key variable in epidemiology of alcoholic liver cirrhosis. *Acta Medica Scandinavica, Suppl. 703*, 157-84

— (1985c) Hva bestemmer omfanget av alkoholskader? In O. Arner, R. Hauge and O.-J. Skog (eds), *Alkohol i Norge*, Universitetsforlaget, Oslo

Skulberg, A. (1974) Utredning om drukningsulykker for Sosialdepartementet, Mimeograph, Sosialdepartementet, Oslo

Teige, B. and E. Fleischer (1981) Medikament- og alkoholdodsfall undersøkt ved Rettsmedisinsk institutt, Universitetet i Oslo, i årene 1977-1979. *Tidsskrift for den Norske Laegeforening, 101*, 1563-66

Tuyns, A.J., J. Esteve and G. Péquignot (1984) Ethanol is cirrhogenic, whatever the beverage. *British Journal of Addiction, 79*, 389-94

Tuyns, A.J., G. Péquignot and J.S. Abbatucci (1979) Oesophageal cancer and alcohol consumption. Importance of type of beverage. *International Journal of Cancer, 23*, 443-8

19

Sex Differences in Alcohol-Related Casualties: The Case of Self-Destructive Behaviour

Roberta G. Ferrence

> The important part played by alcoholism in the causation of suicide has been abundantly recognized by all observers of both these social phenomena; and so far as debate now touches the question, it is merely to deal with points of detail. (Sullivan 1898)

The relationship between alcohol and self-destructive behaviour has been studied extensively, but few investigators have subjected the issue of causality to empirical test (e.g. Whitehead 1972; Frankel *et al.* 1976; Maris 1981); even fewer have tried to specify the conditions of the relationship (e.g. Rushing 1968). Sex differences are often reported, but rarely has the effect of gender on the relationship been the central research question.

There is good reason to believe that the relationship between alcohol and self-destructive behaviour varies by sex. Women are less likely than men to drink, to drink heavily and to be diagnosed as alcoholic (Ferrence 1980). Rates of suicide are invariably higher for men, in part because of the more lethal methods they use. Non-fatal self-injury occurs more frequently among women in the general population, at least in part a reflection of their greater use of prescribed psychoactive drugs (Cooperstock 1973). Because sanctions against deviant behaviour are stronger for women than men, alcohol consumption, alcoholism and self-destructive acts may be under-reported more for women than men.

The purpose of this paper is to address the following issues related to sex differences in the prevalence and reporting of alcohol-related self-destructive behaviour:

1. Does alcohol involvement in self-destructive behaviour vary by sex?

2. Does the reporting of alcohol involvement in self-destructive behaviour vary by sex?

3. Do the causes of alcohol-related suicide and self-injury vary by sex?

4. Can the findings for self-destructive behaviour be generalised to other alcohol-related casualties?

Methods

Measures of alcohol involvement used in this analysis include diagnosed alcoholism, patterns of heavy drinking, drinking or intoxication just prior to the act, and the prevalence of mortality from liver cirrhosis. Forms of self-destructive behaviour include suicide, attempted suicide, drug overdose and other self-inflicted injury. The term 'self-injury' is used to denote non-fatal acts. Sources of data include mortality statistics, alcohol consumption data, studies of alcoholics, studies of suicides and surveys of attempted suicide. Findings from a large set of original Canadian data on self-injury are included (Johnson *et al.* 1975).

Data on suicide attempts could be gleaned from morbidity and mortality statistics, but each source has serious limitations. Cases of poisoning reported to hospitals designated as Poison Control Centres are incomplete and information on alcohol involvement and intention is lacking. Hospital Medical Records Institute (HMRI) data do not always include information on alcohol and exclude patients discharged from emergency services. Mortality data are complete, but alcohol involvement is not reliably reported because only about 30 per cent of all deaths are autopsied. Some correlational studies provide support for a relationship between alcohol and suicide, but sex is not included as a variable (Corey and Andress 1977, Lester 1980).

Results

Morbidity and Mortality Statistics

Canadian statistics on *per capita* consumption of alcohol and suicide mortality were used to examine sex differences in the relationship between drinking and suicide. Total *per capita* consumption of absolute alcohol for persons aged 15 and over for the provinces of Canada and two territories in 1982/3 was compared with the standardised death rates for male and female suicide in 1982 (Statistics Canada 1984a, 1984b). Rank order correlations were significant for females (r_s = .65; $p < .05$) but not for males (r_s = .09, n.s.). Sex-specific standardised death rates from liver cirrhosis were also compared with suicide rates for males and females by province. Correlations were higher for males than females (r_s = .46 versus r_s = .15), but neither was statistically significant, due in part to the small number of cases (Statistics Canada 1984b).

Correlational analyses for liver cirrhosis and suicide mortality were also carried out for a period of 23 years (Statistics Canada 1976). Significant correlations were found for both males and females (males r_s =.95, $p < .01$; females r_s =.68, $p < .01$). When first differences were correlated to remove time trends, the associations were weaker, but sex differences persisted (males r_s =.39; females r_s =.19). Sex ratios for cirrhosis and suicide mortality over time were also compared, but no relationship was apparent (r_s = -.12).

These analyses suggest that liver cirrhosis is related to suicide, at least for males, whereas consumption of alcohol is related to suicide for females. Time series analyses may be required to determine the effect of drinking on suicide and variations by sex. While ecological studies are useful for exploratory analyses to suggest further tests using individual data, the findings presented here require further investigation and specification.

Clinical Studies and Surveys

Most studies examining the relationship between drinking and self-destructive behaviour use clinical or survey data on individuals. Several research designs have been employed. Cohort studies of alcoholics have measured suicide mortality after a follow-up period. Case studies of suicides have looked at a history of alcoholism or heavy drinking, or at blood alcohol levels determined at autopsy. Cross-sectional surveys of attempted suicide and self-injury have included questions on usual drinking habits and drinking just prior to the act. In some cases, medical records were obtained to determine previous alcohol-related diagnoses. In this section, sex-specific rates and sex ratios for alcohol-related self-destructive behaviours are discussed.

Alcoholics

Rates of suicide among alcoholics vary by study, but are substantially higher than rates for the general population (Table 19.1). The length of follow-up and population studied clearly influence these rates. Sex ratios are low in three of four studies, suggesting that female alcoholics are at disproportionate risk of suicide compared to male alcoholics (see Schmidt and Popham 1980). Alcoholics of both sexes were equally likely to have previously attempted suicide.

Suicides

Rates of alcoholism and heavy drinking among persons who commit suicide are substantial, ranging from 14 to 34 per cent in men and 9 to 33 per cent in women (Table 19.2). Sex ratios are between 1.0:1 and 2.1:1, which is considerably lower than for suicides generally (3.5:1).

Rates and sex ratios for drinking just prior to suicide by alcoholics are similar to those for alcoholism among suicides, which suggests that heavy drinkers account for most of those who drink just prior to suicide.

Table 19.1: *Sex differences in self-destructive behavior among alcoholics*

Source/location	Category/N	% Male	% Female	Sex ratio
Nicholls *et al.* (1974)	Suicides	26.5	18.4	1.4
Schmidt and de Lint (1972) (Toronto)	Suicides	7.4	4.0	1.8
Schmidt and Popham (1980) (Toronto)	Suicides (N = 150/2119)	7.1	7.1	1.0
Berglund (1984) (Sweden: 1980 follow-up)	Suicides (N = 88/537)	7.2	2.5	2.9
Smith (1982)	Previous Attempted suicide	17.0	21.0	0.8

Attempted Suicide and Self-Injury

Rates of alcoholism and heavy drinking appear to be somewhat higher among males who attempt suicide than among those who commit suicide; among females, those who drink heavily are over-represented among suicides compared to attempted suicides (Table 19.3). Sex ratios for alcoholism and heavy drinking are considerably higher among attempters than suicides, with those for three to four studies over 4:1. Drinking prior to suicide attempts is more common than alcoholism among attempters, with 38 to 72 per cent of males and 25 to 45 per cent of females reporting prior drinking in the five most recent studies. Sex ratios for drinking prior to self-injury are similar to those for suicides and range from 1.4 to 2.6 in recent studies.

Mean sex ratios for rates of suicide, alcoholism and drinking prior to the act were calculated for samples of alcoholics, suicides and suicide attempters (Table 19.4). Sex ratios for alcohol-related attempts parallel those for alcohol use in the general population, whereas sex ratios for alcohol-related suicide are lower than expected on the basis of rates of alcoholism and heavy drinking in the general population (Ferrence 1980).

Table 19.2: *Sex differences in alcohol-involvement among suicides*

Source/location	Category/N	% Male	% Female	Sex ratio[a]
a. *Alcoholism or heavy drinking pattern*				
Krupinski *et al.* (1965) (Victoria: 1963)	Diagnosed alcoholic (N = 449)	33	22	1.5
Burvill (1971) (Australia)	Alcoholic/heavy drinker	14	9	1.6
Barraclough *et al.* (1974) (Portsmouth)	Diagnosed alcoholic	19	9	2.1
Chynoweth *et al.* (1980) (Brisbane: 1973-74)	Heavy drinker (N = 135)	34	33	1.0
Maris (1981) (U.S.)	Usually drink 3+, Spirits (N = 242)	29	14	2.1
b. *Drinking prior to act*				
Schneidman & Farberow (1961) (Los Angeles)	Had been drinking	24	11	2.2
James (1966)	Had been drinking (N = 107)			
	(BAC $\geq$ .05)	48	18	2.7
	(BAC < .15)	22	13	1.7
Ford *et al.* (1979) (Cleveland: 1969-74)	Had been drinking			
	BAC Positive	29	22	1.3
	BAC > .10 (N = 864)	22	15	1.5

[a] Male to female

These findings suggest that although prior drinking and alcoholism are higher than expected among cases of self-injury, men and women are not differentially affected. Among suicides, however, women are more likely than men to be alcoholic, compared to the general population. These conclusions are only tentative and require further testing with appropriate meta-analytic procedures (e.g. Kessler and McRae 1983), which would allow for more conclusive results (Rosenthal 1984).

Methodological Issues

There are several possible sources of sex bias in the reporting of alcohol-related self-destructive acts:

1. Female suicides may be less likely than males to be tested for blood-alcohol levels.

2. Female attempters may be asked less frequently about alcohol involvement in the attempt or about usual drinking patterns.

Table 19.3: *Sex differences in alcohol-involvement among cases of attempted suicide or self-injury*

Source/location	Category/N	% Male	% Female	Sex ratio[a]
a. *Alcoholism or heavy drinking among cases of attempted suicide*				
Buckle *et al.* (1965) (Melbourne)	Chronic alcoholic/ suspected suicide attempt	52	12	4.3
Krupinski *et al.* (1965) (Victoria: 1963)	Diagnosed alcoholic after attempt	13	3	4.3
Koller and Castanos (1968) (Edinburgh)	Alcoholic	39	8	4.9
Johnson *et al.* (1975) (London, Canada: 1969-71)	Usually drink 6 +/ Self injury (N = 647)	48	19	2.5
b. *Prior drinking among cases of attempted suicide*				
Krupinski (1965) (Victoria)	Had been drinking	25	12	2.1
Freeman *et al.* (1970) (Hobart)	Had been drinking (N = 335)	42	12	3.5
Patel *et al.* (1972) (Glasgow: 1971-72) capital	Had been drinking $\overline{X}$ BAC level	72 .15	40 .10	1.8 1.5
Morgan *et al.* (1975) (Bristol)	Had been drinking	55	25	2.2
Johnson *et al.* (1975) (London, Canada: 1969-71)	Had been drinking (N = 731)	58	37	1.6
Holding *et al.* (1977) (Edinburgh: 1968, 1974)	Had been drinking 1968 1974	64 64	25 45	2.6 1.4
Kaplan *et al.* (1980) (Toronto: 1975)	Had been drinking/ Drug overdoses (N = 3548)	38	28	1.4

[a] Male to female

Table 19.4: *Mean sex ratios for types of alcohol-related self-destructive behaviour and for drinking practices of the general population*

Population/sample	Alcohol measure	$\overline{X}$ Sex ratio[a]	Range	No. studies
Alcoholics	Suicide	1.8	1.0 - 2.9	4
	Attempted suicide	0.8	-	1
Suicides	Alcoholism	1.6	1.0 - 2.1	4
	Prior drinking	2.1	1.3 - 2.7	3
Attempted suicide/	Alcoholism	4.5	4.3 - 4.9	3
self-injury	Usually drink 6 +	2.5	-	1
	Prior drinking	2.1	1.4 - 3.5	8
	Prior heavy drinking	2.4	-	1
Studies of drinking	Any use of alcohol	1.2	1.1 - 1.6	35
habits of general	Daily use	3.0	1.6 - 4.3	9
population, Canada	Heavy use	4.0	2.2 - 7.4	26
and U.S. (Ferrence, 1980)				

[a] Male to female

3. Female heavy drinkers may be less likely than males to have been diagnosed as alcoholic.

4. Female drinkers may be more likely than males to seek help after attempting suicide.

5. Differential changes in methods of suicide or self-injury could produce bias if certain methods were more associated with alcohol than others.

There is little research that can be brought to bear directly on the matter of sex bias. Ford *et al.* (1979) analysed blood-alcohol levels for suicides dead on arrival in Metropolitan Cleveland between 1958 and 1974. Female suicides were almost as likely as male suicides to be tested (75 to 76 per cent versus 79 to 81 per cent).

Taylor *et al.* (1982) examined death certificates of 50 cases of suicide among alcoholics in St. Louis, Missouri to determine the validity of information on alcohol-related conditions. Only 36 per cent of death certificates mentioned alcohol, whereas 72 per cent of autopsies did. Although death certificates were biased by marital status, health status, type of hospital and social class, under-reporting did not vary by sex or race. If these data are representative of other jurisdictions, it is unlikely that sex differences in testing significantly influence reported alcohol involvement in suicide.

There are also indirect ways of estimating the likelihood of sex bias. One way is to look at sex ratios for deaths that are possible cases of

349

suicide. Sainsbury and Jenkins (1982) compared trends in rates of suicide with 'estimated' rates of suicide that included accidental poisoning and undetermined deaths as well. They reported that rates of suicide increased by about half with the addition of the accidental and undetermined deaths, but that the effect was similar for males and females.

Malla (Personal Communication 1985) examined sex differences in reported, unreported and undetermined suicides in Newfoundland (1974/9). The sex ratio for reported suicide was 5.8:1 compared to 1.8:1 for unreported cases. Since this latter group comprised only 15 per cent of the total (N = 14), their inclusion would produce little change in the overall sex ratio. The sex ratio for undetermined suicides was similar to that of the reported group (6.2:1). Burvill (1971) calculated that Australian suicide rates are underestimated by 5 to 10 per cent for males and 10 to 20 per cent for females because poisoning deaths are more often misclassified, and females are over-represented in this category.

Canadian data on specific cause of death can be examined to determine whether sex ratios vary according to classification of death as suicide, accident or undetermined. Death rates and sex ratios for those causes of death usually associated with suicide are compared according to category (Table 19.5). Cases aged 0 to 14 years have been excluded to eliminate childhood poisonings and accidents. Some categories of accidents are more likely to contain suicides than others. For example, accidental drowning is more plausible than accidental drug overdose or hanging. Accidental falls have been omitted because the largest proportion involves the elderly.

Table 19.5: *Death rates per 100,000 population aged 15+ and sex ratios for suicides, undetermined injuries and accidents, by selected causes, Canada, 1983*

Cause of death	Suicides			Undetermined			Accidents		
	M	F	SR	M	F	SR	M	F	SR
Psychoactive drugs	2.23	2.79	*.80*	0.89	0.71	*1.25*	0.81	0.64	*1.27*
Other gases and vapours	2.17	0.75	*2.89*	0.09[a]	0.00	-	0.76	0.16[a]	*4.75*
Hanging	7.34	1.66	*4.42*	0.07[a]	0.05[a]	*1.40*	0.19[a]	0.04[a]	*4.75*
Submersion	1.35	0.98	*1.38*	0.46	0.17[a]	*2.71*	0.78	0.12[a]	*6.50*
Firearms	12.03	0.84	*14.32*	0.35	0.00	-	0.29	0.00	-
Cutting	0.51	0.16[a]	*3.19*	0.04[a]	0.00	-	0.02[a]	0.00	-
Jumping/falling	1.20	0.61	*1.97*	0.09[a]	0.02[a]	*4.50*	-	-	-

[a] Number of cases < 20

Source: Statistics Canada, *Causes of Death, Vital Statistics*, Vol. IV, 1983, Catalogue 84-203, Ottawa, 1985

Comparing the three categories that are most open to interpretation — drug overdose, gas and hanging — we find similar sex ratios across categories and, in fact, a lower sex ratio for suicide by drug overdose. The number of cases of undetermined hanging is too small to conclude anything. Sex ratios for other methods are lower for suicides. These data suggest that males may be under-represented in the suicide by drug category. In most other categories, the proportion of cases classified as undetermined or accidental is small and unlikely to make much difference.

Studies that ask in detail about prior drinking should elicit more accurate information than those that do not probe. If there are sex differences in reporting of alcohol consumption, we should find lower sex ratios in those studies that ask for more detail. Data from the London, Ontario self-injury study provide an opportunity to test this hypothesis (Johnson *et al.* 1975). The sex ratio for prior drinking in this study was 1.6, slightly lower than the average of 2.1 for the eight studies examined, but higher than two studies conducted during the same period (Table 19.4). This test does not support the hypothesis that prior drinking is under-reported more for women. More definitive comparisons would involve controls for age and sex-specific drinking patterns of the general population in the study community.

The issue of under-reporting can be examined in a different way. Interviewers in the London self-injury study were asked to estimate the accuracy of responses to the interview schedule. Slightly more males than females (16.5 per cent versus 13.9 per cent) were judged to have given inaccurate responses.

The question of differential changes in methods over time has been raised by McIntosh and Santos (1982). They suggest that an increase in the proportion of female suicides involving firearms may result in greater reporting of alcohol involvement because firearm deaths are more often fatal and more often classified as suicides than poisonings. Data from the London study on prior use of alcohol by method used show no significant sex difference. Since the number of self-injury cases involving firearms was small, data on alcohol involvement in fatal cases should be used.

To summarise, evidence for differential under-reporting of drinking by sex among suicides and self-injury is weak. If such under-reporting does occur, it appears to be greatly outweighed by real sex differences in the drinking behaviour of these groups.

Conclusion

In this paper, several types of data have been applied to questions on the role of alcohol in self-destructive behaviour. No one source is adequate for testing hypotheses about the relationship, but the use of multiple sources of data strengthens the case.

On the basis of the analyses performed and evidence from other studies, certain conclusions may be drawn:

1. Alcohol involvement in self-destructive behaviour varies by sex, but in most cases these differences reflect sex differences in drinking habits in the general population. Female alcoholics appear to be at greater risk of suicide compared to other women than are male alcoholics to other men.

2. It was not possible to conclusively test our hypotheses, however. Those data sets which are sufficiently large, comprehensive and lengthy to carry out appropriate tests do not provide systematic reporting of alcohol involvement. Official statistics on mortality and morbidity are of this type. Most studies that provide good information on prior drinking and usual pattern of drinking are single cross-sectional studies of a single community or hospital. Only coroner's reports offer relatively consistent data on prior drinking among suicides that could be analysed over time, but even here, low rates of testing results in under-reporting in some communities.

2. There is no evidence that alcohol involvement in self-destructive behaviour is under-reported for women.

3. The question of sex differences in the etiology of alcohol-related self-injury and suicide cannot be answered on the basis of the data presented here. Because sex differences in drinking associated with self-destructive acts reflect those in the general population, there may be nothing special about this particular form of deviant behaviour. Sex differences in causes of drinking behaviour, such as drinking contexts, social expectations about drinking or physiological factors, probably apply to self-destructive behaviour as well.

4. Findings from this research may apply to other alcohol-related casualties. Since sex differences in drinking associated with self-injury and suicide reflect those for drinking in the general population, it would likely be true of other casualties. Since there was no evidence of sex differences in under-reporting of alcohol-involvement in self-destructive behaviour, there is no reason to believe that this would differ for other casualties.

References

Aaren, M., and R. Roizen (1978) Drinking problems among suicide attempters: A comparison of drinking problems seen in a population of suicide attempters with those found in a general population survey, Working Paper F76, Social Research Group, Berkeley, California

Barraclough, B., J. Bunch, B. Nelson and P. Sainsbury (1974) A hundred cases of suicide: Clinical aspects. *British Journal of Psychiatry, 125,* 355-73

Berglund, M. (1984) Suicide in alcoholism. A prospective study of 88 suicides: I. The multidimensional diagnosis at first admission. *Archives of General Psychiatry, 41,* 888-91

Buckle, R.C., J. Linnane and N. McConachy (1965) Attempted Suicide presenting at the Alfred Hospital over two months. *Medical Journal of Australia, 1,* 754

Burvill, P.W. (1971) Suicide in Western Australia, 1967: An analysis of coroner's records. *Australian and New Zealand Journal of Psychiatry, 14,* 37-45

Chynoweth, R., J. Tonge and J. Armstrong (1980) Suicide in Brisbane - a retrospective psychosocial study. *Australian and New Zeland Journal of Psychiatry, 14,* 37-45

Cooperstock, R. (1973) Sex differences in the use of mood modifying drugs: An explanatory mode. In P.C. Whitehead, C.F. Grindstaff and C.L. Boydell (eds.), *Alcohol and other drugs: Perspectives on use, abuse, treatment, and prevention,* Holt, Rinehart and Winston of Canada, Toronto, pp. 173-81

Corey, D.M. and V.R. Andress (1977) Alcohol consumption and suicidal behavior. *Psychological Reports, 40,* 506

Ferrence, R. G. (1980) Sex differences in the prevalence of problem drinking. In O.J. Kalant (ed), *Alcohol and drug problems in women: Volume 5, Research advances in alcohol and drug problems,* Plenum, New York, pp. 69-124

Ford, A.B., N.B. Rushforth, N. Rushforth, C.S. Hirsch and L. Adelson (1979) Violent death in a metropolitan county: II. changing patterns of suicides (1959-1974). *American Journal of Public Health, 69,* 459-64

Frankel, B.G., R.G. Ferrence, F.G. Johnson and P.C. Whitehead (1976) Drinking and self-injury: Toward untangling the dynamics. *British Journal of Addiction, 71,* 299-306

Freeman, J.W., C.A. Ryan and R.R. Beattie (1970) Epidemiology of drug overdosage in Southern Tasmania. *Medical Journal of Australia, 2,* 1168-72

Holding, T.A., D. Buglass, J.C. Duffy and N. Kreitman (1977) Parasuicide in Edinburgh - A seven-year review 1968-74. *British Journal of Psychiatry, 130,* 534-43

James, I.P. (1966) Blood alcohol levels following successful suicide. *Quarterly Journal of Studies on Alcohol, 27,* 23-9

Johnson, F.G., B.G. Frankel, G.K. Jarvis and P.C. Whitehead (1975) Self-injury in London, Canada: A prospective study. *Canadian Journal of Public Health, 66,* 307-16

Kaplan, H.L., E.M. Sellers, J.A. Marshman, H.G. Giles, S.M. MacLeod, B.M. Kapur, C. Stapleton, F. Sealey and U. Busto (1980) Alcohol use by patients admitted to hospital emergency rooms for treatment of drug overdose and misuse. *Journal of Studies on Alcohol, 41,* 882-93

Kessler, R.C., and J.A. McRae Jr. (1983) Trends in the relationship between sex and attempted suicide. *Journal of Health and Social Behavior, 24,* 98-110

Koller, K.M., and J.N. Castanos (1968) Attempted suicide and alcoholism. *Medical Journal of Australia, 2,* 835-7

Krupinski, J., P. Polke and A. Stoller (1965) Psychiatric disturbances in attempted and completed suicides in Victoria during 1963. *Medical Journal of Australia, 2,* 773-8

Lester, D. (1980) Alcohol and suicide and homicide. *Journal of Studies on Alcohol, 41,* 1220-3

Malla, A.K. (1985) Personal communication

Maris, R.W. (1981) The physical context of suicide: Alcohol, drug use, and physical illness. In R.W. Maris (ed), *Pathways to suicide. A survey of self-destructive behaviors,* Johns Hopkins University Press, Baltimore, Maryland, pp. 170-204

McIntosh, J.L., and J.F. Santos (1982) Changing patterns in methods of suicide by race and sex. *Suicide and Life Threatening Behaviour, 12,* 221-33

Morgan, H.G., C.J. Burns-Cox, H. Pocock and S. Pottle (1975) Deliberate self-harm: Clinical and socioeconomic characteristics of 368 patients. *British Journal of Psychiatry, 127,* 564-74

Nicholls, R., G. Edwards and E. K· le (1974) Alcoholics admitted to four hospitals in England. *Quarterly Journal of Studies on Alcohol, 35,* 841-55

Patel, A.R., M. Roy and G.M. Wilson (1972) Self poisoning and alcohol. *Lancet, 2,* 1099-102

Rosenthal, R. (ed) (1984) Meta-analytic procedures for social research. *Applied Social Research Methods Series, Volume 6,* Sage Publications, Beverly Hills

Rushing, W.A. (1968) Alcoholism and suicide rates by status set and occupation. *Quarterly Journal of Studies on Alcohol, 29,* 399-412

Sainsbury, P., and J.S. Jenkins (1982) The accuracy of officially reported suicide statistics for purposes of epidemiological research. *Journal of Epidemiology and Community Health, 36,* 43-8

Schmidt, W. and J. de Lint (1972) Causes of death of alcoholics. *Quarterly Journal of Studies on Alcohol, 33*, 171-85

Schmidt, W. and R.E. Popham (1980) Sex differences in mortality: A comparison of male and female alcoholics. In O.J. Kalant (ed), *Alcohol and drug problems in women, Research advances in alcohol and drug problems, Volume 5*, Plenum Press, New York, pp. 365-84

Schneidman, E. and N. Farberow (1965) Statistical comparisons between attempted and committed suicides. In N. Farberow and E. Schneidman (eds), *The cry for help*, McGraw-Hill, New York, pp. 19-47

Statistics Canada (1976) *General mortality, 1950-1972*, Government of Canada, Ottawa, Catalogue 84-531, Occasional

— (1984a) *Statistics Canada Daily*, Government of Canada, Ottawa, Catalogue 11-001

— (1984b) *Mortality, summary list of causes, Vital statistics Volume III, 1982*, Government of Canada, Ottawa, Catalogue 84-206

— (1985) *Causes of death, Vital statistics Volume IV, 1983*, Government of Canada, Ottawa, Catalogue 84-203

Sullivan, W.C. (1898) Alcoholism and suicidal impulses. *Journal of the Mental Sciences, 45*, 259-71

Taylor, J.R., S.J. Holmes, T. Combs-Orme and E.B. Scott (1982) Alcohol and death certificates. *Journal of the American Medical Association, 248*, 3096

Whitehead, P.C. (1972) Notes on the association between alcoholism and suicide. *International Journal of Addictions, 7*, 525-32

20

Opportunities and Problems in Conducting Research on Alcohol and Casualties in Developing Countries

Judy Roizen

Adequate health planning in every country depends on the ability to track and document patterns of consumption of alcohol and consequent social and health problems. However, countries differ radically in their ability to monitor these patterns and problems.

This paper looks at some of the problems and opportunities of gathering 'alcohol statistics' in developing countries, especially in relation to injury, including self-injury. In the first section, it is argued that many developing countries lack the critical 'infrastructure' of alcohol research which, in developed countries, gives meaning to the rates and proportions of alcohol-present casualties. The second section looks at five case studies of alcohol's involvement in casualties which were prepared for the 1985 Toronto International Symposium on Alcohol-Related Casualties (*referred to below as the casualty symposium; see* Giesbrecht and Fisher, 1987). The third section explores the consequences of the absence of an 'infrastructure' of alcohol research and provides recommendations for future work on alcohol and casualties in developing countries. The purpose of this paper is to offer an interpretation of regional differences in work on alcohol-related casualties in order to provide a sound basis for suggestions regarding efforts in the future.

The Need for a Research Infrastructure: The Validity of the 'Developed' Research Model

In contrast to most developing countries, most developed countries have a long tradition of research on the adverse social and health consequences of drinking alcohol and on the consequent morbidity and mortality. Both developed and developing countries suffer from a paucity of data on the acute consequences of drinking alcohol. The 35th World Health Assembly highlighted the 'lack of accurate data on the nature and extent of alcohol-related problems' and noted a strong 'appeal for sound basic information as a foundation for developing national policies and programmes.' In a series of meetings of national and international organisations, the task was defined as follows:

1. start with an area described as statistics on alcohol-related casualties;

2. emphasize the etiological aspects;

3. seek to improve methods of measuring the alcohol dimension among casualty cases.

A question we will ask here is whether this task is possible or useful in most developing countries, given the limited data on other aspects of drinking alcoholic beverages: including availability, patterns of consumption, long term consequences and social control for the populations as a whole or for key groups within them.

To illustrate the dilemma, research on alcohol problems might be contrasted with contemporary research on infant mortality in developing countries. The level of infant mortality is widely regarded as a useful indicator of the state of health of a society, and often used as one indicator of development. Rates of infant mortality are widely researched, with the current research strongly funded by the developed countries and international organisations. Leading universities in many industrialised countries offer courses in demography and population studies which directly facilitate the research in the developing countries.

There has been particular interest in some of these programs in developing methods of estimating infant mortality from deficient and defective data. In particular, there is interest in adapting the methodology of survey research which has seen such rigorous work in developed countries. Further, considerable work exists on measurement and analysis of infant mortality which takes account of conditions prevalent in developing countries.

The disciplines of anthropology, medicine and epidemiology in developing countries and, equally important, the understanding of the causes of infant mortality in developed countries have contributed to research on infant mortality. The result is a solid base of work created, in part, by the World Fertility Surveys, which in the mid-1970s investigated infant mortality, fertility and family in 50 developing countries under common auspices. This forms the basis for on-going cross-cultural research and research in individual countries on many aspects of maternal and child health. In short, the work already carried out on infant mortality has delimited the most important areas of investigation.

In contrast, in most developing countries, alcohol research on patterns of consumption or related problems is made up of an eclectic array of studies, coming from a number of different disciplines. This research takes a wide variety of theoretical perspectives. The quantitative research, where it exists, is in many cases decades old. In most developing countries, the work will have been unfocussed, reflecting the fortuitous interests of visiting anthropologists and sociologists, colonial administrators, medical personnel and, much more rarely, local researchers and health administrators.

Few developing countries will have had any recent large-scale social surveys of the kind that are routine in most developed countries. Work in any given country will have been carried out under a variety of different auspices, in most cases without any clear, overall research strategy for the investigation of patterns of consumption of alcohol or its adverse consequences. One result of this is that existing work will be of little use for cross-cultural comparisons. (There are notable exceptions, such as the work by Puffer and Griffith, 1981, and the WHO Community Response Study, *see* R. Roizen, 1981.)

However, much of the work may be important and interesting in its own right. The alcohol-related ethonographic work, of which there is a great deal, offers an important window for viewing cultural patterns generally, as well as both the benefits and adverse consequences of alcohol consumption. Nevertheless, in most countries it will prove of limited value in estimating the rates of alcohol-present casualties and in understanding the contribution of alcohol to the occurrence of these serious events.

There is little available research funding for the study of alcohol problems, either from developing countries themselves, from developed countries or from international organisations. In large part, the limitations in funding and paucity of data on alcohol problems create an impasse in relation to new research. There is unlikely to be substantial funding for alcohol problems in developing countries until there is some recognition of the size of the problem; but it is impossible to estimate the size and severity of the problem without substantial research funds. And in light of the other pressing social and health problems (both chronic and acute) facing developing countries, it is perhaps not surprising that neither the provision or seeking of research funds for alcohol-related casualties has received high priority in the past.

Developed countries, in contrast, have spent substantial amounts of money to provide what might be called the 'infrastructure' of research on alcohol problems — the 'roads and bridges' which have facilitated work on a large number of alcohol problems, including alcohol-related casualties and crime. This infrastructure includes: 1) the very important general population surveys of drinking practices which are now old enough and often enough repeated to allow for analysis of trends; 2) surveys of important components of the population—e.g. blacks and Hispanics in the United States; 3) historical research which allows contemporary problems to be put into a longer perspective; 4) medical research; and 5) anthropological and survey research on indigenous groups and psychosocial research.

It is the 'infrastructure' of alcohol research which creates a mosaic in which the statistics gathered in emergency rooms, morgues and prisons begin to have some meaning. Simple facts of emergency life such as '80% of those coming to an emergency room had been drinking alcohol in the six hours preceding their visit' must be set against the background of knowledge from general population studies, studies of labelled alcoholics, single studies of particular alcohol-related problems such as traffic crashes or criminal assault, and more general research on the delivery of medical care in emergency rooms. In most developing countries, an 'infrastructure' is not yet in place.

To document this absence one needs only turn to some of the recent reviews of the research literature. Caetano notes that:

> Once the general population surveys of the late 1950's and 1960's were developed (in those countries which had them), and the prevalence of alcoholism was established, epidemiologically-oriented research just ground to a halt in many (Latin American) countries.
>
> Outside (those populations on which ethnographic studies have been carried out), which are concentrated in small towns and rural areas, little is known about reasons for drinking, drinking contexts, norms, attitudes, and beliefs associated with alcohol use in Latin America.
>
> By using only such indicators (as 'inability to stop' or 'inability to abstain'), along with amount and frequency of drinking, to identify 'at risk' drinkers, the broader range of alcohol-related problems remains largely unexamined (in Latin America) ... and by identifying a population of alcoholics ... or ... excessive drinkers ... epidemiological surveys in Latin America provide only a very limited picture of the target population for prevention strategies and of the kinds of problems that should be prevented. (Caetano 1982)

Casswell states that:

> Few data are available on the consumption of alcohol in the less developed countries of Oceania.
>
> It is apparent from what little ethnographic and survey data are available that commercial alcohol use is less widely distributed in

the less-developed countries in the region. (*see* Chapter 4, pp. 114, 116)

Haworth reports that:

There is a lack of information from Africa on alcohol-related problems generally....

It appears from the figures given that there are either massive differences in the drinking habits of various African countries (Nigeria, for example, has a predominantly Muslim population) or that the means of collecting data are so disparate that no comparisons can be made. (*see* Chapter 3, pp. 85, 88)

In contrast, a look through the table of contents for the Fifth Special Report to the US Congress on Alcohol and Alcoholism (1983) demonstrates the abundance of riches to be found in countries with a well-established, well-funded alcohol research tradition. Hundreds of US studies are cited in this report alone, extending back over several decades. Reports such as this one represent a consensus that the consequences of drinking create health and social problems considered serious enough to be worthy of the expenditure of millions of dollars to understand, document, and prevent.

It must also be recognised that there are many countries and sub-cultures in developing parts of the world in which drinking is not recognised as a cause of conflict, crime or health problems. Equally, there are many anthropologists who have studied these cultures who also do not identify serious social and health problems as a consequence of drinking or 'addiction' to alcohol — even where there is heavy drinking. Whether or not other investigators might find problems where none or few have been recognised is the subject of some debate (*see, for example,* Room *and responses to* Room, 1984). As long as there is a lack of consensus as to whether or not problems are actually or possibly alcohol-related, research funds and energy are unlikely to be forthcoming.

The recognition of the importance of alcohol problems to total health care is but a first step in the development of a research programme. Equally important is the recognition that patterns of consumption and drinking behaviour are as varied, if not more varied, than those found in developing countries. It is likely that the patterns of drinking and associated problems among the middle classes in the capital cities of many developing countries will be much more like those in developed countries. However, among groups in rural areas, *patterns* of consumption may vary widely within the same geographical area or show marked similarities even in quite different cultural settings. The *effects* of drinking vary, as well. The Kofyar of Nigeria and the Tiriki of Kenya 'use beer as a constant medium and social interchange for men ... [which] induces physical and social mellowness' (Mandelbaum 1979). Drinking is apparently not accompanied by aggressive behaviour nor does it apparently result in 'addiction'. The Camba of eastern Bolivia and those living in Lunahuanc in the Andean foothills in Peru regularly drink themselves into a drunken stupor—a pattern of consumption shared by proportionately few men in developed countries (Mandelbaum 1979). In these cultures, whatever havoc is wreaked on the body, the result is 'safe interaction' among one's fellow men. Lemert (1979), looking at drinking patterns in three Polynesian societies—Tahiti, the Cook Islands and Western Samoa—identifies three decidedly different patterns of drinking and its consequences. Beverages, drinking rhythms and adverse consequences differ in the three cultures—despite the many similarities in aspects of everyday life, diet and availability of fermentable fruits. However, in all of these societies, patterns of consumption are changing in proximity to Western drink and drinking styles.

Further, there is no simple model of research with sampling schemes and validated measures which sensibly can be carried over to most developing countries and quickly adapted for local use. In this respect, alcohol research is very different from research on infant mortality, to continue our previous illustration. Babies are born and some of them die. When they die and how they die are seen as important in most societies and, relative to 'alcohol addiction', are open to reasonably objective empirical investigation. The utility of modelling alcohol research in developing countries on research from developed countries is itself a question for research. Therefore, a first-order question is whether a culture-specific 'infrastructure' of alcohol research is to be created in every country.

It may well prove to be the case that many of the techniques and measurements routinely used in developed countries may not provide useful data in developing countries. Let us consider the common measurement of quantity and frequency of drinking. In many countries, quantity of drinking will be exceedingly difficult to measure at the individual level, that is, as compared to many indicators of national consumption. Within the same drinking group, drinking may involve the use of a jar, a glass, a coconut shell, a coffee cup, a bottle—in short, any container at hand. There is no metric against which an individual drinker can estimate quantity, such as the 1-1/2 ounces of spirits, six ounces of wine, and twelve ounces of beer used in many developed countries. This common metric, therefore, has no meaning to most drinkers in most of the developing countries. Not only is quantity difficult to measure, the amount of alcohol in alcoholic beverages will vary depending partly on whether the drink is commercial or home brew.

Frequency, too, will involve very considerable problems of measurement involving rhythms and patterns of drinking different from those in developed countries. Adequate estimates will depend on a sensitive understanding of the patterns of regular drinking (if any), as well as festive and ritual drinking in a society.

Survey research on most social and economic problems in developing countries is most often confined to the use of simple and straightforward interview schedules and questionnaires—in contrast to those in developed countries. There are a number of reasons for this parsimony in developing countries including: the need in many countries to use highly trained interviewers—teachers, university students or medical personnel—the people who most often have many other competing demands on their time. Additionally, work in developing countries is inevitably carried out with considerable constraints on resources—small overall research budgets which have to buy expensive paper for printing, petrol, consultants, office equipment and computer time. Perhaps most important, the information gathered will need to be limited because of the difficulties of obtaining it: enormous amounts of time will be spent devising sampling frames or finding interviewees who are 'not on the phone', who work irregular hours, who may be migrant or in relatively inaccessible places.

Motivation is yet another problem. For most of the people in these countries, there will be no evening news and no morning newspaper which underscores the importance of citizen participation in social surveys by describing the latest political poll, survey of smoking or dietary fibre content in the diet. In many countries, the presence of a stranger with a clipboard will be threatening or, at the least, odd.

The study of alcohol problems has generated a number of models for research, each with its own complex array of measures and indices. The development of new culture-specific theoretical and empirical research, whether on patterns of consumption or problems such as alcohol-related casualties, is an expensive and demanding undertaking. Without laying the necessary ground work, limited efforts to improve health statistics are likely to prove of little value.

Alcohol, Casualties and Crime in Developing Countries

The review papers in this volume by Casswell, Haworth, Medina-Mora and González and the earlier review by Caetano (1982) point to the paucity of data on alcohol problems generally and alcohol-related casualties specifically in developing countries. Medina-Mora and González (*see* Chapter 2) point to the difficulties in understanding the role of alcohol in casualties in Latin America: the scarcity of published literature, the low concern for and variation in the registration of alcohol-related casualties, the low priority given the alcohol component, the under-recording of alcohol data, and the under-analysis of such data when they are reported. Casswell's review (*see* Chapter 4) notes that for a number of reasons, including the lack of technology, there are few data from Oceania focusing on the role of alcohol in casualties. Haworth (*see* Chapter 3) refers to the lack of reliable statistical information, and the under-reporting and under-estimating of alcohol-related casualty incidents in African contexts. With these reviews in mind, we consider in some detail the five case studies from developing countries which were prepared for the casualty symposium.

The countries differ from each other in many relevant respects. They differ in size, accessibility, rural populations, linguistic homogeneity, religious homogeneity, attitudes toward drinking, drinking culture, availability of alcohol and types of alcohol commonly used. The Sudan is a predominantly Muslim country of about 2.5 million square kilometres, with a population of about 20 million. It is the largest country in Africa and it is among the poorest countries in the world. Since 1983 it has come under strict Sharia law which has had a pronounced effect on drinking practices. However, as it shares borders with eight African countries, considerable variations in attitudes toward drinking and drinking practices are expected throughout the country.

Nigeria, in West Africa, is a federal republic with an estimated population of 80 million in an area of 1 million square kilometres. The population consists of three main ethnic groups—the Hausa, Yorubas and Ibos. The north and west are predominantly Muslim. The country has benefited from petroleum earnings until quite recently.

Costa Rica, with a population of 2.5 million, is the second smallest country in Central America and the most prosperous. As Caetano (1982) notes, 'Costa Rica is one of the few Latin American countries with a constant output of alcohol studies.' The country is predominantly Roman Catholic. With no standing army, it has considerably more revenue to devote to problems of social welfare than do most developing countries.

Argentina is the second largest country in South America, with an area of nearly 3 million square kilometres. The 1976 population was estimated at nearly 26 million, the majority of European descent. The Indian population is small, as is the mestizo population. The population of Buenos Aires, the venue for the study reviewed here, is estimated at over 8 million, approximately equal to that of New York City.

Mexico has a population estimated at 80 million in an area of 2 million square kilometres. The vast majority of the population are mestizo and about 10 per cent are Indian. While Spanish is the official language, an estimated 6 million Indians speak only one of their own languages, of which there are over 50.

The countries considered here differ widely from one another and, indeed, differ as much from each other as some of them do from more developed countries. The five case studies on alcohol-related casualties were prepared by the following researchers in their own countries (extended abstracts are provided in Giesbrecht and Fisher 1987):

The Sudan: Dr El-Tigani A. Hammad, Faculty of Medicine, University of Gezira, Wad Medani

Nigeria: Professor A.O. Odejidi, with the assistance of Mr. B. Ikuesan, Department of Psychiatry, University College Hospital, Ibadan

Costa Rica: Dr Enrique Madrigal Segura, National Institute of Alcoholism (now with the Pan American Health Organization, Washington, DC).

Argentina: Dr Juan Carlos Garcia Fernandez, Dr Heraldo Donnelwald, and Dr Manuel Guatelli. (Drs Fernandez and Guateli, Chemical Experts of the Forensic Medical Body, National Judicial Power; Dr Donnewald, Medical Director, Judicial Morgue.)

Mexico: Dr Haydee Rosovsky, Mexican Institute of Psychiatry.

These case studies will be summarised and cited liberally in the following paragraphs; unless otherwise noted, the quoted material is drawn from the case study in question.

The Sudan (El Tigani A. Hammad 1985)[1]

With respect to the social control of alcohol in the Sudan toward drinking, recent history is divided into several distinct periods:

> Until the end of the Mahdist State in 1898 the Sudan always had a Muslim State during the times of national rule to conform with Islamic teachings. Sharia law was implemented and alcohol categorically prohibited. The British rule in the Sudan (1898-1955) created a dichotomy between religion and the state. The government legalized the sale of alcohol against public opinion thus encouraging non-conforming Muslims to drink under the cultural influence of a Western life-style. Religious and health education remained strong antagonists to alcohol but with a varying degree of influence. The community exhibited a negative attitude towards alcohol. This persistent anti-drink campaign remained an influential force in prevention. However, alcohol-related problems occasionally appeared along all axes of the alcohol dependence syndrome.

More recent research and clinical experience show that the size of the problem in the country is by no means negligible as it presented itself as a major health and social problem among males in Khartoum Province (Salik 1977, Nadim and Rahim 1980). The situation, however, did not lead to the formation of any specialized helping agency as a response.

In 1983 a historical decision in the history of alcohol in the Sudan in recent times was taken by the government. Prohibition of alcohol was announced with an immediate ban on its production and import. Dealings in alcohol were stopped in hotels, restaurants and shops, public houses and the few breweries in the country were closed. Sharia law was applied. Native alcohol production was seriously limited. Short though this experiment is, its consequences were dramatic. Personal experience of casualty doctors, psychiatrists, police officers, law men and the public at large agreed that alcohol-related problems and casualties have been cut down seriously. This remains the case so far, but all are worried that relaxation of the situation may cause a rebound.

There are no reliable statistics on the prevalence of alcoholism in the Sudan (Nadim and Rahim, 1984). The problem does not seem to be a priority and therefore no specialist services have been established and no special training is offered. However, certain services have an obligation to handle alcohol-related problems. These are mainly the medical profession, the psychiatric services, the Social Welfare Department, the Police and the Law.

The alcohol dimensions measured and the services provided are not enough which reflects negatively on the information collected. Few personnel are actually aware of this. The secondary role of alcohol and its indirect involvement in casualties is generally not documented...

Currently, the availability of alcohol is seriously limited following the recent move to ban alcohol. Despite reduction in the clinical load of alcoholics other problems have arisen in the few who have persisted in drinking. It now costs more effort and money to obtain alcohol from the black market. The stuff obtainable is likely to be adulterated with toxic and sedative substances leading to poisoning and overdose. Some alcoholics have substituted drugs for alcohol. Sedatives, tranquilizers and hypnotics are now widely known and abused. Research in this field is urgently needed along with research in alcohol-related problems.

In the Sudan, three agencies keep some statistical data on alcohol-related problems. However, the fact that 'alcohol-related problems are not a priority in their work' leads to erratic results which are largely uninterpretable. The Division of Health Statistics and Research (numbers apply only to the Muslim North) reported 1,079 cases of admission to hospital for 'alcoholism' or 'accidental poisoning by alcohol' between 1979 and 1983. However, admissions vary from 23 to 369 annually; 23 admissions were recorded in 1983, the year of the turn to Sharia law. The single psychiatric hospital reported alcohol-related admissions between 1979 and 1982 at 598. Yet the number of admissions to this single hospital for 1979 greatly exceeded the Division of Health Statistics estimates for total alcohol-related admissions for the whole of the North in that year—suggesting serious problems of definition and record keeping. Men between the ages of 15 and 44 make up the majority of cases in both series.

Variable quality in the investigation of suicide and homicide also make police reports unreliable for research purposes; 210 homicides were reported to have had either a drinking victim or offender. This is of little use without full reporting on the total number of homicides, especially given the inadequate reporting in many jurisdictions. Just over 1 per cent (N = about 1,000 per year) of all traffic charges are argued to be 'drunk and driving'. Without appropriate breath-testing capabilities, this figure is probably markedly too low. Offences related to alcohol control suggest a greater degree of alcohol use than other statistics. The number of violations of the law prohibiting 'local drinks' is given in Table 20.1, along with the number of licensing offences.

Table 20.1: *Alcohol-related charges for possession and licencing offences, 1979-1983, inclusive (northern Sudan)*

Year	Possession of local drinks	Licencing offences
1979	20,121	352
1980	20,056	560
1981	16,860	571
1982	13,132	698
1983	14,824	380

Source: El-Tigani Hammad, 1985

An important opportunity for a natural experiment was missed in the Sudan with the 1983 imposition of Sharia law. It would have been of considerable value to strictly monitor alcohol-related casualties in the months prior to and after the change in law in a sample of the jurisdiction.

El-Tigani argues that 'alcohol abuse presents serious problems in Southern Sudan where alcohol is an indispensable daily commodity and drunkenness a commonplace ritual'. However, there is a 'lack of information' on these problems.

The study of alcohol problems among Muslims — one-sixth of the world's population — is a clear priority for world health research. A Cape Town study (Midgley, 1979) of drinking among Muslims provides an interesting model of the sort of research which would provide valuable baseline data on alcohol consumption and problems in Muslim societies. The groups studied were orthodox Sunnis, strict observers of the tenets of Islam. Despite the strong religious sanctions, 12 per cent of those interviewed (one-quarter of the men) reported drinking. Nearly all the drinkers lived in a resettlement community in close contact with non-Muslim families, rather than in the Muslim area. The drinkers had also been poor *madressa* attenders (afternoon religious classes for children).

A study such as this, on a larger scale and with strict adherence to norms of anonymity, would be a useful base on which to build further data collection on alcohol-related problems in both Northern and Southern Sudan. Without a clear understanding of the prevalence and patterns of alcohol use, information from existing reporting systems related to alcohol problems is of little value. Upgrading current systems and encouraging new problem-oriented research requires considerable groundwork which will take account of the sensitivity of this social problem under Sharia law.

Nigeria (Odejide et al. 1985)[2]

Alcohol is produced and used in the Nigerian community traditionally. Some examples of the alcoholic beverages produced locally are palmwine, native gin (*ogogoro*) and *burukutu*.... As far as local production is concerned, there is no government control of production, no statistics of producers and production level, and as such records of the quantities produced do not exist.

Apart from the traditional production, many alcoholic beverages are now being produced industrially, while a significant amount is being imported. Beer, stout and other distilled alcohols are not only being produced locally, but are also imported. Breweries have sprung up in many parts of the country with the number increasing from about 8 in 1977 to 31 in 1985. Twenty-five of the 31 breweries are sited in eight of the nine States constituting Southern Nigeria. The preponderance of breweries in the South as opposed to the North is attributable to the ban on the production and consumption of alcohol enjoined by Islamic religion which prevails in that part of the country.

Importation of beer in 1970 was about 1.3 million litres compared with 132 million litres in 1976 (FOS 1977) and from January to August, 1977, importation of beer and stout amounted to 62.6 million litres while production stood at 86.7 million litres. Since

December 1983, the present Federal Military Government has imposed restrictions on the importation of alcoholic beverages. The current statistics on the quality of alcoholic beverages allowed to be legally imported is not available.

However, when the present number of local breweries is used as an index of the quantity of beverage alcohol consumed, it would appear that alcohol consumption is on the increase.

The several studies of alcohol use cited by Odejide *et al.* are typically very small and limited in geographic area. Half of the men in a small rural community study report drinking (Odejide *et al.*, 1977). Beer and palm-wine are the most common drinks. In urban areas, moderate drinking is common. School surveys show alcohol to be the 'most abused drug'. Increasing proportions of female students drink.

Clinical samples show few alcohol-related psychiatric problems. A recent review by Odejide and his colleagues of admissions to the psychiatric unit of the University of Ilorin Teaching Hospital over a three-year period turned up only eleven alcohol-related cases. However, it is noted, 'inadequate record keeping made our task almost impossible'. Again looking at case records of a representative sample of general practitioners, no diagnosis of an alcohol-related problem was found in the 2,189 cases studied. A study of a single month's hospital casualty admissions (N = 1,441) showed no cases where alcohol was 'implicated as a causal factor' among 50 casualty cases sampled. In a review of 35 casualties, known to be alcohol-related, a third were the result of road traffic accidents.

Given the substantial availability and consumption of alcohol in Nigeria, the limited numbers of alcohol-related problems clearly demonstrate massive under-reporting. In large part, this is a function of the failure to define alcohol as responsible for substantial numbers of health and social problems. 'There are no laws in respect of drunkenness *per se* except when it leads to a breach of the law...there is no law concerning the blood alcohol level above which one is not permitted to drive.' 'Police final records' do not reflect alcohol presence in assaults and road traffic accidents.

Medical doctors were preoccupied with the treatment of life-threatening situations almost to the exclusion of history taking on the use of alcohol prior to the accident...Information is currently inadequate or poorly disseminated on the danger of alcohol abuse...There is no government or non-governmental programme in Nigeria specifically designed for the rehabilitation of people with alcohol-related problems.

There are as yet no in-depth national epidemiological surveys and reports on alcohol-related problems have largely relied on the review of case-records. This report shows clearly the increasing trend of alcohol production and use in Nigeria. Therefore, it can be predicted that in the next decade with increased education and urbanization, cases of alcohol-related problems may become a major problem in Nigeria. Thus far, cases are not identified early until the complications are severe enough to warrant hospitalization. Odejide (1978) attributed this observation to the lack of information in the Nigerian society of the dangers associated with prolonged and/or excessive alcohol use. Therefore there is the urgent need in Nigeria to intensify research activities especially in the area of epidemiology of alcohol abuse. Basic data gathering on this subject should be a continuous process. Furthermore, instruments for determining breath or plasma alcohol levels are urgently required. These will help to confirm diagnostic impressions.... The highlight of this study is the lack of information on contribution of alcohol to non-psychiatric casualties.

Costa Rica (Madrigal Segura 1985)[3]

Taken together, recent general population studies of drinking practices have covered nearly 70 per cent of the country. The categories of drinkers typically include abstainers, moderates and excessives (defined by sex-specific consumption) and 'alcoholics'. Based on a national representative sample, in the population of 2.5 million, an estimated '75,000 persons 15 and older are addicted to alcohol, whereas nearly 155,000 are "excessive drinkers", that is, they get intoxicated with alcohol at least twice a month' (Miquez 1983).

A relatively low mortality by cirrhosis of the liver (4.6 per hundred thousand) and a reported mortality rate of alcoholism of 2.5 per hundred thousand, match a relatively low level of consumption: 4.28 litres of absolute alcohol per person 15 and older (1984).

In spite of these data, it is generally agreed, among staff at the National Institute on Alcoholism, that Costa Ricans, especially male, drink in considerable amounts, episodically and that there are specific 'cultural crises', where there is a degree of societal permissiveness, allowing higher consumption such as weekends, national festivities, etc.

There is, at present, a dearth of indicators and data, aimed to reflect that particular situation. In addition, general hospitals, major insurance companies and law enforcement agencies, have mainly emphasized case studies related to driving under the influence of alcohol, but they have neglected other areas such as family and public violence, accidents in the working premises, non-traffic accidents, intoxications and even some acute medical complications caused by alcohol consumption.

The study, presented to the Symposium was carried out in a major city hospital emergency room in San Jose, and focussed on a sample of 2,130 subjects seen over ten days in one month. Interviews were carried out by physicians and other health professionals.

'Alcohol intoxication and/or alcohol as a cause-related agent' was observed in 13 per cent of the cases. Alcohol was 'seen as an underlying' factor or etiologic agent in 11 per cent of the cases. Among men, 21 per cent of the cases were alcohol-related (as defined above) as compared to only 4 per cent of the women. Of the alcohol-related causes, 28 per cent were medical cases and 72 per cent were surgical. Alcohol-related cases were disproportionately drawn from the age group 30 to 49; 47 per cent of the alcohol-related cases fall within this age group compared to 29 per cent of the others. Unfortunately, no analysis of types of events was included.

No measures of drinking patterns and history were taken. Therefore, it is impossible to analyse whether the proportion of alcohol-related cases is high or low in relation to consumption patterns in the general population. Similarly, a comparison of the demographic characteristics of alcohol-related and other cases with general population data would have been valuable.

Argentina (Fernandez et al. 1985)[4]

Argentina is a leading wine-producer; *per capita* wine consumption ranks among the highest in the world. Several studies have documented patterns of alcohol consumption in Buenos Aires and in an industrial suburb of Buenos Aires.

There are few studies of alcohol and unnatural death in developing countries which are based on autopsy. Lack of trained personnel, appropriate technology and the need to use scarce resources for the care of the living explain this limited effort. The case study carried out by Drs Fernandez, Donnewald and Guatelli on a series of 1981 fatalities is, therefore, a useful contribution. The study includes a detailed analysis of the different techniques for analysing blood. Although gas-liquid chromatography methods are to be preferred, the instruments are expensive and are not commonly available in many developing countries. An enzymatic technique is used in the majority of cases in the work on which this study is based.

Alcohol-positive results were found in 11 per cent of the males and 3 per cent of the females. The series, unfortunately, included an unknown number of children which should have been excluded in analysis. There is considerable variation in the proportion of alcohol-positive cases, with the highest proportions in the age groups: 26 to 30, and 41 to 50. These proportions would be considerably higher if females were removed from the base. Of the alcohol-positive cases (N = 163) in the series of 1981 cases, 20 per cent were accidents; 14 per cent were suicides, 32 per cent were homicides; 34 were 'doubtful deaths' (*muerte dudosa*). The majority of this latter group were apparently 'natural deaths'. If homicides 'not deliberately produced, without the wish to kill' (most commonly, traffic deaths) are removed from the homicide category, the proportions are changed to 43 per cent accidents and 10 per cent homicides. Unfortunately, no analysis of the non-alcohol deaths in the series is included.

In a city of 8 million people, it would be expected that the number of unnatural deaths in a year would greatly exceed the numbers in this series. Therefore, the criterion for selection of the examined cases is needed.

The blood-alcohol levels of the cases were relatively high: 87 per cent of the alcohol-present series had BACs greater than or equal to 0.49 mg/ml; with the following distribution:

Table 20.2: *Distribution of blood-alcohol concentration in a sample of fatalities, Buenos Aires, Argentina, 1981*

BAC mg/ml	Per cent	BAC mg/ml	Per cent
0-0.49	13.4	1.50 -1.99	20.1
0.50-0.99	20.7	2.00 -2.49	14.0
1.00-1.49	11.7	2.50 -2.99	11.7
		> = 3.00	8.4

Source: Fernandez *et al.*, 1985

A roadside breath-testing survey near 'leisure zones or facilities either in the city of Buenos Aires or in Mar del Plata' in 1977 reported high levels of alcohol-positive cases. Testing was carried out between midnight and 5 a.m. in 2,500 cases on working days, Saturdays and public holidays; the percentage positive were respectively 39.3 per cent, 50.1 per cent and 43.6 per cent. These data, coupled with research on consumption, suggest that the reported alcohol presence in this series may be a significant underestimate.

Mexico (Rosovsky, 1989)

The Rosovsky study, reported in this volume (*see* Chapter 14), is a model of the type of study that is needed in developing countries. Mexico can be distinguished from many developing countries in the attention given to alcohol research. Studies have been carried out both in the general and in clinical populations. Smart *et al.* (1980) and Natera *et al.* (1981, 1982) have reported drinking patterns in a rural community. Several surveys of drinking practices have recently been carried out in urban areas by the Instituto Mexicano de Psiquiatria and earlier as part of the WHO Community Response Study. In contrast to most developing countries, new work on alcohol-related casualties and crime is based on substantial knowledge of drinking patterns and alcohol-related problems.

The study had three objectives:

1. To take a single district – in this case the Federal District – and determine the procedures for recording alcohol use in the casualties and crimes 'that reach the knowledge of the medical and justice authorities'.

2. To develop a methodology with which to explore alcohol use in these events and evaluate the role drinking may play in contributing to them.

3. To gather data to analyse the social and demographic characteristics of those who are injured or involved in crimes and to analyse their drinking practices and problems.

Reviewing this study suggests the following guidelines for future research:

1. Grounding casualty research in studies of drinking practices in the general population is a necessary first step in alcohol-related casualty research. Without a clear idea of drinking patterns and problems — demography, epidemiology and social psychology of drinking patterns and problems – work on alcohol-related casualties is of very limited value. Measurement of alcohol use must be related to the patterns of consumption in the jurisdiction under investigation.

2. A careful evaluation of existing registration systems needs to be made which considers such factors as under-registration in rural and outlying areas; under-registration of those with money or social status to keep themselves out of the public registration systems; antiquated categorisation of demographic and other variables. The research for this study used both usual agency registration forms and a purposely designed questionnaire. This facilitated not only analysis of the adequacy of current record keeping in the area, but also more extensive analyses of the casualty events and drinking patterns.

3. Given constraints on resources, a geographically delimited area is essential — areas chosen should have had a recent study of drinking patterns and be located in jurisdictions for which social, economic and demographic characteristics are also known. In this study, the research was limited to the Federal District — still a very large and heterogeneous area — but less so than the country as a whole. Importantly, the Federal District had seen considerable other social research which could be analysed alongside the current work.

4. As in this case study, close attention will need to be paid to the choice of sites and sampling frame. These need to be chosen and designed with attention to the representative character of the events; knowledge of the temporal variation in the events studied; and the socioeconomic characteristics (i.e. the selective recruitment) of those who attend the agencies or hospitals under investigation.

5. The study design called for both measurement of drinking in the event, alcohol consumption on the day of the event and previous drinking problems. For analytic purposes, measuring drinking patterns and problems is of equal importance to measuring drinking at the time of admission or arrest. The ability to compare the drinking variables of the clinical sample with those in the general population will allow the analyst to make some judgement about the characteristics of the population which is captured by the clinical sample. For example, 29 per cent of the alcohol-present cases in the Mexico study reported that when they drank they 'always or almost always get drunk', compared to 12 per cent of the others. This suggests that a very close analysis of drinking patterns and problems is necessary before attributing criminal behaviour or injury to alcohol or to an amount of alcohol. Clearly, a substantial proportion of cases, when they drink, drink heavily. Yet, presumably no adverse consequences occur in most instances.

6. An attempt was made to include a comparison or control group. The importance of having such a group has been emphasized elsewhere (*see* Chapter 1). In this case, all those presenting themselves to the emergency service at a shift were interviewed. The comparison groups were those cases immediately following an alcohol-present case (alcohol-present cases included those drinking on the day of the event, as well as those examined by a physician). This was judged a 'methodological error'; a preferred sample would have been based on a systematic selection of those with no alcohol present.

Future Work on Alcohol-Related Casualties in Developing Countries

As the case studies show, countries are in different states of readiness to carry out research on alcohol-related casualties and crime. The Sudan, with little research on alcohol problems, is entering a new period of social control which will have, as yet, undetermined consequences for empirical work on alcohol problems. Nigeria, with a large, pluralistic population, a federal political structure and with a substantial Muslim population, faces many hurdles in the development of a coherent program of alcohol studies at a national level. The Latin American countries which are represented suggest a different picture. These countries have a base of research on alcohol problems which includes epidemiological research, at least in some urban areas. However, if the countries chosen had been Bolivia or Peru, countries with less epidemiological research, the picture would be a different one.

It can be concluded that there is a developmental or evolutionary process that occurs in relation to research on alcohol problems; a process which also applies to most other social and health problems as well. This means that countries, states within countries, even cities and hospitals within cities, are differentially able to carry out meaningful research which may be seen as important, even vital, to those outside. As a consequence, a call for a particular type of research in all countries may lead to a meaningless mimicry of the research in developed countries.

The first step in developing a national programme of research on alcohol problems is clearly the recognition that there are adverse consequences of drinking alcohol. There is enormous cultural variation (within and across cultures) in the degree to which alcohol is seen as a 'problem', and also variation in perceptions of the severity of the problems, especially in relation to other health problems. As in developed countries, alcohol problems must be evaluated in relation to other problems competing for the same resources. However, in developing countries, health ministers and administrators are too often confronted with health problems of enormous magnitude: the sequelae of famine, drought and hurricanes; epidemics of infectious disease; endemic malnutrition; poor and declining hospital facilities; shortages of trained personnel; and most important, a shortage of money. A first-order problem in establishing a research program related to statistics on alcohol-related casualties and crime is to establish that alcohol problems generally are recognised as problems sufficient in importance to command attention and resources.

The study of alcohol use and problems presents a distinct research challenge in relation to other types of health problems. There is, for example, an increasing body of theory to suggest that the concept of dependence itself is largely a product of a specific pattern of general cultural beliefs and norms. There is, as well, considerable debate about the way alcohol problems should be understood. Whereas, as Caetano points out, there has been a shift away from the disease model to one which focuses on 'problems related to alcohol consumption', there is by no means cross-cultural consensus among researchers in respect of models and theories which explain alcohol problems.

As well, the study of alcohol use and problems relies on a great variety of measures of consumption and problems; as a consequence, there is no simple set of indicators which can be parsimoniously applied to establish rates and types of alcohol problems and to describe patterns of consumption.

Further, the analyst of data on alcohol-related casualties is explicitly or implicitly asking questions of the clinical data in relation to other data on the events under investigation or in the general population. Therefore, in the absence of formal control groups, casualty studies need to be related to the types of measures of consumption and drinking rhythms and patterns that are the stock-in-trade of general population studies. A poorly-designed study of alcohol presence in an emergency room (and even in developed countries most are poorly designed) is of no value in assessing etiological factors. A well-designed study offers little more if the conclusions are of the order '20 per cent of assault victims had BACs greater than 0.05 mg/ml'. In the Sudan, 20 per cent would, no doubt, be considered a very substantial proportion; in some Scandinavian countries the proportion would be considered so low as to constitute an error in measurement.

On the other hand, an analysis of the level of alcohol in a casualty event linked with other drinking variables and demographic variables places the work in a broader and more valuable analytical context, addressing questions such as: Are alcohol-present casualty cases a fairly random sample of drinkers? Are they drawn from particular ethnic and demographic groups? What other drinking, social, and health problems are associated with alcohol-related casualties?

Given the limited resources of most developing countries, where should work on alcohol-related casualties begin?

1. Emergency room and related studies should begin in areas where there has been other work on alcohol problems and should be limited in scope.

2. They will need to be part of an overall strategy for the study of alcohol use and problems, however limited in initial resources and scope that may be.

3. Studies of alcohol-related casualties will need to make use of appropriate technology. This will differ from country to country.

4. Developed countries should commit energy and resources to help develop strategies suited to the different circumstances and resources of particular countries. In particular, more work in developed countries should be devoted to collaboration with researchers in developing countries on the sorts of culture-specific measures which are needed to create an appropriate base to build research on alcohol-related casualties.

An example of productive collaborative work is found in the Chilean study prepared by Drs Florenzano, A. Pemjean, P. Orpinas and J. Manzi (1985)[5] for the casualty symposium. In this small emergency room study the alcohol tape ('dipstick'), designed by researchers at the Addiction Research Foundation (Kapur and Israel 1983) to measure the amount of alcohol in the saliva or other body fluids, was used to establish its reliability in relation to other alcohol measures. The 'dipstick' provides appropriate technology for the study of alcohol-related casualties in developing countries – it is relatively inexpensive, easy to use and portable.

Keeping in mind the need for the development of a research infrastructure in relation to alcohol problems and constraints on resources in most developing countries, there are very considerable opportunities for the development of research programmes on alcohol-related casualties. Injury is the leading cause of death in developed countries for those between one and 40 years and a leading cause of death and disability in all age groups. Injury is rapidly becoming a leading cause of death in developing countries also. Wintemute (1983) has observed: 'the secular increase in injury mortality and morbidity from several causes, coupled with the profound decrease in morbidity and mortality related to infectious disease, has produced a striking alteration in the relative importance in many developing countries'. With the increasing worldwide recognition of the significance of accidents as a cause of death, especially among young men and women, there is growing interest in the discovery of causal factors.

The considerable anthropological work on drinking practices also provides a base for the development of research programmes. In many countries, it will be the case that rural areas best suited for inclusion in an on-going research programme will be those which have been the object of anthropological investigation into drinking patterns and practices. Here again, there is the opportunity for collaboration between developed and developing countries.

Despite the problems outlined above, there are enormous opportunities for research on alcohol-related problems in developing countries. Few countries have, as yet, a fully developed alcohol research programme. In the development of such programmes in developing countries new dimensions of the relationship between drinking and casualties will emerge, as well as new research techniques. These differences across societies and cultures will benefit other developing countries as well as developed countries. In particular, research in developing countries will be of great importance in increasing our understanding of the drinking problems of ethnic minorities in developed countries, e.g., the Maori in New Zealand, Mexican-Americans and American Indians in the US. Making the most of these opportunities depends both on the availability of material resources and on researchers in developed and developing countries not making the assumption that what applies in the one necessarily applies in the other.

In a growing number of developing countries, there is awareness of how important alcohol-related problems are, and increasing prominence is given to the issue of casualties. Furthermore, there is a growing willingness to collaborate in research. Opportunities exist for the development of programmes of research on alcohol-related casualties, if resources both within and outside developing countries are made available in greater amounts than currently exist. In achieving these greater resources, it is essential that international organisations such as WHO continue their work to raise awareness of the alcohol dimension in understanding and coping with a wide variety of social and health problems — of which alcohol-related casualties are one important example.

© 1989 Judy Roizen

Notes

1. An abstract of this paper appears in Giesbrecht and Fisher (1987).

2. *Ibid.*

3. *Ibid.*

4. *Ibid.*

5. *Ibid.*

Acknowledgements

Contributions from the following organisations to the International Symposium on Alcohol-Related Casualties (August 12-16, 1985, Toronto, Canada) made the preparation of this paper possible: Addiction Research Foundation of Ontario, Health and Welfare Canada, the U.S. National Institute on Alcohol Abuse and Alcoholism and the World Health Organization. Staff of the Alcohol Research Group, Berkeley, California, provided assistance in collecting material and preparing this manuscript.

References

Caetano, R. (1982) Manifestations and perceptions of alcohol-related problems in the Americas. In M.K. Kaplan (ed), *Legislative approaches to prevention of alcohol-related problems: An inter-American workshop*, Institute of Medicine, National Academy Press, Washington, DC, pp. 64-126

Casswell, S. (1989) Alcohol-related casualties in Oceania. In N. Giesbrecht, R. González, M. Grant, E. Österberg, R. Room, I. Rootman and L. Towle (eds), *Drinking and casualties: Accidents, poisonings and violence in an international perspective.* Routledge, London, pp. 112-29

El-Tigani Hammad (1985) Alcohol-related casualties in the Sudan. Paper presented at the International Symposium on Alcohol-Related Casualties, Toronto, August 12-16, 1985

Fernandez, J.C.G., H. Donnewald and M. Guatelli (1985) Blood alcohol levels found in a forensic laboratory; possible relation to casualties. Paper presented at the International Symposium on Alcohol-Related Casualties, Toronto, August 12-16, 1985

Florenzano, R., A. Pemjean, P. Orpinas and J. Manzi (1985) Prevalence of alcohol use and alcohol-related diagnoses and casualties in Santiago de Chile emergency services. Paper presented at the International Symposium on Alcohol-Related Casualties, Toronto, August 12-16, 1985

Giesbrecht N. and H. Fisher (eds), (1987) *Alcohol-related casualties: proceedings of an international symposium,* Addiction Research Foundation, Toronto

Hall, M. (1980) Research in violent crime in Lusaka, 1972, Zambia Police Force Mimeo, University of Zambia, Lusaka

Haworth, A., M. Mwanalushi and D. Todd (1981) Community response to alcohol-related problems in Zambia. *Historical and Health Research Reports*, No. 1, Institute for African Studies, Lusaka

Haworth, A. (1989) Alcohol-related casualties in Africa. In N. Giesbrecht, R. González, M. Grant, E. Österberg, R. Room, I. Rootman and L. Towle (eds), *Drinking and Casualties: Accidents, poisonings and violence in an international perspective*, Routledge, London, pp. 84-111

Lemert, E.M. (1979) Forms and pathology of drinking in three Polynesian societies. In M. Marshall (ed), *Beliefs, behaviors and alcoholic beverages: A cross-cultural survey,* University of Michigan Press, Ann Arbor, pp. 192-208

Kapur, B.M. and Y. Israel (1983) A dipstick methodology for rapid determination of alcohol in body fluids. *Clinical Chemistry, 29,* 1178

Madrigal Segura, E. (1985) Alcohol consumption and emergencies: An emergency room study. Paper presented at the International Symposium on Alcohol-Related Casualties, Toronto, August 12-16, 1985.

Mandelbaum, D. (1979) Alcohol and culture. In M. Marshall (ed), *Beliefs, behaviors and alcoholic beverages: A cross-cultural survey,* University of Michigan Press, Ann Arbor, pp. 14-30

Medina-Mora, M.E. and L. González (1989) Alcohol-related casualties in Latin America: A review of the literature. In N. Giesbrecht, R. Gonzalez, M. Grant, E. Österberg, R. Room, I. Rootman and L. Towle (eds), *Drinking and casualties: Accidents, poisonings and violence in an international perspective*, Routledge, London, pp. 68-83

Midgely, J. (1979) Drinking and attitudes toward drinking in a muslim community. In M. Marshall (ed), *Beliefs, behaviors and alcoholic beverages: A cross-cultural survey*, University of Michigan Press, Ann Arbor, pp. 341-51

Miquez, H. (1983) Alcohol consumption levels in Costa Rica. *Bulletin of the Pan-American Health Organisation, 17,* 4

Nadim, A.A., S.I. Rahim and O.B. Salik (1980) Clinical aspects of alcohol addiction in the Sudan: July, 1975 – June, 1977. *British Journal of Addictions, 75,* 32-2

Nadim, A.A. and S.I. Rahim (1984) Clinical aspects of alcohol addition in the Sudan. *British Journal of Addictions, 79,* 449-50

National Institute on Alcohol Abuse and Alcoholism (1983) *Alcohol and health: Fifth special report to the U.S. Congress*, US Department of Health and Public and Public Services, Washington, DC

Natera, G. and C. Orozco (1981) Opiniones sobre el consums de alcohol en una comunidad semi-rural. *Solid Publico de Mexico, 23,* 473-82

Natera, G., M. Renconco, R. Almendares, H. Rosovsky and J. Almendares (1983) Comparacion transcultural de las constumbres y actitudes asociadas al uso de alcohol entre Honduras y Mexico. *Acta Psiquiatrica y Psicologica de America Latina, 29,* 2, 116-27

Odejide, A.O. and M.O. Olatawura (1977) Alcohol use in a Nigerian rural community. *African Journal of Psychiatry, 1,* 69-74

Odejide, A.O. (1978) Alcoholism: a major health hazard in Nigeria. *Nigerian Medical Journal, 9*, 230-232

Odejide, A.O., B.A. Ikuesan and J.U. Ohaeri (1985) Alcohol-related casualties: The Nigerian experience. Paper presented at the International Symposium on Alcohol-Related Casualties, Toronto, August 12-16, 1985

Owosina, F.A.O. (1981) The traffic scene in Nigeria—an African example, Document prepared for a conference on traffic accidents in developing countries, Mexico City, November, 1981

Puffer, P.R. and G.W. Griffith (1967) *Patterns of urban mortality*, Pan American Health Organization, Scientific Publication No. 151, Washington, DC

Roizen, R. (1981) *The World Health Organization study of community responses to alcohol-related problems: A review of cross-cultural findings*, Alcohol Research Group, Institute of Epidemiology and Behavioral Medicine, Berkeley, California

Room, R. (1984) Alcohol and ethnography: A case of problem deflation? *Current Anthropology, 25*, 2, 169-91

Rosovsky, H. (1989) Alcohol-related casualties and crime in Mexico: Description of reporting systems and results from a study. In: N. Giesbrecht, R. González, M. Grant, E. Österberg, R. Room, I. Rootman and L. Towle (eds), *Drinking and casualties: Accidents, poisonings and violence in an international perspective*, Routledge, London, pp. 260-74

Salik, O.E. (1977) Alcoholism in Khartoum Province, unpublished M.D. thesis, Khartoum University

Smart, R.G., G. de Natera and J.A. Bonilla (1980) A trial of a new method for studying drinking and driving problems in three countries of the Americas. *Bulletin of the Pan American Health Organization*, 14, 318-26

Tongue, E. (1976) Alcohol-related problems in some American countries. *African Journal of Psychiatry, 3*, 351-63

Wintemute, D. (1983) The size of the problem. In G. Wintemute *et al.* (eds), *Injury prevention in developing countries*, World Health Organization, Geneva, pp. 1-10

Section V:

RESEARCH AND POLICY

21

Research on Alcohol-Related Casualties and Public Policy Information Needs

Ron Draper

Solid empirical data on alcohol-related casualties are a prerequisite to rational and effective policy formulation. While necessary, however, existing data on alcohol casualties are by no means sufficient as a basis for public policy decision making. There are a great many shortcomings of such data—some of which are intrinsic to data collection itself, and others which are peculiar to the subject matter of interest. If data on alcohol-related casualties are to be responsive to the needs of policymakers, it is important to be aware of these limitations and to make efforts to overcome them.

Although issues relating to the identification, definition and measurement of alcohol-related casualties are intimately related to any discussion of the deficiencies of existing data, these are not the major shortcomings from a policy maker's perspective. The major shortcomings arise from the particularly narrow focus of much research into alcohol-related casualties, which is preoccupied with enumeration of events.

Simple enumeration of events provides only a limited and biased description of the problem, and one that is of comparatively little use to the policy maker. Alcohol-related casualties are a manifestation of social, institutional, political and economic relationships within society. They are an outgrowth of societal, cultural and group norms, public knowledge, attitudes, beliefs, values and perceptions relating to the these phenomena, and to a great many other factors. All are relevant data; all are required for adequate descriptions of the problem; all are important determinants of public policy outputs. At present, little of this information is available to the policy maker who is expected to deal with the problem. Not only does the information available from studies of alcohol-related casualties fail to satisfy the needs of policy makers, but the situation is unlikely to improve unless the present scope of research is expanded considerably. If studies of alcohol and casualties are to be useful adjuncts to the policy development process, they must expand the scope of enquiry to describe the phenomena in its entirety, including the set of social, political, institutional and economic relationships within which they exist. This requires a substantial effort to reconceptualise the problem from the perspective of policy makers.

Who Are the Policy Makers?

The relevant policy makers can be ministers of particular departments, senior bureaucrats, hospital administrators or public interest groups. If the purpose of research is to stimulate action in the form of policies designed to reduce the magnitude of the problem, the starting point of the research enterprise should be an identification of research issues from a policy perspective. At present, this is rarely the case—policy implications, if addressed at all in the course of a study, tend to be addressed at its conclusion rather than at its outset.

This frequently results in policy recommendations that are incomplete, devoid of context and directed towards no readily identifiable group of decision makers. If data on alcohol-related casualties are to be useful to policy makers, they must be generated with the needs of this particular target group clearly in mind. It is also important to have a clear understanding of the nature of public policy decision making in order to define research questions whose answers may be of practical assistance to policy makers. Policy making involves politics, values, issues, people and their perceptions as well as costs.

What Does Public Policy Decision Making Involve?

Policy Making Involves Politics

In many ways, politics and policies are inseparable. Etymologically, the same Greek root, *polis* appears in both 'policy' and 'politics'. In French, the word *politique* applies to both policy and politics. The term policy can be used to refer to the intentions of politicians, to the actions of government or even to the impact of government. Nevertheless, to speak of public policy concentrates attention upon issues that concern government, and political considerations. If information on alcohol-related casualties acquires meaning in a socio-political context, then it is within this context that data are 'interpretable' to a policy maker; in other words, data are primarily of social value through their link to politics and to issues.

Accordingly, if research on alcohol-related casualties is to be of value to policy makers, it must be recognised that not only alcohol-related casualties but also research on this subject are political phenomena. The need for research is the consequence of the political dimensions of the problem; the conduct of research is influenced by social, political and cultural restraints and biases; the use of research results occurs through their entry into the arena of public political debate.

Thus, for research results to be useful to a policy maker, the role of research within the political process must be clearly delineated—not only by the policy maker but also by the researcher. At present, researchers, under the guise of 'value-free' research, tend to divorce themselves from the political processes that give rise to and influence the need, the conduct, and the use of their research information. At the extreme, this attitude constitutes an abdication of responsibility on the part of the scientific community. Scientists are more than technicians—they are also experts whose input into the debates on, and resolution of, important social problems is essential.

Policy Making Involves Values

Policy making involves values and, often, the need for decision makers to mediate between conflicts of competing values. For example, the decision maker may seek to balance the positively valued privilege of drinking with the negatively valued consequences of alcohol-related damage. Unfortunately, these underlying values are rarely articulated, which diminishes greatly the use of the information from a policy perspective. If public policy decision making requires information, then decisions regarding what information is generated are intrinsically decisions about values. More important, perhaps, is the information that tends not to be generated in the course of normal research.

Research on alcohol-related casualties often focuses on the behavioural rather than the social, political, economic or cultural aspects of the problem. For example, research on impaired driving has focused attention disproportionately on the impaired driver at the expense of emphasis on these other considerations. Partly as a consequence of this emphasis, there is, perhaps, ample public support for more stringent penalties for impaired drivers, but little support for other social measures. Similarly, in areas such as spousel abuse, rape, assault and accidents on the job, emphasis upon the behavioural aspect of alcohol's involvement provides an extremely biased and limited portrayal. At the extreme, such an emphasis may even be detrimental to the victims and result in a 'blame-the-victim' mentality.

Not only does research on alcohol-related casualties have an implied explanatory bias, so do the related data collection mechanisms. The reluctance of women to report rape to the authorities is well-documented; this tendency may be exacerbated when alcohol is involved. These biases affect not only the reporting of violent acts to the police, but also the nature and extent of the victim's interaction with the medical and legal systems. In addition, social acceptability, vested interests and taboos often influence what is asked or what is recorded, as well as the validity of the responses, and so on.

Policies Arise from Issues

The intention of policy is to alleviate a certain state of affairs or to maintain a *status quo*. Understanding this entails identification of the factors that have produced a current state of affairs, identification of a desirable future state of affairs and the means through which this may be accomplished. Are the factors that give rise to alcohol-related casualties predominantly behavioural, social or structural? In most circumstances, this is a contentious issue that must be the subject of a social consensus if effective public policies are to be developed. Even if societal consensus can be attained regarding the existence of a problem and its fundamental determinants, there is always considerable debate regarding the effectiveness and acceptability of alternative means for dealing with it.

Although research on alcohol-related casualties implies these issues and indeed adopts a perspective on them, it does so only in a vague and indirect manner. This is insufficient since the underlying issues must be articulated explicitly and placed on the agenda of political controversy if public policy changes are to come about. For example, the problem of impaired driving had remained largely unchanged for over ten years and relegated to the back burners of public policy issues. Recently, however, it has again been elevated to the status of an issue, placed on the agenda of controversy and, consequently, has become the subject of a marked flurry of policy-making activity.

Policies Involve People and Perceptions

Who perceives alcohol-related casualties to be a problem? This is a key question since it conditions the nature and extent of the public policy response, in so far as it determines the demand for action, and the support for specific measures. It is immediately evident that public policy responses vary markedly across the spectrum of casualty events, from rape and spouse abuse, through violent crime, fire and accidents. To a large degree, these different responses are shaped by varying public and institutional perceptions of these problems, and of the range of 'acceptable' measures. Even more so, they are conditioned by the size, nature and characteristics of the groups who perceive themselves as having a vested interest in these problems and their eradication. Who are (or who perceive themselves to be) real or potential victims? This question involves the value of the group being harmed, their power to mobilise and fight for change, their size and their ability to advance demands upon the political system.

To whom is responsibility for existence of the problem assigned? Alcohol producers, distributors, advertisers and servers could be assigned responsibility for the problem. The existence of the problem could be linked to prevailing social and economic conditions or could be largely focused on the individuals who commit violent acts. Which groups accept or claim responsibility for dealing with the problem? The alcohol regulatory agencies, the legal system, the medical system all have a part to play. Again, data on alcohol-related casualties can be valuable if they are used to shape public perceptions of the problem, to further the advancement of demands for action, to mobilise support for specific initiatives and to legitimise the involvement of societal institutions. Otherwise, there is a danger that existence of data may be largely irrelevant, or may actually work against the injured group.

Policies Involve Costs

All policies whether of allocation, redistribution or regulation entail not only potential benefits, but also costs to individuals or groups, either through the imposition of direct costs on specific groups or the transfer of costs from one group to another. A good policy is not necessarily defined as one in which the benefits are greater than the costs, but one in which there are a few, if any, visible or controversial costs. Politicians are understandably reluctant to implement policies that impose visible or controversial costs upon groups capable of mobilising and articulating political opposition to the policy. Unfortunately, the costs of public policy initiatives are rarely considered carefully or within a political context by researchers. This results in policy recommendations that are often untenable to policy makers, and have little chance of adoption.

This failing is particularly characteristic of studies focused upon alcohol-related casualties and a logical consequence of their narrow focus. In particular, there is a tendency to articulate policy recommendations on the basis of their benefits (damage reduction) without adequate consideration of the costs of these measures, the groups upon whom these costs will be imposed, and so on.

Thus, studies of alcohol-related damage tend to draw attention to perpetrators of the damage (e.g. the impaired driver, the wife beater or child abuser), resulting in public support for stringent measures directed against these groups. Within this climate, which can be attributed in part to the narrow behavioural focus implied in research on alcohol casualties, it is difficult to generate public and political support for proposals to reduce this damage by reducing the availability of alcoholic beverages, since such proposals impose costs predominately upon those who do *not* perpetrate the damage.

Conclusions

Alcohol involvement in casualties is intrinsically a social and political phenomenon implicating politics, issues, people, perceptions, values and difficult decisions of allocation, distribution and regulation. Data on alcohol-related casualties that are generated independent of this context or that fail to address these areas explicitly are of limited value to the policy maker. Research on alcohol-related casualties is itself an inherently political undertaking, since it is the perception that a problem exists and that information is required for public policy measures that generally gives rise to research. The data themselves are of limited use outside of describing the problem fully in its social and political context, conditioning public perceptions about the problem, stimulating demands for action, and mobilising support for specific and politically viable alternatives which will result in realistic, implementable and effective policies acceptable not only to the decision makers, but also to the vast majority of the public.

A great deal of time and effort has been devoted by the research community to improving the accuracy of measurement of alcohol's involvement in casualties. It is only when the study of alcohol-related casualties is expanded to include consideration of the phenomenon in its entirety that it will fulfill the needs of the policy maker and contribute to societal consensus regarding acceptable means for its control.

What is implied here is the need for 'more research' not just on societal values, but on public perceptions, structural, economic and social determinants of alcohol-related problems, and a better definition of the environment within which alcohol-related problems emerge and are dealt with societally. The following are needed as well:

1. A redefinition of research within a socio-political context, including a clear definition of the role of research in the identification of and response to public problems. In other words, research on alcohol-related casualties is ultimately a political and social undertaking, rather than a technological, functional and neutral activity, and must be recognized as such.

2. A redefinition of the roles and responsibilities of researchers within a socio-political context. The researcher is inescapably more than a technocrat. The researcher is part of a political process linked to the need for information and expertise, public debate and problem resolution. Ultimately, the researcher cannot divorce the research function from the values implied in the problem. Attempts to do so inhibit efforts at problem resolution and are an abdication of the responsibility bestowed upon the researcher by society.

At present, when viewed from a policy maker's perspective, the information we have on alcohol-related casualties is not the information that we need for policy formulation. Unfortunately, there is little likelihood that this information will ever exist unless the research community is willing to adopt a greater share of the social responsibility for problem resolution.

Acknowledgement

The assistance of Reg Warren in the preparation of this paper is gratefully acknowledged.

22

Alcohol and Casualties: Divergences and Convergences in the Researcher's and Policy Maker's Agenda

Jacek Moskalewicz and Ignacy Wald

The relationship between alcohol and casualties has aroused much interest among researchers and policy makers because of its link to major issues and hazards facing contemporary society. The progress of civilisation via technology, communication and chemistry has increased the possibility of violent events hazardous to man. Injuries are becoming one of the major causes of morbidity and mortality, especially among young people and people of productive age. This increase is even more apparent when the decline of infectious disease and other causes of death is taken into account. Alcohol, for its part, plays an important role in many world affairs and issues of contemporary life, both in social and health-related terms. The relationship between alcohol and casualties reveals various essential problems and leads to questions of immense practical purport, even though these questions are often perceived differently by adherents of various disciplines.

It seems from the range of papers in this volume that policy makers and scholars from the social, medical, biochemical and legal sciences are equally interested in this subject. This is the fundamental convergence in policy makers' and researchers' agendas. However, this is only a superficial indication of a deeper convergence. There are many convergent points that can be found useful and acceptable for policy makers, and, more precisely, there are many issues where convergence enhances effective performance. Let us briefly review those points where the convergence between the policy makers' and researchers' point of view is most important.

The first is the very selection of the subject. It seems to be particularly vital that the policy maker and the researcher come to a general agreement regarding the established needs, as well as the general values, involved. The process of coming to an agreement ties in with a common system of values and with what both the policy maker and the researcher, as members of the same society, consider to be important. Researchers and policy makers are linked by their mutual desire to improve the quality of life in society. There must first be agreement that the number of injuries and accidents in society should diminish. But preventive policies recommended in recent years do not always find approval in the eyes of the public. To be further developed, these policies need to employ arguments more convincing than those used thus far. This may involve drawing society's attention to the relationship between alcohol consumption and such dramatic events as casualties in which victims are wounded or killed. Alcohol researchers, too, while looking for ways of raising their prestige among scientists and the general public, may find that research on accidents and injuries will provide strong evidence that the problems they study are serious and worthy of concern and support.

Another important point of convergence is that both policy makers and researchers expect the effects of these activities to be used in practical application. This is the significance for the policy maker, as it justifies his decisions and consequent actions. For the researcher it is an important social gratification since success in this field contributes to his prestige and paves the way for resources for further studies. Prevention of injuries and casualties and, by the same token, the elimination of the number of fatalities is particularly gratifying from the point of view of social utility. There are opportunities here for researchers and policy makers to cooperate. The role of research is to define the scope of hazards, risk groups and risk situations and work out general and specific proposals for preventive measures. Provided with such data, the policy makers can take steps towards reducing accidents and their adverse effects.

The third and very significant point of convergence is the need for evaluation of policy measures. The politician or policy maker needs the researcher to prove that a given measure is effective or to prompt the direction which should be taken. In achieving this, the researcher is likely to encounter many issues of interest for himself. Developing evaluative research, he not only performs useful services, but also joins the critical current in science.

It does not, however, follow that the situations and perspectives of the policy maker and researcher are identical. There is no such thing as a single point of view or a single value system among policy makers. A finance minister and health minister usually work according to different value systems; as do ministers of agriculture and home affairs. While all of these ministers serve society, they see social responsibilities in different perspectives which are determined by their particular agencies. A similar divergence occurs among researchers. For a biological or medical researcher, reduction of direct biological and health detriments is most important in the formulation of aims; for social researchers, it is social factors that are most crucial.

However, if we compare policy makers and researchers in more general terms, it becomes clear that policy makers are more concerned with social expectations and the proliferation of social stereotypes. Hence, in many societies, measures aimed at preventing alcohol-related accidents are treated within the convention of 'combating alcoholism'. It is necessary to ensure that these divergences do not reduce the breadth of perspective. Narrowly specialised research on the role of alcohol in casualties is certainly useful, but it should not over-shadow the real size and nature of hazards. Although the role of alcohol in casualties is quite considerable, many surveys show that its share in lesions is even higher than routine statistics would suggest. It has to be borne in mind that there are a few other independent sources of accidents aside from alcohol. These sometimes tend to be overlooked by policy makers, researchers and the general public when the role of alcohol is articulated too strongly, often because these other sources of injuries and accidents are politically embarrassing and harder to manipulate. When alcohol is identified as the main cause of an accident, it is a specific individual who is found guilty. This individualisation of the cause, combined with the neglect of other causes, can lead to ineffectiveness of practical preventive measures.

Another source of divergence involves the fact that policy makers most often tend to expect swift research results, while the quality of the research may be in substantial cognitive values which will bear fruit only in the long-term future. Thus a very important factor is the independence of the researcher in the process of evaluation of practical measures. It is quite natural for an author of an innovation to expect the best results possible. Here the obedience to the rigorous rules of scientific research can hardly be over-emphasized. Any deviation from the autonomy of scientific research can produce dangerous consequences, both moral and practical. It is in the interest of the policy maker to foster both the professionalism and the autonomy of the researcher. At the turn of the nineteenth century, there lived a Polish painter, very popular but perhaps not of the highest calibre, called Jan Styka. He was very religious and a story has it that he was kneeling when painting one of his pictures of Jesus. When Jesus appeared to him and said: 'Listen Styka. Don't paint me on your knees. Do paint me well.' The same recommendation applies to the researcher.

A potential source of conflict can arise with the formulation of research directions and their findings. The policy maker who pays for the study can come to the researcher with a ready-made diagnosis of the situation based on his own ideology, common sense or a mixture of both.

All he wants from the world of science is to confirm his convictions. A good example is a belief, not too rare in socialist countries, that alcoholism is a relic of the old system and should gradually disappear with the advancement of socialism. Consequently, the fight against alcoholism is considered a part of the political struggle with the relics of the past. Such views have more than once borne heavily on what was expected of the researcher.

The role of ideology in defining the problems to be dealt with in scientific research projects is most manifest in the times of significant political change or when financial resources become scarce. This was, for instance, the case in the United States in 1980, when the share of spending on social research was drastically cut, the priority having shifted to biological and medical projects. This particular attempt at changing the social definitions of the problem seems to have proved a failure, since social research came back to favour under the name of 'epidemiological investigations'.

Similar reactions can occur when appraising research findings. Upon receiving research results for assessment, the policy maker may select those results which tally with his convictions and ignore those which are at variance with his expectations. Quite often, the policy maker has a vision of the measures that have to be taken to solve a given problem. If he expects them to be unpopular or meet with resistance from some part of public opinion, he turns to the researcher to provide him with scientific legitimisation of his scheme. Under these circumstances, the money earmarked for the research will find its way to where the likelihood of meeting the specific demand of the commission is greater.

It must not be forgotten that, like the policy maker, the researcher is also a member of society. And like the policy maker, he is exposed to certain pressures and to similar stereotypes. The choice of a problem area for research, the methodology used, conclusions and practical recommendations are not free from the effects of the value system accepted by the researcher. The solution seems to be not to attempt to detract or avoid these values and thus, as it were, rise above society, but to become aware of this peculiarity so very apparent in social sciences. It is by all means honest and desirable for the researcher, while presenting the findings of his study, to inform his readers about the system of values he subscribes to.

In conclusion, it is difficult to write a simple, precise and all-embracing prescription for a good relationship between policy makers and scientific researchers. It can be said with great certainty that their mutual understanding, common goals, and concern with the social utility of science are among the most important areas of convergence. It is, however, indispensable to maintain and protect the autonomy of the researcher, to pay attention to his findings and to the professional quality of his services. These complex relations can and should themselves constitute a field for scientific reflection.

POSTSCRIPT

Postscript

Future Directions in Research and Policy

Norman Giesbrecht, René González, Marcus Grant, Esa Österberg,
Robin Room, Irving Rootman and Leland Towle

The work of the policy maker, administrator of service or practitioner can be facilitated by information that is accurate, comprehensive, representative, relevant and where the context of the casualties can be interpreted. Conversely, the policy maker, administrator of service and practitioner can initiate or support new procedures or projects that will facilitate the work of the researcher and directly or indirectly lead to preventive actions.

Directions for research, noted below, reflect or build on the other chapters in this volume. Several suggestions are offered, involving a combination of research lines and methodology.

General Prevalence and Social Impact of Casualties

We propose that the conventional scope of research into alcohol-related casualties be expanded by devoting greater attention to the general population. This attention should not only involve victims, or perpetrators, but also 'third parties' — others who were affected. Greater attention should also be devoted to casualties *per se* in order to better understand the relative importance of drinking along with many other factors. Key questions for these lines of inquiry would include: How many have experienced accidents, poisonings or violence over a recent time period (e.g. twelve months)? What were considered the key contributory factors? What actions were taken by the subjects, by others?

General population social surveys are a key vehicle for providing information on more common disruptions or events such as accidents or fights, and provide an important contrast to the more specific foci of studies based on emergency service clientele, in-patient statistics or mortality data.

Another approach, discussed in more detail elsewhere (Room 1987), focuses on the institutions which typically respond to casualties. Here repeated sampling of the caseload of a number of institutions over short periods on, say, an annual or biannual basis provides information on the differences across institutions (case-load characteristics, information and storage arrangements, case-management, etc.) and an opportunity to document changes over time.

Studies which combine several sources of information, for example, data from general population surveys and from emergency service clientele, provide unique opportunities to address both substantive and methodological questions.

Studies of High-Risk Populations or Situations

Research into the groups or populations with above-average casualty rates and/or a higher proportion involving alcohol should be encouraged. This may involve studies into certain groups of heavy drinkers, e.g. heavy drinking among single adult males, or related to certain occupations or activities.

Although aggregated data from hospital or police records can provide some indication of the characteristics and circumstances, special studies involving primary data and case-control or comparisons need to be encouraged. Also, ethnographic techniques, such as unobtrusive observation or participation in the sub-culture or group, are key approaches to understanding casualty events and the responses to them, and serve as a basis for developing suggestions for prevention or more effective emergency management techniques.

Natural Experiments

For a number of reasons, such as gradual secular changes, covariation of series data and confounding variables, it is usually difficult to investigate the relationships among aggregate rates of consumption, drinking styles and casualties. Natural phenomena which involve the dramatic manipulation of one of the variables provide unique opportunities in this respect. In the past casualties have not typically been a focus of the studies, except, in some cases, motor vehicle accidents.

Future work in this area should strive to give a more central place to observations involving both primary and secondary data on casualties, including domestic, work and transportation events. Natural experiment opportunities may involve not only dramatic changes in the availability of alcohol, via, for example, strikes, price shifts or changes in the distribution arrangement, but also changes in occupational or leisure activities which lead to a convergence or separation of drinking and risk-taking opportunities.

In order to encourage these studies and increase the potential for findings to be obtained from them, further work is required on design options and the minimal data set required. Unfortunately, since these opportunities cannot be predicted long in advance and arise with little notice, finding and mobilising resources quickly enough to establish baseline information and do an adequate study are major hurdles. Hence the jurisdictions where these studies can effectively be conducted are limited by these practical matters.

Prevention Demonstration Projects

An underlying assumption in casualty research is that a better data base will be a useful resource in prevention or treatment responses. This can be explored through various routes, including experimental or quasi-experimental studies where the manipulated variable is the level and/or type of information provided to the subjects. For example, some patients (victims or perpetrators) could be provided with information on their BAC, or other aspects of the casualty, and see if in follow-up there was any difference in the risk-taking or drinking of this group compared to a similar group that was not provided with this information. Similarly, medical doctors could be told about the BAC of clients, and their actions studied in contrast to those physicians who did not have this information.

At a broader level, community-based information on casualty rates could provide a basis for health promotion and problem prevention initiatives. Demonstration projects might be undertaken on enhancing prevention initiatives via using local information about levels and patterns of casualties: for example, does the monitoring of — and dissemination of information on — local casualty rates, severity of casualties and/or types of events lead to more effective action?

Also, more naturalistically oriented studies might be undertaken — communities with a high interest in casualties and their prevention could be examined in comparison to jurisdictions where there is little interest in this topic.

Policy Issues

Three generic policy issues warrant greater attention in the future: information and research, education and prevention.

Promoting Documentation and Research

With regard to the former, casualties need to be given a more prominent place in data systems of health care institutions. As indicated in various chapters of this volume, casualties are a major contributor to potential years of life lost and to person-days in hospital. In order to facilitate both epidemiological study and preventive action, basic information on the event and the person involved might be collected in a form amenable to aggregation. Steps should also be taken toward routine monitoring of BAC or apparent ethyl sign among emergency service patients. The jurisdiction, the resources on hand and the procedures already in place will have a bearing on the route that should be chosen. In some cases, a repeated sampling approach, for example all clients seen in one week, may be the most effective. In others, procedures piloted in a few key health facilities may lead the way to more routine implementation. Or, placing the procedures on the agenda of networks, such as associations planning a trauma registry, could be another route. However, policy changes will likely be required before routine information is available about the alcohol component in casualties.

Facilitating Education and Training

Policy initiatives should also be undertaken in the areas of education and training. Health professionals, including doctors and nurses, should be provided with up-to-date information about the roles of drinking in casualties, the characteristics of the patients most likely to be presenting with alcohol-related trauma, and the confounding impact of alcohol on diagnoses and treatment. This information can be provided in the course of initial training and/or, on a more local basis, from the results of on-site studies at a hospital or clinic that investigate drinking and casualties.

Education initiatives aimed at the general population and especially at those groups that are most at risk of experiencing trauma should also be encouraged in the interests of public health. This would involve innovative and highly focused efforts, considering the wide range in the types of incidents and the differences in ages and other demographic characteristics of those affected by casualties.

Prevention Initiatives

Finally, prevention initiatives such as policies controlling drinking in connection with certain sports or in connection with work activities, or more general alcohol regulatory measures, provide an avenue for reducing the rates of drinking-related casualties. Exploratory or trial initiatives are warranted in a number of areas, including, for example, documentation of drinking-related accidents involving mass public transportation, or major work-related accidents in which multiple deaths or injuries occurred. Consideration should also be given to prevention strategies oriented to effective handling and treatment of the casualty once it has occurred, including temporary self-care procedures and efficient contact with emergency services.

In some populations, such as among aboriginal peoples, which, on average, have extremely high rates of casualties, a large proportion of which involve drinking, dramatic changes in socio-economic living conditions and mores about alcohol use and drunken comportment will likely be required in order to realize a significant reduction in casualty rates.

In conclusion, one can safely predict that research on drinking and casualties will continue even if adequate routine data collection arrangements are not available, or the research findings are not applied in educational and prevention programs. It is also highly likely that policy decisions will be made even if the research to justify them has not been undertaken, or if they run contrary to the available research findings. Nevertheless, perhaps from time to time, there will be greater opportunities in the future for complementary initiatives in research and policy in order to curtail drinking-related casualties.

© 1989 Norman Giesbrecht

References

Room, R. (1987) Models for future work on alcohol's role in casualties. In N. Giesbrecht and H. Fisher (Eds), *Alcohol-related casualties*, Addiction Research Foundation, Toronto, pp. 85-94

APPENDICES

APPENDICES

Appendix A

The Alcohol Dimension in Casualty Reporting Systems

Honey Fisher

In all countries around the world, casualties play a major role in morbidity and mortality. In both Canada and the United States, casualties are a leading cause of death. The largest number of deaths and injuries are the result of motor vehicle accidents and, consequently, a great deal of research and public concern has focused on the relationship between drinking and driving. Other causes of fatal and non-fatal unintentional injury include falls, burns, fires, drownings, recreational accidents, and occupation-related accidents. Although these accidents occur in a variety of settings, alcohol is frequently a common element.

Unfortunately, under-reporting of alcohol involvement and other difficulties involved in obtaining accurate data make the precise extent of alcohol's role in casualties unknown. Because this role is an unknown quantity, the significance of alcohol-related casualties is underestimated compared to chronic alcohol disorders. Systematic procedures for reporting and recording alcohol involvement are necessary in order to identify the scope of alcohol-related problems and effectively manage and reduce them. Current data collection and reporting practices, for the most part, are scattered and fragmented. The development of a finely tuned, centralised system that integrates information from various sources and jurisdictions would facilitate decision-making, policy initiatives and preventive programming for alcohol-related injury, and would be a national investment.

The Casualty Reporting Systems Questionnaire was developed with the intention of examining the state of casualty reporting systems especially as they relate to alcohol within different countries around the world.

The design of the questionnaire was a group effort: various people, some of whom were from the planning committee for the International Symposium on Alcohol-Related Casualties (*see* Giesbrecht and Fisher 1987), offered suggestions as to the content and format.

It was clear from the completed questionnaire that it was not nearly as detailed as it could have been, once the complexity of the actual reporting systems became apparent. Efforts to complete the questionnaires highlighted the difficulties in locating the necessary information.

The tables that follow present a brief overview of the reporting systems from the ten jurisdictions that returned the questionnaire. The responses range from within North and South America, the Caribbean, Africa, Europe, Australia and New Zealand.

Table A.1 presents a list of various casualty reporting systems and the jurisdictions that indicated having such systems. In addition, the table indicates the jurisdictions in which it is mandatory to report any involvement of alcohol in casualties.

Table A.2 outlines what methods of alcohol detection would be used for various reporting systems in different jurisdictions.

If examined closely, we would probably find that no country has a fully adequate reporting system for every health and social institution, but that nearly every country has some type of reporting system, albeit simple. It is a rarity to find a system that has both a broad scope and a deep information base. The breadth should cover a range of reporting systems and the depth should include casualty-specific and alcohol-related casualty requirements. In those countries with relatively good reporting systems, it may be best to emphasize improving the existing systems and enhancing the collection of alcohol statistics, while in those countries with few or no reporting systems, the emphasis should perhaps be placed on setting up such systems.

Although data for a reporting system may be collected in a systematic fashion, there are often gaps and considerable variation in the quality of the data both between and within jurisdictions. As a result, there are few indicators with widely accepted validity and international comparability. Of greatest concern is that these data are widely used to estimate the types and extent of alcohol-related damage and to provide direction for control policies and prevention programmes.

The data on which reporting systems rely are collected by those who deal in the course of daily work with health and social problems (i.e. doctors and other health workers, police, fire departments, etc.). For many reasons, however, alcohol's involvement in health and social problems appears to be systematically under-reported in the statistics. Although, in theory, it is often mandatory to include any alcohol dimension within a reported casualty, the reporting of any alcohol involvement is usually (or generally) discretionary.

Table A.1: *The alcohol dimension in casualty reporting systems for different jurisdictions*

Casualty reporting system	Jurisdiction	Alcohol dimension reported
Traffic accident statistics (police)	1 +: 12 (all)	2, 3, 4, 5, 6, 7, 9, 10, 12
Mortality reporting systems	1, 2, 4, 5, 6, 7, 8, 9, 10, 11, 12	2, 4, 5, 6, 7, 9, 10, 12
Hospital utilisation/ discharge statistics	2, 3, 4, 5, 6, 7, 8, 10, 11, 12	2, 5, 6, 7, 8, 10, 11, 12
Police case reports/statistics	1, 3, 4, 5, 7, 8, 9, 10, 11, 12	4, 5, 7, 9, 10, 12
Poison control centres	1, 4, 5, 6, 7, 8, 9, 12	1, 5, 6, 7, 12
Workers' compensation/ employee health systems	1, 3, 5, 6, 7, 8, 9, 10, 12	9, 12
Fire department statistics	4, 5, 7, 9, 10, 11	5
Casualty/emergency service systems	4, 5, 6, 8, 9, 10, 12	5, 8, 10, 12
Traffic accident statistics (health)	1, 3, 4, 5, 7, 11, 12	5, 12
Treatment clinics	5, 7, 8, 10, 11, 12	5, 7, 8, 10, 12
Health, life and casualty insurance reporting systems	1, 5, 6, 8, 9	6, 9
Ambulance service statistics	5, 7	5
Others		
Addiction research centre	5, 10	10
Aviation accident statistics	1, 12	1, 12
Consumer product safety commission	12	
Coroner's Reports	5, 7	5
Drug abuse warning system	12	12
Surf lifesaving association resuscitation statistics	1	1
Women's refuges	7	

Key:
1.	Australia	7.	New Zealand
2.	Western Australia	8.	Nigeria
3.	New South Wales	9.	Poland
4.	Buenos Aires[a]	10	Sudan
5.	Canada	11.	Trinidad and Tobago
6.	Finland	12.	U.S.A.

[a] Buenos Aires reporting systems (no general systems for Argentina as a whole)

Table A.2: *Methods of alcohol detection in reporting systems for different jurisdictions*

Jurisdiction	Hosp.	Mort.	Police	Poison	Fire	MVA	OTA	Work	Rx clinic	Emerg.	Other
Australia	3	2	1, 5, 6	1, 2, 3, 5, 6		1, 5, 6					1, 5, 6
Buenos Aires		1, 2, 3, 4, 6									
Canada	1, 2, 3, 4, 5	1, 2, 3, 4, 6	1, 2, 3, 4, 5	1, 2, 3, 4, 5		1, 3, 5, 6					
Finland	7	1, 7		5, 6		1, 3, 5				3	
New Zealand	1, 3, 6, 7	1, 3, 6, 7	2, 3, 5, 6			1, 3, 5, 6					
Nigeria	2, 6								2, 6		2, 6
Poland		1	1, 3, 5, 6				1, 3, 5, 6	1, 3, 5, 6			
Sudan			1, 3, 5, 6						2, 3, 5, 6		
United States	3, 4	1, 6, 7	5, 6	3, 5	1	1, 3, 6, 7	1, 2, 3, 4, 5, 6		1, 2, 5, 6	2	

[a] Abbreviations for hospital morbidity, mortality, police, poison control centres, fire departments, motor vehicle accidents, other transport accidents (i.e. aviation), workers' compensation agencies, treatment clinic, emergency departments, others

Key:
1. blood-alcohol concentration
2. drinking history
3. notation on form
4. other reference on form
5. self-report
6. witness
7. other method of detection

There are several aspects which confound a simple relationship between an alcohol-related event and the record that appears in official statistics (Giesbrecht *et al.* 1985). These intervening aspects do not render these statistics worthless, however they should be kept in mind when assessing the utility and meaning of these data.

One early source of deflation in the number of recorded cases with alcohol-specific involvement is the fact that not every alcohol-related event or condition which might warrant official intervention (i.e. hospitalization, police, workers' compensation, etc.) does in fact do so. Many go unnoted by institutions or agencies and accordingly do not result in a recorded event.

Biases in reporting can also occur when decisions are made as to the circumstances under which alcohol involvement is to be tested and/or recorded following an injury. In occupational-related injuries or deaths, alcohol involvement is seldom determined and/or reported because of potential complications for employees, management, medical and legal professionals, and insurance claims.

Cultural mores and social pressures are strong influences on reporting practices. If heavy drinking is the typical pattern in a community, then physicians and other health professionals may pay little heed to a patient's drinking behaviour and there may be a tendency not to note secondary diagnoses that are alcohol-specific.

Classification policies present a potential source of deflation in the incidence of alcohol-specific diagnoses. Reporting systems tend to shy away from assigning alcohol as a sufficient cause and lean more toward alcohol involvement as a conditional cause, or a residual category when no other cause seems apparent.

Further error can occur during the stages of information transfer and conversion, critical steps in the chain of events beginning with a medical condition and culminating in an official medical record. During these stages, medical record coders must make subjective decisions when translating information from patients' files into International Classification of Diseases (ICD) categories and this process can lead to error in general.

As discussed earlier, the best reporting systems will offer both breadth and depth. The model proposed by Aitken and Zobeck (1989, *see* Appendix B) has both these qualities and serves as a good reference tool for jurisdictions wanting to improve their reporting systems.

References

Aitken, S.S., and T.S. Zobeck (1989) A proposed model establishing an alcohol-related casualty surveillance system. In N. Giesbrecht, R. González, M. Grant, E. Österberg, R. Room, I. Rootman and L. Towle (eds), *Drinking and Casualties: Accidents, poisonings and violence in an international perspective*, London, Routledge, pp. 409-22

Giesbrecht, N. (1986) Alcohol and injuries: Quality of information and research agenda. Prepared for the Conference on Research Issues in the Prevention of Alcohol-Related Injuries, Prevention Research Center, Berkeley, California, March 2-4, 1986

Giesbrecht, N., and H. Fisher (eds) (1987) *Alcohol-related casualties*, Toronto, Addiction Research Foundation

Giesbrecht, N., G. Conroy and H. Fisher (1985) Collecting and reporting alcohol-related morbidity statistics. In R.B. Cromier and B. Reimer (eds), *Alcohol, drugs and tobacco: An international perspective—past, present and future. Proceedings of the 34th International Congress on Alcoholism and Drug Dependence, August 4-10, 1985, Calgary*, Alberta Alcohol and Drug Abuse Commission, Edmonton

Appendix B

A Proposed Model Establishing an Alcohol-Related Casualty Surveillance System

Sherrie S. Aitken and Terry S. Zobeck

Background

There is a momentum building to support the epidemiologic investigation of morbid and mortal outcomes of accidental injury and suicidal and homicidal acts. The force of this momentum comes from the great strides made by the developed nations in the eradication of chronic disease.

Improvements in productivity, standards of living, environmental sanitation, personal sanitation, public health measures and the capacity for medical intervention, coupled with a decrease in internecine warfare, and the invention and use of pesticides and chemotherapy (Kitagawa and Hauser 1973) have affected what Omran (1977) has called the 'epidemiologic transition' Infant and childhood infectious diseases have largely been conquered. As a result, chronic disease has become the focus of scientific research. In 1901, 46 per cent of all deaths in the United States were attributable to chronic disease. By 1955, the level had risen to 81 per cent (Lilienfeld and Gilford 1966). Age-specific mortality for the elderly, i.e. those most susceptible to death from chronic disease, showed a substantial decline during the past decade (Brody 1983). With the understanding that injury, like disease, occurs through manipulatable non-random patterns of events, has come an effort to erode it as a prominent cause of death.

Americans die at the rate of 140,000 per year and are disabled or disfigured at a cost of $75 to $100 billion per year through injury. Injury may account for as much as 41 per cent of the total number of years of potential life lost (YPLL), almost as much as is attributable to heart disease, cancer, and all other diseases combined. A lower estimate of 39 per cent

411

was reported in 1983 (MMWR Annual Summary). The YPLL from all causes was reported as 9,429,000, with accidents accounting for 2,367,000, and homicides and suicides for 1,314,000 of the total. Non-fatal injury results in personal, family and societal loss. Up to the age of 44, injury is the leading cause of death (Committee on Trauma Research 1985).

Falling birth rates and declining mortality rates among older persons conspire to squeeze the economically productive middle-aged population. A measure of the non-productive segment of the population is the dependency ratio, defined as the proportion of the population under age 15 and over 65, divided by the number remaining in between. As a society matures, the ratio increases with a growing majority of the dependents being elderly (Espenshade and Braun, 1981). The cost of financing public transfers to youth is about one-third that of the cost of financing transfers to the elderly. Furthermore, whereas public transfers to youth increase human capital, public transfers to the elderly have been regarded economically as maintenance costs (Clark and Spengler 1978). In an aging society, the United States must safeguard the health and longevity of its working population or it will cost the well-being of every member of the society. The greatest threat to that well-being today is the high incidence of casualties.

The 1990 Public Health Service Objectives were developed by the US Department of Health and Human Services. They provide a mandate for high priority research focussing upon the role of alcohol as a risk factor in injury prevention and in the control of stress and violent behaviours. Furthermore, they seek to develop detailed plans for a uniform system of reporting injuries for 75 per cent or more of the states by the year 1990 (NIAAA n.d.)

Justification for a National Reporting System

The development of an adequate epidemiologic data base is dependent upon answers to two questions:

1. Why might national level epidemiologic data on alcohol-involved casualties be needed?

2. What kind of data would be desirable?

The answers to each depend upon the level of effort made to associate alcohol, casualty events, and outcomes. At the most basic level of inquiry, the simple incidence and prevalence of alcohol-associated casualty would be determined. At an intermediate level, populations at special risk would be identified. The investigation of associated ecological factors would require a third level of analysis. At the point where the effect of intervention strategies would be evaluated or where monitoring of alcohol-involved casualties would be undertaken, a surveillance system would have to be implemented.

In response to the first question, we propose that a national epidemiologic investigation of injury is needed because injury is a prominent cause of death and curtails many lives. A complex interdisciplinary research effort is required to identify and eventually to intervene in injury mechanisms and injury outcomes. A national investigation of casualties will require the integration of currently fragmented casualty data collection and analysis efforts as well as the development of a fine-tuned mechanism for integrating information from various sources and jurisdictions. The lack of a cohesive, comprehensive data base at this point requires our use of ranges to describe the risk of alcohol involvement, which is a term that has been defined differently from study to study. Studies may differ in the way in which alcohol use is determined and whether alcohol use data are collected on non-victims involved in the casualty event. The overall level of risk of alcohol involvement has been estimated at between 30 and 50 percent (Roizen 1982). Wide ranges of estimates for specific casualty events, currently available, suggest that national estimates cannot be attained without a national effort and that such an effort should provide for geographic disaggregation.

Key considerations include what data should be collected and how alcohol involvement can be measured. The Fatal Accident Reporting System (FARS) serves as good model for the assessment of alcohol involvement in a casualty. FARS obtains observational data on the investigating officers' judgment of alcohol involvement (yes or no) and ratio level data on blood alcohol concentration (BAC) in fatal motor vehicle accidents. Having both allows the use of one in lieu of the other or as a check against the other. Both have limitations.

The observational assessment of alcohol involvement on fatal motor vehicle accidents has been associated with higher BACs. This suggests a threshold effect. If only observational data were recorded, low level alcohol involvement would probably be missed. The literature on injuries including, but not limited to, traffic fatalities suggests that low to moderate BACs are associated with an excess of fatal outcomes involving, for example, cardiac injury (Brodner *et al.* 1981) or CNS damage (Liedtke and DeMuth 1975). Thresholds of levels of BAC for excess injury involvement or increased damage resulting from injury may vary by person factors and casualty type and severity. Therefore, BAC would be both a more sensitive indicator and one which could be used to explore ideas about dose-response or threshold.

The practical limitations of relying upon BAC have to do with the relationship between the time of the serious event, the time of the test and the rate of its being administered. If the test is delayed for a person who is alive, it can underestimate the blood-alcohol concentration at the time of the event. If delayed in a person who has died, the methane produced by decaying tissue (MEOH) can give an erroneously high BAC (ETOH), although these can be distinguished if care is taken to do so (Aarens and Roizen 1977).

The rate of being tested varies with person and environmental factors, casualty type and severity, source of information (e.g. emergency room data, medical examiners' office data, police report data) and the state in which the casualty occurred. Therefore, it seems prudent to use both observational and BAC measurements of alcohol involvement.

Data adequate for estimating the incidence and prevalence of alcohol-associated casualties would minimally contain information on the time of day, the day of the week, the location of the casualty event, the type of casualty event (by agent, place of occurrence, type of injury, degree of injury, duration of injury and intention) and whether alcohol use at the time of the incident was suspected or confirmed. Relatively rare casualty events could be oversampled to increase the validity and reliability of the estimates.

The identification of particular populations at risk for alcohol-associated casualties of various types would require a sophisticated data collection effort. In addition to the information required for simple estimates of incidence and prevalence, socio-demographic information would have to be collected and the sampling scheme would have to allow for description of risk by geographic unit.

Another level of inquiry identified earlier would analyse the association of casualty events with other variables thought to be within the complex causal nexus surrounding them. Ideally, the data collection process would provide for the data to be matched for casualty and non-casualty events by person, casualty and environmental factors, alcohol involvement, situational context, the time of day and the day of the week.

Review of the Data Systems Currently in Operation

A wide range of casualty categories is represented by the current data bases that routinely collect information on casualties (*see* Table B.1).There is, however, a tremendous amount of variation among the systems with respect to their usefulness in tracking casualties, in general, and alcohol-involved casualties, in particular.

The Fatal Accident Reporting System (FARS), the National Accident Sampling System (NASS), the Mortality Data System (MDS) — from which the multiple cause mortality data base is constructed — and the

Table B.1:   *U.S. national level casualty data bases*

Data base	Operating agency	Coverage	Alcohol determination	Percentage of cases in which alcohol involvement is determined	Requirement of reporting
Fatal Accident Reporting System	National Highway Traffic Safety Administration	Census[a]	BAC, police reported	42	mandatory
National Accident Sampling System	National Highway Traffic Safety Administration	Probability Sample[b]	BAC, DWI citation, police reported	?	mandatory
Aviation Accident Data System	National Transportation Safety Bureau	Census[a]	BAC (dead pilots only)	100	mandatory
Hospital Discharge Survey	National Center for Health Statistics	Probability Sample[b]	ICD codes	?	voluntary
Occupational Safety and Health Administration Injury & Insurance Form	Bureau of Labor Statistics	Census (fatalities only)[a]	Not required, seldom reported	?	mandatory (deaths only)
Mortality Data System (Multiple Cases)	National Center for Health Statistics	Census[a]	ICD codes	?	mandatory
American Assoc. of Poison Control Centers National Data Collection	Poison Control Center	Sample (non-probability)[c]	Self-reported	100	voluntary
American Assoc. of Railways Monthly Frequency Report	Railway Companies	Sample (non-probability)[c]	None	N/A	voluntary
Drug Abuse Warning Network	National Institute on Drug Abuse	Sample (non-probability)[c]	Self-reported (only associated with drug mention)	?	voluntary
National Electronic Injury Surveillance System	Consumer Product Safety Commission	Sample (non-probability)[c]	None	N/A	voluntary

[a] 100 percent of cases are collected
[b] Cases are statistically selected and weighted to produce national estimates
[c] Nonstatistically selected cases, not suitable for producing national estimates

Hospital Discharge Survey (HDS) have proven to be the most useful to epidemiologists.

FARS reports annually on approximately 40,000 fatal traffic accidents while NASS collects data on a probability sample of 10,000 fatal accidents which are then weighted, producing a national estimate of 5.8 million yearly traffic accidents. The FARS and NASS contain a wealth of data on the circumstances surrounding traffic accidents and those individuals involved in them, including possible alcohol involvement, which is measured with a BAC test or by the judgement of the investigating officer. However, the determination of alcohol involvement is not routinely and consistently made in either fatal or, especially, non-fatal traffic accidents. This under-reporting makes it difficult to accurately estimate the prevalence of alcohol in these events. These two data bases also lack crucial demographic and socio-demographic variables, particularly race and ethnic origin.

The HDS is a probability sample of 225,000 short-stay hospital discharges which is weighted, producing a national estimate of over 30 million annual discharges. The MDS is a census of the nearly 2 million registered deaths occurring each year in the United States. They record alcohol involvement as either the underlying or contributing cause of death with the standard International Classification of Disease (ICD) codes (e.g. cirrhosis of liver - 571, alcoholic psychosis - 291, alcohol dependence syndrome - 303). But like the FARs and the NASS, they are deficient in their reporting of alcohol involvement in discharges (HDS) and deaths (MDS). Physicians and medical examiners are reluctant to code alcohol as a cause of death either because they want to avoid stigmatising the victim or they do not fully appreciate the importance of identifying the role of alcohol in illness and disease. Such under-reporting of alcohol involvement hinders accurate estimation of prevalence and incidence rates.

The remaining systems are even more seriously flawed for use in alcohol studies than those described above. The US Occupational Safety and Health Administration's insurance form system requires employers to collect data on all work-place injuries and fatalities, but only requires that the fatality data be reported (although the Bureau of Labor Statistics does estimate rates of injury for full-time workers). There is no specific entry made for alcohol involvement in either case; therefore, it is seldom mentioned.

Reporting to the American Association of Railways monthly frequency report, the Poison Control Center and the National Electronic Injury Surveillance System (reporting on product-associated injuries) is voluntary and, therefore, coverage is incomplete. Because reporting to these systems is voluntary and varies in completeness from year to year, national-level prevalence and incidence rates of these events cannot be determined. Additionally, the Railway and Product Injury Systems do not report involvement while the Poison Control Center's system relies upon self-reports of alcohol involvement.

The Drug Abuse Warning Network is a non-random sample of emergency room episodes of drug abuse (including abuse-associated casualties). Alcohol is self-reported only in association with drug usage. Approximately 740 hospitals and 80 medical examiner's offices in 27 standard metropolitan statistical areas report on about 100,000 drug episodes (3,500 of which are deaths) each year. Because reporting is voluntary and unrepresentative of the country as a whole, national-level prevalence and incidence rates cannot be calculated with these data.

Some of the limitations inherent in these data systems can be overcome by merging or matching two or more systems. An NIAAA (DuFour *et al.* 1984) study conducted in Oklahoma that matched traffic fatalities from FARS files with those from multiple cause mortality files is an example of this procedure. By matching the two files it was possible to combine multiple cause data on race and ethnicity with FARS' detailed accident data.

Several states maintain their own accident/casualty systems. The state of Maryland, for example, operates several reporting systems that collect data on general mortality, motor vehicle accidents, traumatic injury, boating accidents, industrial accidents, fires and criminal acts (Table B.2). The majority of the systems are independently operated by state agencies. However, the Mortality Data System and the Maryland Automated Accident Reporting System function as part of the nationwide efforts of NCHS' vital statistics program and FARS, respectively.

While these national and state-level data bases exist, the majority of epidemiologic studies have traditionally approached the problem of alcohol involvement in serious events by conducting independent analyses of specially selected sample data. These studies have produced estimates of alcohol involvement in such serious events as fires, falls, industrial accidents, homicides, suicides and drownings, as well as motor vehicle accidents. The majority of the recent studies of this kind have been reviewed by Roizen (1982).

Some measure of the inadequacy of these various data sources for estimating the extent of alcohol involvement in serious events is provided by the figures presented in Table B.3. These are crude estimates and probabilities of the occurrence of serious events and alcohol involvement. They are derived from data drawn from the various national data sets and specialised epidemiologic studies.

For each category of serious event the table presents information on the frequency of the event, the probability of the event's being reported to the authorities, the probability of an alcohol involvement determination being made, the probability of such a determination yielding

417

Table B.2: *Maryland casualty data bases*

Data base	Operating agency	Coverage	Alcohol determination	Percentage of cases in which alcohol involvement is determined	Requirement of reporting
Report: Boat Accidents and Recreation	Maryland Marina Police	Census[a] (fatalities only)	BAC, self-report	100	mandatory
Mortality Data System	Maryland Center for Health Statistics	Census[a]	ICD codes	100	mandatory
Maryland Shock Trauma Records	Univ. of MD Shock Trauma Center	Census[a]	BAC, self-reported	?	mandatory
Annual Autopsy Report from County Sheriff-Coroner	County Sheriff-Coroner's Office	Census[a]	BAC, witnesses	100	mandatory
Hospital Management Information System	Maryland Dept. of Health and Mental Hygiene	Census[a]	?	?	mandatory
Universal Crime Reporting System	Maryland Police	Census[a]	Self-reported, witness, police reported	1	mandatory
Maryland State Workers Compensation Accident Fund	Employers	Census[a]	None	N/A	mandatory
Maryland Automated Accident Reporting System	Maryland Police	Census[a]	BAC, self-reported, police reported	?	mandatory
DWI Assessment Data	Maryland Alcohol Control Administration and Motor Vehicle Administration	Non-probability[b] sample	BAC, police reported	100	mandatory
Fatal Fire Victim Report	Baltimore County Fire Department	Census[a]	BAC	?	mandatory
Alcohol Related Injury Project	Johns Hopkins University	Non-probability	BAC	56	mandatory

[a] 100 percent of cases are collected
[b] Nonstatistically selected cases, not suitable for producing state-level estimates

a positive result, the rate of alcohol involvement in the event and the frequency of alcohol involvement in the event.

The reported frequency of the event is taken from various published reports (*see footnotes for* Table B.3). The probability of an event being reported to the authorities depends on the nature and severity of the event. Nearly all fatalities come to the attention of the authorities with the exception of a small proportion of concealed homicides. Non-fatal injuries, depending upon their severity, have much lower probabilities of being reported. The rate of alcohol involvement in motor vehicle accidents is calculated directly from the available data (FARS and NASS). For the remainder of the events, the rate is represented by the midpoint of the range of alcohol involvement for each event presented by Roizen (1982). Multiplying the rate by its associated reported frequency produces the frequency of alcohol involvement.

The rationale for determining the remaining two probability categories is based upon studies of drunk driving (e.g. Mercer 1984). These studies have found that police are reluctant to make a determination of

Table B.3: *Estimated frequencies, rates and probabilities of alcohol involvement in serious events*

Casualty Type	Reported frequency	Probability of being reported	Probability of a determination of alcohol involvement being made	Probability of obtaining a positive result	Rate of alcohol involvement (percent)	Frequency of of alcohol involved casualties
Fatal						
Motor Vehicles	45,000[a]	1.00	0.42	0.90	38	17,000
Industry	12,000[b]	1.00	0.35	0.73	25	3,000
Drowning	6,000[b]	1.00	0.50	0.87	43	2,600
Fire	4,900[b]	1.00	0.60	0.78	47	2,300
Fall	12,000[b]	1.00	0.40	0.75	30	3,600
Homicide	22,000[c]	0.95	0.60	0.87	51	11,200
Suicide	28,000[c]	1.00	0.70	0.57	40	11,200
Non-fatal						
Motor Vehicle	1,200,000[d]	1.00	0.15	0.74	11	135,000
Industry	2,100,000[b]	0.70	0.30	0.90	27	567,000
Fire	1,125,000[e]	0.95	0.42	0.93	39	438,000
Fall	15,000,000[e]	0.75	0.40	0.95	38	5,700,000
Assault	500,000[f]	0.50	0.60	0.80	48	240,000
Rape	55,000[f]	0.50	0.55	0.69	38	20,900

[a] Department of Transportation (1985a)
[b] National Safety Council (1982)
[c] National Center for Health Statistics (1984)
[d] Department of Transportation (1985b)
[e] Wingard and Room (1977)
[f] Roizen and Schneberk (1977)

alcohol's role in an accident, yet when they do so they are correct in their assessment of alcohol involvement in over 90 per cent of the cases. Based upon these findings of low probabilities of determination – high probabilities of a positive result, the remaining two probabilities are assigned to each type of serious event in proportions that keep them consistent with their associated reported frequency, alcohol involvement rate and resulting frequency of alcohol involvement.

The estimates and probabilities from Table B.3 reveal several significant features of alcohol involvement in serious events. First, many serious injuries go unreported, particularly violent criminal acts. If unreported they will not enter into the data collection system, thereby potentially biasing any subsequent analyses. Second, the probability of a determination of whether alcohol is involved is alarmingly low even for fatalities. In all likelihood, if the chances of an alcohol determination's being made were to rise it is also quite probable that the rate of alcohol involvement would rise. Third, when a determination of alcohol involvement is made there is a high probability that the result will be positive. Fourth, even conservative estimates of alcohol involvement produce disturbingly high frequencies of alcohol-related casualties; casualties that could perhaps be prevented.

Proposed Model for a National Casualty Surveillance System

A model injury surveillance system would have the following features:

1. centralisation of notification, command and control;

2. centralisation of integration of information and reporting;

3. immediacy of information;

4. simplicity of key surveillance information;

5. true surveillance by generating continuous statistics and reports;

6. on-line report generation with data input to a central unit.

The kinds of information which ought to be collected on publicly known casualty events would include an event ID number, event type, location, time, the number injured, and the number dead. For each injured or dead casualty victim the event ID would link information coming from various sources. For each injured or dead person information on the nature and severity of injury, the BAC level, apparent (tested) or reported alcohol involvement, blood pressure and/or their disposition or destination would be collected as well as some demographic information.

Links would be made between the data derived from several reports, including:

1. the original event report, to which an event number would be assigned;

2. a supplemental initial diagnostic report assigned a victim number;

3. a supplemental diagnostic, evaluative or treatment report;

4. other agency reports.

Reports sources would include fire, police emergency, trauma units, Federal Aviation Administration, Coast Guard and others responsible for identification and diagnosis, and disposition. Other reports would be generated by local emergency units, medevac units (shock trauma unit, burn unit, specialized trauma units and others) and the morgue. Well-defined data linkages are crucial. This requires the identification of key points of intersection and data development:

One model for a pilot county-level alcohol-related injury surveillance project is a study presently being conducted in the city of Baltimore, Maryland and its five surrounding counties. The Alcohol-Related Injury Surveillance (ARIS) Project, sponsored by the US National Institute on Alcohol Abuse and Alcoholism, the Centers for Disease Control and the Association of Schools of Public Health, has established a procedure through which information on the injury type and severity, circumstances surrounding the injurious event, the injured person and the injured person's blood-alcohol concentration (BAC) are collected.

Data were collected from hospital emergency rooms, Maryland's Shock Trauma Center and from medical examiners' offices. Two study members work in the emergency rooms, approaching patients, obtaining consent using a certificate of confidentiality, administering the breathalyzer test (when blood has not been taken to perform a BAC), interviewing patients and abstracting medical records. BAC is routinely determined and recorded in both cases.

Data analysis of ARIS will involve an assessment of the distributions of selected variables by population type, the determination of population based rates and a comparison of the profiles of the estimated 13 per cent who do not enrol in the project and the remainder who do.

There are several construct impediments to putting a county-based pilot injury surveillance system into place. The first is resistance to the idea itself, although it will save lives through more appropriate treatment, serve as a basis for public concern, lead to public awareness, prevention programmes, the identification of high risk situations, locations and persons, and enhanced law enforcement, surveillance and interdiction. Finally, a county-based pilot surveillance will allow a more complete assessment of the costs of injury, and especially alcohol-involved injury, to society.

A second impediment to putting a county-based pilot injury surveillance system into place is resistance by those countries first implementing it. This can be countered by drawing attention to the funding source (direct grant), the technical sophistication of the effort, which can be expanded to other service delivery systems, and the opportunity to build, test and refine injury surveillance. This survey is a 'test bed' for other critical reporting systems, such as those developed for use by fire and police departments. Most importantly, this pilot project is a precursor to a national level system of emergency aid. Entering the project at this point would give particular countries direct input into the development of the national injury surveillance system.

The final construct impediment is legal and other barriers to measuring alcohol involvement. It will be important to get the American Bar Association's support. The data will have to be treated as inviolate, requiring consent and confidentiality. The American Medical Association should be asked to embark on a program to advocate and insure proper diagnosis and treatment of alcohol-involved injury. Finally, public support groups should be enlisted to pressure legislators to make the measurement of alcohol involvement in injury mandatory when publicly funded emergency assistance is provided.

References

Aarens, M., and R. Roizen (1977) *Suicide and alcohol.* Berkeley, Social Research Group

Brodner, R.A., J.C. Van Gilder, and W.F. Collins (1981) Experimental spinal cord trauma: Potentiation by alcohol. *Journal of Trauma, 21,* 124-129

Brody, J.A. (1983) Research priorities in the epidemiology of aging. Scientific Group on the Epidemiology of Aging, January 11-17, Geneva

Clark, R.L., and J.J. Spengler (1978) Changing demography and dependency costs: The implications of future dependency rations. In B.R. Herzog (ed), *Aging and income: Essays on policy prospects.* Human Sciences Press, New York, pp. 55-89

Committee on Trauma Research, Commission on Life Sciences, National Research Council and the Institute of Medicine (1985) *Injury in America: A continuing public health problem.* National Academy Press, Washington, DC

Department of Transportation, National Highway Traffic Safety Administration, Fatal Accident Sampling System 1983 (1985a) *A review of information on fatal traffic accidents in the US in 1983.* DOT Pub. No. DOT-HS 806 699, Washington, DC

Department of Transportation, National Highway Traffic Safety Administration (1985b) *National accident sampling system 1983. A report on traffic accidents and injuries in the US.* DOT-HS 806 699, Washington, DC

DuFour, M., H. Malin, D. Bertolucci, and C. Christian (1984) Alcohol-involved traffic fatalities among Native American Oklahomans. Paper presented at the American Public Health Association Conference, Anaheim, California

Espenshade, T.J., and R.E. Braun (1981) Economic aspects of an aging population and the material well-being of older persons. In *Leading edges: Recent research on psychosocial aging.* The National Institute of Aging, U.S. Dept. of Health and Human Services, National Institutes of Health, Public Health Service, NIH Publication No. 81-2390, November, Bethesda, Maryland

Haberman, P.W., and M.M. Baden (1978) *Alcohol, other drugs and violent death.* Oxford University Press, New York

Kitagawa, E., and P.M. Hauser (1973) Differential mortality in the United States: A study in socioeconomic epidemiology. Harvard University Press, Massachusetts

Liedtke, A.J., and W.E. DeMuth (1975) Effects of alcohol on cardiovascular performance after experimental non-penetrating chest trauma. *American Journal of Cardiology, 35,* 243-50

Lilienfeld, A.M., and A.J. Gilford (1966) *Chronic diseases and public health education.* Johns Hopkins Press, Baltimore

Mercer, G.W. (1984) Counter attack: Traffic research papers 1984. British Columbia, Canada· Police Services Branch, Ministry of Attorney General, 1985.

National Center for Health Statistics (1982) *Vital Statistics of the United States, 1979: Volume II. Mortality Part A.* DHHS Pub. No. (PHS) 84 1101, Washington, DC

National Safety Council (1982) *Accident facts: 1982 edition.* National Safety Council, Chicago

National Institute on Alcohol Abuse and Alcoholism (NIAAA) (n.d.) 1990 Objectives for the Nation: Mid-Course Review. Alcohol and Drug Misuse Prevention, Objectives No. 1, No. 4, No. 12; Occupational Safety and Health Series, Objectives No. 1, No. 2, No. 3, No. 5; Injury Prevention Series, Objectives No. 1, No. 2, No. 3, No. 4, No. 5, No. 6, No. 7, No. 8; Control of Stress and Violent Behaviors, Objective No. 1. Unpublished paper.

Omran, A.R. (1977) Epidemiologic transition in the United States: The health factor in population change. *Population Bulletin, 32,* 2, May, Population Reference Bureau, Washington, DC

Roizen, J. (1982) Estimating alcohol involvement in serious events. *Alcohol and Health Monograph 1: Alcohol consumption and related problems.* US Government Printing Office, Washington, DC

Roizen, J. and D. Schneberk (1977) Alcohol and crime. In Aarens, M., and T. Cameron, R. Roizen, D. Schneberk and D. Wingard (eds) *Alcohol, Casualties and Crime.* Final Report No. 18, Social Research Group, Berkeley

Wingard, D., and R. Room (1978) Alcohol and home, industrial and recreational accidents. In Aarens, M., and T. Cameron, R. Roizen, D. Schneberk and D. Wingard (eds) *Alcohol, Casualties and Crime.* Final Report No. 18, Social Research Group, Berkeley

Authors and Editors

Manuella Adrian
Head, Statistical Research Program
Prevention Studies Department
Addiction Research Foundation
33 Russell Street
Toronto, Ontario, Canada M5S 2S1

Sherrie Aitken
President
CSR, Incorporated
1400 Eye Street NW, Suite 600
Washington, DC, USA 20005

Sally Casswell
Director
Alcohol Research Unit
University of Auckland
Auckland, New Zealand

Cheryl J. Stephens Cherpitel
Scientist
Alcohol Research Group
1816 Scenic Avenue
Berkeley, California USA 94709-1399

Yvon Chich
Institut National de Recherche
sur les Transports et leur Sécurité
2, Avenue du Général Malleret Joinville
94114 Arcueil Cedex, France

Ron Draper
Consultant
World Health Organization
Regional Office for Europe
8, Scherfigsvej
AK-2100 Copenhagen O, Denmark

Roberta G. Ferrence
Research Scientist
Prevention Studies Department
Addiction Research Foundation
33 Russell Street
Toronto, Ontario, Canada M5S 2S1

Honey Fisher
Fisher and Associates
110 Erskine Avenue
Suite 1902
Toronto, Ontario, Canada M4P 1Y4

Norman Giesbrecht
Research Scientist
Prevention Studies Department
Addiction Research Foundation
33 Russell Street
Toronto, Ontario, Canada M5S 2S1

Yves Goehrs
Caisse Nationale d'Assurance Maladie
des Travailleurs Salariés
66, Avenue du Maine
75682 Paris Cedex 14, France

Laura González
Researcher
Division of Epidemiology and Social Sciences
Intituto Mexicano de Psiquiatría
Antiguo Camino A, Xochimilco No. 101
México DF, México

René González
Former Regional Advisor on Mental Health
Pan American Health Organization
PO Box 2275-1000
San José, Costa Rica

Claude Got
Chef de Service d'Anatomie et Pathologie
Hôpital A. Paré
9, avenue du Général de Gaulle
92104 Boulogne Cedex, France

Marcus Grant
Senior Scientist
Division of Mental Health
World Health Organization
1211 Geneva 27, Switzerland

Alan Haworth
Professor and Head
Department of Psychiatry
University of Zambia School of Medicine
PO Box 30043
Lusaka, Zambia

Harold D. Holder
Director
Prevention Research Center
2532 Durant Avenue
Berkeley, California, USA 94704

Bhushan M. Kapur
Director
Clinical Laboratories
Addiction Research Foundation
33 Russell Street
Toronto, Ontario, Canada M5S 2S1

Jean L'Hoste
Institut National de Recherche sur
les Transports et leur Sécurité
Autodrome de Linas/Montlhery
91310 Linas, France

John B. Macdonald
Former Chairman and President
Addiction Research Foundation
33 Russell Street
Toronto, Ontario, Canada M5S 2S1

Maria Elena Medina-Mora
Head, Division of Epidemiological and Social Sciences
Instituto Mexicano de Psiquiatría
Antiguo Camino A, Xochimilco No. 101
México 22 DF, México

Jacek Morawski
Assistant Professor
Institute of Psychiatry and Neurology
1/9 Sobieskiego Str.
02-957 Warsaw, Poland

Jacek Moskalewicz
Researcher
Institute of Psychiatry and Neurology
1/9 Sobieskiego Str.
02-957 Warsaw, Poland

Richard Müller
Director
Swiss Institute for the
Prevention of Alcoholism
Case Postale 1063
CH 1001 Lausanne, Switzerland

Robyn Norton
Visiting Research Fellow
Academic Department of Medicine
The Royal Free Hospital
Pond Street, Hampstead
London NW3 2QG, England

Esa Österberg
Researcher
Social Research Institute of Alcohol Studies
Kalevankatu 12
SF-00100 Helsinki, Finland

Laure Papoz
Institut National de la Santé et
de la Recherche Médicale, U21
16, Avenue Paul Vaillant Couturier
94807 Villejuif Cedex, France

Kai Pernanen
Research Scientist
Institute of Social Medicine
University of Uppsala
Uppsala, Sweden

Kari Poikolainen
National Public Health Institute
Mannerheimintie 166
SF-00280 Helsinki, Finland

Judy Roizen
University of the South Pacific
P.O. Box 1168
Suva, Fiji

Robin Room
Director
Alcohol Research Group
1816 Scenic Avenue
Berkeley, California, USA 94709-1399

Irving Rootman
Director
Program Resources Division
Health Promotion Directorate
Health and Welfare Canada
Jeanne Mance Building, Tunney's Pasture
Ottawa, Ontario, Canada K1A 1B4

Haydeé Rosovsky
Instituto Mexicano de Psiquiatría
Antiguo Camino A, Xochimilco No. 101
México 22 DF, México

Ole-Jørgen Skog
Director
National Institute for Alcohol and Drug Research
Dannevigsveien 10
0463 Oslo, Norway

Leland Towle
Director
International and Intergovernmental Affairs
National Institute on Alcohol Abuse and Alcoholism
5600 Fishers Lane
Rockville, Maryland, USA 20857

Ignacy Wald
Director for Research
Institute of Psychiatry and Neurology
1/9 Sobieskiego Str.
02-957 Warsaw, Poland

Jacques Weill
Laboratoire Biochimie
Hôpital Trousseau
CHR de Tours
37044 Tours Cedex, France

Terry Zobeck
CSR, Incorporated
1400 Eye Street NW
Suite 600
Washington, DC, USA 20005

Author Index

431

Subject Index